Multicultural Counseling Applications for Improved Mental Healthcare Services

Anasuya Jegathevi Jegathesan
HELP University, Malaysia

Siti Salina Abdullah
University Malaysia Terengganu, Malaysia

A volume in the Advances in Psychology, Mental Health, and Behavioral Studies (APMHBS) Book Series

IGI Global
DISSEMINATOR OF KNOWLEDGE

Published in the United States of America by
IGI Global
Medical Information Science Reference (an imprint of IGI Global)
701 E. Chocolate Avenue
Hershey PA, USA 17033
Tel: 717-533-8845
Fax: 717-533-8661
E-mail: cust@igi-global.com
Web site: http://www.igi-global.com

Library of Congress Cataloging-in-Publication Data

Names: Jegathesan, Anasuya Jegathevi, 1974- editor. | Abdullah, Siti Salina, 1978- editor.
Title: Multicultural counseling applications for improved mental healthcare services / Anasuya Jegathevi Jegathesan and Siti Salina Abdullah, editors.
Description: Hershey, PA : Medical Information Science Reference, [2019] | Includes bibliographical references.
Identifiers: LCCN 2018010753| ISBN 9781522560739 (hardcover) | ISBN 9781522560746 (ebook)
Subjects: | MESH: Community Mental Health Services--methods | Counseling--methods | Cultural Diversity | Religion and Psychology | Malaysia
Classification: LCC RA790.55 | NLM WM 30.6 | DDC 362.2/2--dc23 LC record available at https://lccn.loc.gov/2018010753

This book is published in the IGI Global book series Advances in Psychology, Mental Health, and Behavioral Studies (APMHBS) (ISSN: 2475-6660; eISSN: 2475-6679)

British Cataloguing in Publication Data
A Cataloguing in Publication record for this book is available from the British Library.

All work contributed to this book is new, previously-unpublished material. The views expressed in this book are those of the authors, but not necessarily of the publisher.

For electronic access to this publication, please contact: eresources@igi-global.com.

Advances in Psychology, Mental Health, and Behavioral Studies (APMHBS) Book Series

Bryan Christiansen
Global Research Society, LLC, USA
Harish C. Chandan
Argosy University, USA

ISSN:2475-6660
EISSN:2475-6679

Mission

The complexity of the human mind has puzzled researchers and physicians for centuries. While widely studied, the brain still remains largely misunderstood.

The **Advances in Psychology, Mental Health, and Behavioral Studies (APMHBS)** book series presents comprehensive research publications focusing on topics relating to the human psyche, cognition, psychiatric care, mental and developmental disorders, as well as human behavior and interaction. Featuring diverse and innovative research, publications within APMHBS are ideally designed for use by mental health professionals, academicians, researchers, and upper-level students.

Coverage

- Eating Disorders
- Mental Health & Disorders
- Cognition
- Psychiatry
- Substance Abuse
- Human Behavior
- Anxiety
- Trauma & Stress
- Treatment & Care
- Socialization

IGI Global is currently accepting manuscripts for publication within this series. To submit a proposal for a volume in this series, please contact our Acquisition Editors at Acquisitions@igi-global.com or visit: http://www.igi-global.com/publish/.

The Advances in Psychology, Mental Health, and Behavioral Studies (APMHBS) Book Series (ISSN 2475-6660) is published by IGI Global, 701 E. Chocolate Avenue, Hershey, PA 17033-1240, USA, www.igi-global.com. This series is composed of titles available for purchase individually; each title is edited to be contextually exclusive from any other title within the series. For pricing and ordering information please visit http://www.igi-global.com/book-series/advances-psychology-mental-health-behavioral/110200. Postmaster: Send all address changes to above address.

Titles in this Series

For a list of additional titles in this series, please visit: www.igi-global.com/book-series

Handbook of Research on Psychosocial Perspectives of Human Communication Disorders
Sanjeev Kumar Gupta (All India Institute of Speech and Hearing, India) and Srinivasan Venkatesan (All India Institute of Speech and Hearing, India)
Medical Information Science Reference • copyright 2018 • 465pp • H/C (ISBN: 9781522549550) • US $275.00

Deconstructing Stigma in Mental Health
Brittany A. Canfield (Southern New Hampshire University, USA) and Holly A. Cunningham (CPES Inc., USA)
Medical Information Science Reference • copyright 2018 • 307pp • H/C (ISBN: 9781522538080) • US $225.00

Social, Psychological, and Forensic Perspectives on Sexual Abuse
Rejani Thudalikunnil Gopalan (Gujarat Forensic Sciences University, India)
Information Science Reference • copyright 2018 • 374pp • H/C (ISBN: 9781522539582) • US $195.00

Raising Mental Health Awareness in Higher Education Emerging Research and Opportunities
Melissa Martin (State University of New York at Plattsburgh, USA) Jean Mockry (State University of New York at Plattsburgh, USA) Alison Puliatte (State University of New York at Plattsburgh, USA) Denise A. Simard (State University of New York at Plattsburgh, USA) and Maureen E. Squires (State University of New York at Plattsburgh, USA)
Medical Information Science Reference • copyright 2018 • 136pp • H/C (ISBN: 9781522537939) • US $175.00

Web-Based Behavioral Therapies for Mental Disorders
Sitwat Usman Langrial (Sur University College, Oman)
Medical Information Science Reference • copyright 2018 • 310pp • H/C (ISBN: 9781522532415) • US $255.00

Measuring the Psychological and Electrophysiological Attributes of Human Personality Emerging Research and Opportunities
Sanja Tatalović Vorkapić (University of Rijeka, Croatia)
Information Science Reference • copyright 2017 • 242pp • H/C (ISBN: 9781522522836) • US $130.00

Emerging Research in Play Therapy, Child Counseling, and Consultation
Rheta LeAnne Steen (Loyola University New Orleans, USA)
Information Science Reference • copyright 2017 • 436pp • H/C (ISBN: 9781522522249) • US $205.00

IGI Global
DISSEMINATOR OF KNOWLEDGE

701 East Chocolate Avenue, Hershey, PA 17033, USA
Tel: 717-533-8845 x100 • Fax: 717-533-8661
E-Mail: cust@igi-global.com • www.igi-global.com

Table of Contents

Foreword *by Goh Chee Leong* xiv

Foreword *by Mohan Raj Gurubatham* xvi

Preface xvii

Chapter 1
Challenges Associated With Counselling Multicultural Clients 1
Sindusha Darshini Kanna Dasan, HELP University, Malaysia

Chapter 2
Counseling Chinese Communities in Malaysia: The Challenges and Needs in Mental Health Service Deliverance 23
Rachel Sing Kiat Ting, Monash University Malaysia, Malaysia
Pei Lynn Foo, Penang Association of Counselling and Psychology, Malaysia

Chapter 3
A Case Study of MY Psychology: Malaysia's First Online Psychoeducational Platform 50
Chong Shen Hew, MY Psychology, Malaysia
Mu Yi Hor, MY Psychology, Malaysia
Hou Huai Gary Yap, MY Psychology, Malaysia
Tin Fung Chong, MY Psychology, Malaysia

Chapter 4
Revised Reality Therapy: A New Intervention to Help Boost Self-Esteem in Malaysian Secondary Schools 64
Joo Hou Ng, University of Exeter, UK
Aaron Page, University of Exeter, UK

Chapter 5
Filial Play Therapy Process of a Malaysian Parent 84
Diana-Lea Baranovich, University of Malaya, Malaysia
Cheng Chue Han, University of Malaya, Malaysia

Chapter 6
The Experience of Volunteers and Frontline Workers in Marginalized Communities Across Southeast Asia 93
Chuah Siew Mooi, HELP University, Malaysia
Ann Nicole Nunis, HELP University, Malaysia

Chapter 7
LGBTQ+ Population in Asia Pacific (Malaysia): LGBTQ+ Populace 112
Gianina Ginnie Kon, HELP University, Malaysia
Anne Chong Yuk Ming, Lodge International School, Malaysia

Chapter 8
Counseling Refugees 128
Ann Nunis, HELP University, Malaysia

Chapter 9
Living With Cerebral Palsy in Malaysia: Me, Myself, and Others 150
Rajvin Kaur Randhawa, HELP University, Malaysia
Kiirtaara Aravindhan, HELP University, Malaysia

Chapter 10
Developing Multicultural Counselling in an Australian University: Applying Hinduism to Counselling 168
Carl Vadivella Belle, Independent Researcher, Australia

Chapter 11
Buddhist Approaches to Counselling and Psychotherapy: Exploratory Discussions From Different Traditions 183
Alvin Lai Oon Ng, Sunway University, Malaysia
Ee Mun Hon, HELP University, Malaysia
Ming Tik Chia, HELP University, Malaysia

Chapter 12
Psychotherapy and Christianity: Methods and Challenges 200
Jeremy Lim, HELP University, Malaysia
Ke Hui Chuah, HELP University, Malaysia

Chapter 13
Hinduism and Counseling: Karma, Women Empowerment, Grief and Death, Anger Management, Bhagavad Gita, and Psychotherapies 211
Devi Venashinee Muruges, HELP University, Malaysia

Chapter 14
The Perception of Muslim Clients Towards Non-Muslim Counselors 223
Siti Salina Abdullah, University Malaysia Terengganu, Malaysia
Kamarul Md Shah, University Malaysia Terengganu, Malaysia

Chapter 15
Religion in Therapy: Theravada Buddhism 235
Chandana Namal Kumara, HELP University, Malaysia

Chapter 16
Faces of Grief: Cross-Cultural Bereavement and Support in Malaysia 251
Anasuya Jegathevi Jegathesan, HELP University, Malaysia

Compilation of References 265

About the Contributors 294

Index 300

Detailed Table of Contents

Foreword *by Goh Chee Leong* xiv

Foreword *by Mohan Raj Gurubatham* xvi

Preface xvii

Chapter 1
Challenges Associated With Counselling Multicultural Clients 1
Sindusha Darshini Kanna Dasan, HELP University, Malaysia

The chapter is about different situations that therapists face challenges in and outlines what a therapist can do when faced with these challenging situations. The challenges covered are: challenging the competency of the therapist of color; transferring minority animosity to clients of other cultures; unrealistically viewing the therapist of colour as a super minority therapist; overidentification with the client; encountering clashes in cultural values; encountering clashes in communication and therapeutic styles; multicultural competence in a therapist; therapist of colour needing to prove competence; dealing with expressions of racist attitudes/beliefs/behaviors from clients; receiving and expressing racial animosity; and dealing with the stages of racial and cultural identity of therapists and clients. This chapter is to create awareness in therapist and help build multicultural competent therapist.

Chapter 2
Counseling Chinese Communities in Malaysia: The Challenges and Needs in Mental Health Service Deliverance 23
Rachel Sing Kiat Ting, Monash University Malaysia, Malaysia
Pei Lynn Foo, Penang Association of Counselling and Psychology, Malaysia

This chapter presents the experiences of Chinese in Malaysia (CIM), in the context of mental health services. As the second largest ethnic group in Malaysia, CIM is diverse in its dialectic subculture, education, generation, geography, and degree of assimilation to the mainstream culture. The chapter introduces the ecological characteristics of CIM and how they shape the unique psychological challenges. Though CIM are known for their multilingual ability, strong work ethics, emphasis on education, and family piety, the clashes between tradition and modern values, the marginalized position in the Malaysian political arena, the stereotype of overachiever in education, and the "brain drain" movement of young elite CIM, have all caused a strain in CIM families as well as individuals. Moreover, they face both external and internal barriers in getting quality mental health care. It is therefore imperative to promote a mental health discipline that is open to serve CIM, as well as being sensitive to its cultural and historical backdrop.

Chapter 3
A Case Study of MY Psychology: Malaysia's First Online Psychoeducational Platform 50
Chong Shen Hew, MY Psychology, Malaysia
Mu Yi Hor, MY Psychology, Malaysia
Hou Huai Gary Yap, MY Psychology, Malaysia
Tin Fung Chong, MY Psychology, Malaysia

MY Psychology is an online educational platform currently based in Malaysia, formed with the intention to spread awareness towards the general public of not only on issues related with mental health and those who suffer under mental illnesses, but also to create a place where psychology as a basic knowledge can be taught and learned. This is in order to correct misunderstandings from the public toward psychology. Operating on the internet requires the company to shift towards a marketing-oriented direction, in the meantime, coping with internal and external challenges in order to strive for greater reach and engagement from the audience.

Chapter 4
Revised Reality Therapy: A New Intervention to Help Boost Self-Esteem in Malaysian Secondary Schools 64
Joo Hou Ng, University of Exeter, UK
Aaron Page, University of Exeter, UK

This chapter proposes an intervention – revised reality therapy – that has been developed to help school guidance counsellors treat low self-esteem in Malaysian secondary schools. Revised reality therapy has been developed using literature from a range of fields, including: choice theory, reality therapy, social identity approach, and first-hand experience in Malaysian secondary schools. The proposed intervention uses a simple, easy to use method which - for the convenience of school guidance counsellors and laypeople alike – has been presented as a six-step process. The theoretical background, implementation, and validity of revised reality therapy will be presented in this chapter. Future directions and limitations are also discussed.

Chapter 5
Filial Play Therapy Process of a Malaysian Parent 84
Diana-Lea Baranovich, University of Malaya, Malaysia
Cheng Chue Han, University of Malaya, Malaysia

In Malaysia, some parents leave the duties of child rearing to their domestic helpers. This can cause much trauma to a preschool child who has been raised by his domestic helper if the domestic helper leaves the family. The domestic helper was the primary caregiver of the child; hence, when the domestic helper leaves, the child feels that his "mother" has abandoned him. This in turn cause the child to respond via very negative acting out behaviors. This chapter presents a case study using filial play therapy as a therapeutic intervention for a pre-school child and his mother after the domestic helper left the family. This therapeutic process enhanced the bonding between the child and his mother. As a result of better bonding, the child's negative behaviors subsided.

Chapter 6
The Experience of Volunteers and Frontline Workers in Marginalized Communities Across Southeast Asia 93
Chuah Siew Mooi, HELP University, Malaysia
Ann Nicole Nunis, HELP University, Malaysia

This chapter focuses on the experience of volunteers and frontline workers who serve in marginalized communities across Southeast Asia. More frontline workers and volunteers are taking the initiative to support marginalized communities in the region. With the rise of human rights violations towards marginalized communities in the past decade, frontline workers and volunteers face unique experiences in working with these communities, ranging from stigma and discrimination to unaddressed levels of burnout. Based on the authors' experiences working with these communities and the summary of the interviews with fellow frontline workers, the experience of working with marginalized communities, particularly those affected by HIV/AIDS and refugees, are elaborated in this chapter. Current challenges as well as recommendations are highlighted to ensure that the frontline workers and volunteers are supported throughout their vital work towards society.

Chapter 7
LGBTQ+ Population in Asia Pacific (Malaysia): LGBTQ+ Populace 112
Gianina Ginnie Kon, HELP University, Malaysia
Anne Chong Yuk Ming, Lodge International School, Malaysia

The topic of LGBTQ in Malaysia was chosen as this issue is relatively new (as compared to Western society) and perhaps not as open due to the different religious, cultural, and familial taboo surrounding it. Individuals who face a crisis in their sexuality, hence, face insurmountable challenges and conflicts and may need to seek help from the counselling/helping professionals. This chapter that focuses on LGBTQ+ population in general, and particularly in Malaysia, it is hoped that it would facilitate the relationship between the counsellor with a member of this particular population.

Chapter 8
Counseling Refugees 128
Ann Nunis, HELP University, Malaysia

This chapter discusses the plight of refugees, the challenges faced, and the psychosocial impact of said challenges. It further provides practitioners with a review of coping methods utilized by refugees throughout the refugee journey in order to highlight possible protective factors practitioners may build on in the provision of mental health services. Lastly, the chapter provides an overview of current therapeutic frameworks that are culturally sensitive for counselling refugees, the challenges in the provision of mental health services, and techniques utilized by practitioners in the delivery of mental health services through evidence of research and case-based examples.

Chapter 9
Living With Cerebral Palsy in Malaysia: Me, Myself, and Others.. 150
Rajvin Kaur Randhawa, HELP University, Malaysia
Kiirtaara Aravindhan, HELP University, Malaysia

The authors in this chapter highlights the reality of cerebral palsy in Malaysia. The chapter is a blend experiential account and factual details. The experiential fragment includes a personal case study, providing 32 years' worth of experience and first-hand details on the life of a cerebral palsy individual in Malaysia. The factual fragment provides researched information on the general reality of cerebral palsy in Malaysia, which includes regulations, existing services and support systems, ergonomics, awareness, and inclusion. This chapter also includes an interview with a fellow CP individual. The chapter ends with an interesting take-home message that aims to encourage and motivate those negatively affected.

Chapter 10
Developing Multicultural Counselling in an Australian University: Applying Hinduism to Counselling 168
Carl Vadivella Belle, Independent Researcher, Australia

Lifetime experiences have equipped the author with a broad and diverse background in approaching counselling and problem resolution. This has ranged from grief counselling to management of rural financial counselling and spiritual counselling. In 2004, the author was appointed Inaugural Hindu Chaplain at the Flinders University of South Australia, a position held until late 2007 (although his counselling role has continued until this day). The chaplaincy to which he was appointed was one of several that collectively comprised a multi-faith chaplaincy involving a team approach. The concept was one in which chaplains of different faiths would respect each other's traditions, would eschew proselytization, and would work cooperatively to mount joint educational and community interest projects. However, at the more fundamental level, his role consisted of providing chaplaincy services to Hindu students and staff studying or employed at Flinders University. (Increasingly this role extended to members of the other two universities based in Adelaide, neither of which possessed a Hindu chaplain.)

Chapter 11
Buddhist Approaches to Counselling and Psychotherapy: Exploratory Discussions From Different Traditions 183
Alvin Lai Oon Ng, Sunway University, Malaysia
Ee Mun Hon, HELP University, Malaysia
Ming Tik Chia, HELP University, Malaysia

Three authors from differing Buddhist backgrounds share their approaches to using Buddhism in psychotherapy. The authors argue that Buddhism itself is fundamentally a psychotherapy approach because it is essentially a prescription to end discontent and misery. This chapter provides basic points on how Buddhism can be used in counselling by discussing how different Buddhist traditions might approach counselling. This chapter also brings up reflections on how practice may differ according to experience in the fields of counselling and clinical psychology. Overall, the chapter is subdivided into six parts: (1) introduction; (2) basic tenets of Buddhism relevant to psychotherapy; (3) case study illustrations of applied Buddhism in counselling and psychotherapy; (4) discussion on reconciling differing Buddhist schools of thought in the practice of counselling and psychotherapy; (5) discussion on compatibility of Buddhist principles with applied Western philosophies and therapeutic approaches; and (6) suggestions of future directions given the current research literature patterns.

Chapter 12
Psychotherapy and Christianity: Methods and Challenges 200
Jeremy Lim, HELP University, Malaysia
Ke Hui Chuah, HELP University, Malaysia

Christianity is counted as one of the biggest religious groups in the world, numbering at over 2 billion individuals who identify themselves with this religion. As of the 2010 census, the Department of Statistics Malaysia Official Portal reported that an estimated 9.2% of the population in Malaysia identified themselves as Christians. In numerical terms, this equates to approximately 3 million individuals spread out all over the Malaysian peninsular as well as Sabah and Sarawak who consider themselves part of the Christian church. This chapter intends to do four things: 1) provide a brief history of the church and Christianity, 2) acquaint the reader with basic Christian beliefs, 3) provide insight into the methods and challenges of working with the population in Malaysia drawing from both local as well as international literature, and 4) provide the implications of the methods and challenges of working with the Christian population.

Chapter 13
Hinduism and Counseling: Karma, Women Empowerment, Grief and Death, Anger Management, Bhagavad Gita, and Psychotherapies 211
Devi Venashinee Muruges, HELP University, Malaysia

Indian psychology lays enormous importance on the research of religious experiences and the expansion of approaches by which to accomplish them. In addition to that, it also provides understanding of the different states of consciousness. Hence, it is undeniable that Indian psychology will be able to make a definite therapeutic contribution to many psychological problems. For mental health practitioners dealing with Hinduism, there are teachings within various texts that directly strengthen counseling and mental services. Some of the examples include perceiving the conscious and the unconsciousness aspects of the mind, utilizing meditation to support people with mental health issues, yoga exercises to curb anxiety and stress, and many others. Therefore, this chapter intends to elucidate the application of Hinduism in therapy.

Chapter 14
The Perception of Muslim Clients Towards Non-Muslim Counselors 223
Siti Salina Abdullah, University Malaysia Terengganu, Malaysia
Kamarul Md Shah, University Malaysia Terengganu, Malaysia

Having a counselor with a different religious background from the client might lead to conflicting perspectives. This chapter intends to explore the perceptive of a Muslim client in choosing a non-Muslim counselor. The concept of helping process, which is highly respectable in the teaching of Islam, is explicated. Muslims are encouraged to help each other, especially those who are in need. Preferably, a non-Muslim counselor should have some basic understanding of the Pillars of Islam prior to conducting a counseling session with a Muslim client. The knowledge will facilitate the counselor understanding process of the clients without bias. It is anticipated that the information presented herewith would benefit non-Muslim counselors and help them in understanding their Muslim clients better. This chapter also examines the cultural issues that may influence the effectiveness of a counseling session between Muslim clients and non-Muslim counselors.

Chapter 15
Religion in Therapy: Theravada Buddhism 235
Chandana Namal Kumara, HELP University, Malaysia

The absence of a central holy scripture in Buddhism and myriad manifestations coalesced into indigenous cultural communities across South and South-East Asia, presenting a formidable challenge to define Buddhism and its practices. This complexity may also be manifested in clients of Theravada background, making them elusive candidates in the therapy room. Complexity notwithstanding, Buddhism offers fertile learning ground for any optimistic multicultural counselor. For the purpose of this chapter, several selected fundamentals of Theravada Buddhism are presented with an emphasis on their possible cultural meanings and on therapeutic utility. This chapter is written from the perspective of Theravada school of Buddhism as it is taught, practiced, and seen in South-East Asia. The author's knowledge and personal experience in Buddhism as a former Buddhist monk, experience of Buddhism as a lay practitioner now, and as a practicing counselor inevitably influence, inspire, and may even limit the parameters of this chapter.

Chapter 16
Faces of Grief: Cross-Cultural Bereavement and Support in Malaysia 251
Anasuya Jegathevi Jegathesan, HELP University, Malaysia

Death, bereavement, and grief are natural processes that are experienced by every individual who is born into this world. The level of trauma experienced from such loss can be mitigated by internal factors and the external environment faced by the individual. Spiritual belief systems and culture play a critical role in the experience of bereavement. This qualitative study applies the phenomenological approach to explore the lived experience of bereavement of 15 Malaysians from five different religious groups, namely Buddhism, Christianity, Hinduism, Islam, and Taoism. Rituals and belief systems impact an individual's experience with bereavement. The likelihood of individuals to seek emotional and psychological support depends greatly on individual belief systems, family support, support facilities set up by religious groups, and the perceived availability of professional services.

Compilation of References 265

About the Contributors 294

Index 300

Foreword

The last 20 years has seen a great awakening and growth in Asian counseling and psychology. Communities that in the past were hesitant and wary when it came to matters of mental health and therapy, have started to open up and embrace these concepts and practices. As a result, this region has seen rapid growth in the numbers of counselors and therapists, and the number of students who are training to become mental health professionals.

Part of this awakening has seen practitioners and academics in this part of the world contribute more actively to current debates on the theory and practice of therapy. The focus of these debates have expanded to the environment and the cultural impetus that influences the development, thinking and mental health of individuals.

The truth remains, that much of today's theories and interventions in the arena of mental health come from theories developed in the United States and Europe. With perhaps the exception of Jung who was heavily influenced in his writing from Eastern Philosophies, the dominant names in therapy such as Freud, Adler, Glasser and Neimeyer are indeed from the West. These theories for the most part have been imported wholesale into the East, in the form of Textbooks, Seminars and training sessions. While these theories and models have for a long time been widely accepted and practiced, increasingly more practitioners from the majority world have started to challenge and question their universality. Furthermore, it has become a common assumption among practitioners that the application of these theories must involve some form of modification and localization in order to be appropriate and effective among Eastern communities.

Malaysia with its diverse population and cultural heritage, allows for the study of the modification and application of mental health models to meet the demands of a multi-cultural community.

With a focus on practitioners and applications this book seeks to add to the growing body of knowledge of working with groups of individuals from diverse and unique communities. Snapshot of individuals from different religious and cultural groups have been gathered alongside the voice of other minority groups. From refugees, to LGBTQ, to developing Hindu Chaplaincy in Australia, to the story of an author suffering from Cerebral Palsy the book provides a showcase of the experiences of mental health and therapeutic interventions in the East. It is a tribute to the significant advances in therapy and the richness knowledge, skills, challenges and abilities that practitioners facing diverse populations must bring to bear on a daily basis.

I congratulate the various authors and effort that it took to tackle the issues that have been brought to bear.

As awareness of therapy and the importance of mental health grows in the East it is important to maintain the localization and practical applications of therapeutic modalities to ensure the nurturing, care and continued development of the hearts and minds of the people.

Goh Chee Leong
International Union of Psychological Science (IUPsyS), Malaysia & HELP University, Malaysia

Foreword

It is indeed a special honor to write this forward for this much needed project to forge new avenues of research and practice in counseling by new insights. For a long time we who live in Asia and the West and who synthesize paradigms, theories, models and tools have felt a crying need to reevaluate the frames, bases and paradigms of psychology . Counseling psychology is an intimate endeavor yet professionally disciplined. It demands immeasurable sensitivity and empathy and yet, is disciplined, objective and systematic. Spirituality's ancient dimensions of human life are part and parcel of the inextricable web of life and living in Asia. Spirituality which underpins much of religion in the East is characterized by experientially powerful and subtle streams of influence. 'Hinduism' is a label commonly used to describe Vedic based religion however it is essentially a spiritual path quite unlike other religions. Veda means knowledge in Sanskrit. Faith and more importantly the personal experiential dimension of Being and consciousness are fundamental in this tradition which has been endeared for over 5,000 years. Psychology in Greek means the study of the psyche or 'soul'. Modern psychology in the era of accelerating globalization demands serious attention in learning from counselors working this part of the world who still intimately have to deal with these spiritual issues.

Reflect on this. Over 300 years of the Western industrial revolution and the now the globalized knowledge economy is compressed into 50-60 years of intense transformation in Asia as a diverse continent which is modernizing rapidly. Unpacking the phenomenological bases with the adaptation pressures in such short time frames is unheard of anywhere else the world. This is often glossed over by frames developed from the last century which often seem inadequate. Themes such as approaches to values, relationships, ethics, dying and grief are fundamentally worthwhile to be included in the curriculum-shaping role of the training of generations of counselors in this century. Oftentimes the western frames that we use to address these issues seem to have a strong Western bias.

Given the unrelenting pressures of adaptation accompanied by insidious stress, demands peeling away the layers of human experience and behaviors. At the same time this region is among the oldest civilizations in the world with cultures that have endured and endeared. Malaysia is an auspicious 'crossroads' nation of multicultural influences, geographically and economically poised from the mother lodes of civilization in China, India and Islam yet with conspicuous modernity. This book synthesizes the best of counseling practice drawn from research but is underpinned by spiritual phenomenological - experiential dimensions ancient and modern in the 21st century.

Mohan Raj Gurubatham
HELP University, Malaysia

Preface

INTRODUCTION

It has always been interesting that while multicultural counselling is seen as a critical component of therapy, much of the writings and research then to focus on the experienced of practitioners in the West working with other minority groups. The question of working with individuals from different cultures has very much been work of individuals from the West working with the 'other'. For us therapists in Asia face cultural perspectives of a different kind. Minority groups that have been accepted and supported in the West, still have very little resources and may even be legally persecuted in the East.

Therapeutic modalities and the ideas of integration of culture may clash with actual experiences on the ground. Yet there is little if any compilation of works by Asians from Asia on the topic. This is partly as the field while growing exponentially is still relatively new in the East. There are many barriers to publishing in Asia ranging from language issues, social stigmas and the fact that many who are working in the ground are practitioners not actually researchers.

From its conception this book was aimed at addressing the issues faced by therapists in Asia, addressing multicultural issues that perhaps shifts away from the predominant Western perspectives that dominate the literature. The book would be useful to practitioners, undergraduates and post-graduates in the areas of mental health namely counselling, clinical psychology and welfare workers. The books content especially the latter chapters will also be relevant to individuals from spiritual organizations to see how psychology and therapy may support and help their community.

The book is aimed at being a sharing of experience, cases and skills, with an addition of relevant research in the area of multicultural therapy and interventions. Four main areas were sought as content for the book that is experience of therapists in Asia working with multicultural clients, specific interventions or modalities developed for working in the area of mental health, the issues and challenges faced by specific minority groups and finally issues of religion and spirituality that arise in mental health work. The relevance of this book is to highlight the situation on the ground in tandem with providing ideas and suggestions in managing issues that may arise as mental health in Asian nations increase.

The collections of readings in this book have a wide range, and I would like to sincerely like to thank all the authors and reviewers who took time and effort to support this undertaking. The journey in bring all these works together was a valuable if at times challenging experience. While the contributors are predominantly Malaysian it is possible that the applications may be applied throughout Asia.

ORGANIZATION OF THE BOOK

The first two chapters include the challenges of doing multicultural therapy in Asia as a whole. The third to the fifth chapter are of specific programs and interventions developed for Asian Clients. These interventions are exciting as Asian practitioners take to online platforms, develop their own moralities and modify existing modalities to suit the needs of their specific audience.

The book then addresses mental health realities, challenges and needs of the various minorities and marginalized communities in Asia. From the challenges of being a frontline worker in Mental Health in South East Asia, to working with the LGBTQ community and refugees in Asia both of which are communities that have to contend with mental health issues, while facing harassment and persecution from individuals and the governments of these countries. We than have a very special sharing, a story from an individual with Cerebral Palsy in Malaysia, her unique experience in managing her situation.

The subsequent chapters address the issues of spirituality and religion in therapy. These chapters are written by practitioners of the religion to help support others who provide therapy for individuals of that religion. The religions focused on here were the main four religions in Asia which are Christianity, Islam, Hinduism and Buddhism. The practitioner contributors here focused on issues from their religion that is relevant to mental health and applications of a religious perspective to therapy in supporting the client's needs.

Chapters here involve the development of a very unique Hindu Chaplaincy in Australia, the barriers and challenges in creating a wholly unique method of supporting a minority group in an Australian City known as the City of Churches. There are two chapters on the application of Buddhism in therapy and how the teachings of Buddhism may be applied to support clients, the first chapter presented here, looks at Buddhism in general, the traditions that are applicable in psychotherapy. This is followed by a chapter on the application of Christianity in Counselling from a Malaysian perspective is provided.

A chapter on the Hindu approach to therapy where the author addressed the theory and philosophy of Hinduism and how teachings of the Bhagwat Gita and Vedas may be applied to specific areas in counselling. This is followed by rather interesting chapter on the experiences of Muslim therapist supporting non-Muslim clients and the unique challenges related to the therapists experiences.

Finally we present the second chapter on Buddhism that looks specifically at Theravada Buddhism hailing from Sri Lanka, its relevance and application to mental health work. The final chapter looks at qualitative research done in managing grief work in Malaysia and the sensitivities of working with clients from different beliefs of the afterlife when managing grief. The chapters do focus on experiences of the practitioners and the applications as how they would apply in practice. I feel it is important that the readers understand that this sharing is not exhaustive, and individuals may have different perspectives of their own religions. The works provide a platform for deeper and more engaging work in using religion in therapy from the perspective of the client's own belief system.

CONCLUSION

Once again, I would like to thank all involved in this endeavor and I sincerely hope that this book will be of use to practitioners of mental health to understand multicultural issues from an Asian perspective.

With not a comprehensive digest on all these issues of multicultural therapy, the book is intended to be thought provoking and perhaps an inspiration to others to critically view their work from their unique cultural background and share their applications with the rest of the world.

Anasuya Jegathesan
HELP University, Malaysia

Chapter 1
Challenges Associated With Counselling Multicultural Clients

Sindusha Darshini Kanna Dasan
HELP University, Malaysia

ABSTRACT

The chapter is about different situations that therapists face challenges in and outlines what a therapist can do when faced with these challenging situations. The challenges covered are: challenging the competency of the therapist of color; transferring minority animosity to clients of other cultures; unrealistically viewing the therapist of colour as a super minority therapist; overidentification with the client; encountering clashes in cultural values; encountering clashes in communication and therapeutic styles; multicultural competence in a therapist; therapist of colour needing to prove competence; dealing with expressions of racist attitudes/beliefs/behaviors from clients; receiving and expressing racial animosity; and dealing with the stages of racial and cultural identity of therapists and clients. This chapter is to create awareness in therapist and help build multicultural competent therapist.

CHALLENGING THE COMPETENCY OF THE THERAPIST OF COLOR

Introduction on Being a Therapist

Being a therapist is a delicate and hazardous profession because therapists are entrusted with a responsibility to carry out their highest duty of care to ensure that clients are taken care of to the best of one's ability, skills and expertise in the given area. A therapist will receive clients from all walks of life and one must be prepared mentally as well as emotionally to handle anything that clients may bring with them. Therefore, it is crucial that therapists remember that the most important tool there have in this field is themselves as a person. It is important for therapists to continually work towards getting to know themselves and to develop themselves as they go on. This is because in every therapy session a therapist brings their human qualities and experiences that has the power to influence the therapeutic process. If

DOI: 10.4018/978-1-5225-6073-9.ch001

a therapist is not aware of certain aspects in themselves that could create countertransference it would potentially harm the therapeutic alliance and what's worse is it could cause irreparable damage to the client. As illustrated in this example; a client had come in for sessions due to issues of guilt. Client narrated to his therapist that he had stolen food for his younger brother and himself when he was younger. Overcome by fear of being caught he had opened fire and ran off never knowing what had happened to the guy he shot. The therapist had taken it upon herself to find out what had happened to the guy he shot hoping to help bring some closure to her client's life. However, by doing so the therapist had betrayed the client's trusts. When the client came back for the next session and told the therapist that he was starting to feel much better, the therapist being so caught up by the information she found and what had happened to her personally had unintentionally blurted out to the client asking him if it was too early to feel better and if he thought about the person he shot. This outburst from the therapist brought tremendous harm to the client as it further compounded his feelings of guilt and made him question his past. Therefore, it is vital for therapists to work on their issues and ensure that it does not spill into the session as it can cause irrevocable harm to the client's wellbeing.

Dealing With People of Colour

People of colour come from sensitive backgrounds because they have either been oppressed because of their skin colour, racial differences, ethnic differences, religion or political affiliation. Therefore, dealing with people of colour can sometimes proof to be slightly difficult because they have been looked down upon and treated unequally so coming for therapy sessions may be difficult for them. They may overtly or covertly try to challenge the credibility of the therapist of colour by questioning the therapist competence in an attempt to disprove the therapist's insights to the issues they are facing and undermine the therapeutic process (Sue, 2010a). The challenges that come up may not be conscious to the client. However, they may become apparent through the unwarranted interest from the client in pursuing in depth information about the therapist training and background, types of qualification received, place of training and number of years in clinical practice (Sue, 2010a). It is important for therapist to be able to manage clients views of the therapist they are seeking from because most of the time clients just need assurance that the therapist they have sought out for therapy is capable of holding the space for them to talk about their issues and asking questions about the therapist is a way for them to assess if a therapist is someone who is safe who would not further degrade them. While these inquiries may come across as a personal attack and be uncomfortable for therapist especially therapist who are starting out in the field, it is important for therapist to manage their own comfort in dealing with client's questions about themselves. To be able to do this a therapist needs to remember where their clients are coming from, how would the information that the client is seeking for be beneficial to them and how to provide responses that will uphold their integrity and themselves as a therapist. Example an African-American once asked a therapist of colour if she had worked with similar people in the past to gauge if the therapist was aware of the struggles he went through as an African-American. These challenges are apt to surface during a therapist career so one must be tactful in handling such challenges as it could mean a start to forming a strong therapeutic alliance or an end to an opportunity to support the client in their journey.

Decision to Consider in Confronting or Exploring With a White Client's Resistance to a Therapist of Color

According to David and Gelsomino (1994) they reported that ethnic minority therapists was frequently found to be a recipient of greater hostility, resistance and mistrust in a cross-racial practice compared to their White counterparts. Therefore, for therapist of color, there are no easy techniques or solutions that can be applied in helping therapist deal with challenges that are purported towards their credibility. However, a therapist can take this factors into consideration when making a decision to confront or explore a White client's resistance towards a therapist of colour which largely depends on internal and contextual factors such as; a) the therapists comfort with his or her racial or cultural identity, b) clinical importance of the expressed behavior, c) timeliness of the intervention, d) strength of the therapeutic alliance, e) the manner of which the intervention would be carried out (Sue & Sue, 2016).

What Can Be Done?

First, it is not an easy topic to broach when one's competency is being challenged especially when it is shaded with racial overtones. During this period of time, it is important that a therapist exercises one's highest degree of professionalism in dealing with this situation because becoming upset or allowing one's defensiveness to dictate the flow of the therapeutic session will be counterproductive in nature to helping the client. Other than this, before any intervention can be applied a therapist needs to recognize the purpose of the resistance and not take it personally. This would allow a therapist to sieve through a client's behavior in wanting to know about their competency and other clinical motivations that may be present. Also, it is important that when an intervention is applied a client is ready to receive it. Lastly, the most important facet in addressing racial issues is therapist of color must feel comfortable in engaging in difficult topics regarding race.

TRANSFERRING MINORITY ANIMOSITY TO CLIENTS OF OTHER CULTURES

Being Aware of One's Own Racism, Discrimination and Prejudice

The importance of therapist being aware of one's own animosity towards other cultures who might have privileges status has vast implications in counselling. Without awareness of what is going on in a therapist of colour, a therapist may find it difficult to contain their anger towards clients from the majority group especially when this group is viewed as the oppressor. Therapist in this situation may also find it difficult to understand the worldview of their clients from this group because they may feel a sense of unfairness for the inequality of treatment towards the monitory group. Other than this, it will also make it hard for therapist in this situation to establish rapport with their client because they may be torn between conflicting sides to help and harm their clients. Lastly, the therapist in these situations may feel guilty for imposing the reality of their racial qualms upon client who come from the majority group. Without the awareness of one's own racism, discrimination and prejudice towards another culture who is perceived by a therapist as having the upper hand it would be detrimental to the client's wellbeing to be subjected to the animosity of the therapists.

Managing Countertransference From Therapist of Colour Toward Client of Another Culture

This situation may arise if a therapist experiences countertransference where feelings of bitterness and anger are transferred to a client from another culture (Sue & Sue, 2016). This happens when a therapist is unable to delineate the experiences of racism, discrimination and prejudice he or she might have towards a particular culture. This, this would hamper the therapeutic process. It is important to be able to work this out in a healthy manner because these grudges against another culture may not happen at a conscious level, but they may present themselves in other manners.

In order for therapist to have multicultural competency in counselling a therapist needs to be able to engage with clients from a variety of backgrounds in order to assist themselves in overcoming the challenges they may face. To be able to attain this goal therapist need to be able to work with clients from diverse racial, ethnic and cultural backgrounds. This may be particularly difficult for Black therapist who engage with White clients because their social and political history of this racial group. It is imperative that therapist who face this kind of predicaments to find ways to overcome their struggles because it was shown in a study focusing on counselling that there were significant differences in areas of therapeutic alliance, outcomes and perceived credibility of therapist by clients between therapist who ethically matched and had no match between their clients (Farsimadan, Draghi-Lorenz & Ellis, 2007). In addition to this, Gelso and Mohr (2001) introduced the concept of culture-related countertransference where a therapist who has distorted view of a culture of a client who identifies with the majority group and having inelastic interpersonal behaviors engrained in ones displaced experiences of the member of this racial group was found to experience reactions such as fear, disdain, superiority or comfort.

Given the unique nature of what a Black therapist has experienced due to being oppressed and their racial group negatively stigmatize it may impact the interactions the therapist has with their clients (Chapman, 2006). As such it is imperative that the minority therapist takes steps in achieving an integrated Black racial identity through the 5 stages proposed by Cross (1971) in this model; Pre-encounter; where individuals upheld attitudes that idealized Whites and devalued the Black culture which led Black to look down upon their identity. At the encounter stage Blacks are called to inspect their thinking about their own race and during this stage individuals are no longer able to deny their race because the events or experiences that led them to devalue their own race to begin with begins to show the differences they faced in the racist society. Next stage the immersion-emersion stage where Blacks begin to view heir racial identity differently and form new perspective that allows them to view their Black identity. In immersion Blacks tend to immerse themselves in their culture and adopt an identity based on what they believe to be Black and emersion is where Blacks begin to move from idealization of what is Black to learning the complexities of their history and culture through reading literature, attending organization dedicated to their culture and engaging in different activities to help them have a better understanding of what it mean to be Black. Then at the internalization stage Blacks begin to have an integrated positive Black identity where they begin to recognize the significance of their own identity and are able to appreciate others' identities as well. Lastly at the internalization- commitment stage is where Blacks maintain a continuous effort of internalizing their identity by frequently reflecting on their identity and exploring social activism in their community. Since, the focus is on Asian culture this same model can be applied to therapist who identifies as a minority in the Asian culture. Thus, by looking at the importance of forming a healthy racial identity of a therapist who identifies as a member from a minority group and the implications it has on the therapeutic process it is imperative that therapists are aware that this exists and put it into practice.

UNREALISTICALLY VIEWING THE THERAPIST OF COLOUR AS A SUPER MINORITY THERAPIST

Explanation

Some clients who identify with the majority group may prefer to see a therapist of color because they may have an exaggerated sense of a therapist of color's qualifications, believing that to achieve the status of a therapist one must have extraordinary effort that enabled them to go against the forces of discrimination. Clients may believe that the accomplishments attained by the therapist was due to high intelligence, having exceptional capabilities and high motivation (Sue & Sue, 2016). Thus, therapist of color are seen as superior and perceived by the client to be able to offer them effective help compared to other therapist.

Understanding the Subtlety of the Perceptions of Clients

Clients regardless of race may have faced rejection, invalidation, misunderstood, and suffer from feelings of inferiority and feelings of worthlessness (Sue & Sue, 2016). As such they may have a mistaken belief that a therapist of color might understand their position better thinking that they themselves might have gone through similar things such as racism and discrimination that would enable them to empathize with their situation. Though clients may find comfort in believing that their therapist of colour may be able to offer them the comfort and encouragement they need but it is harmful to allow them to go on believing in their perception of their therapist in this manner. Other than this, therapists of color may be perceived as skilful in dealing with issues on race especially to client who are in the process of dealing with their own racial attitude. While it may be nice to be perceived and regarded in such a light the outcome of such perceptions can be detrimental and unfavourable in the long run as it may harm the therapeutic process and clients may grow to rely on the therapist to give them solutions to their issues thinking that they must know it all since they have similar experiences to them.

Importance of Bringing to Clients Awareness About the Uniqueness of Their Journey

It is crucial for therapist to have a good sense of their own racial and cultural background so that therapist can correct their client's notions they may have of their therapist. It is important for therapist to be firm, honest and authentic when dealing with this matter so that clients are able to readjust their perception and begin taking responsibility for their issues. Other than this, therapist should also be mindful of the possibility of clients returning to their preformed notions of their therapist and be consistent in reminding them of the differences that exists. In doing so the therapist would be carrying out their duty of non-maleficence and beneficence and also being aware of the existence of cultural differences between themselves and their clients.

OVERIDENTIFICATION WITH THE CLIENT

Explanation

Psychodynamic theory has expounded the occurrence of transference and countertransference in counselling and psychotherapy, concepts that are vital in the development of self-awareness. To grasp the essence of this concepts, transference is where a client projects one's feelings of past experiences and relationships onto a therapist whilst countertransference is the opposite where a therapist projects their feelings from past experiences and relationships onto their clients in the present (Urdang, 2010). It is inevitable that therapist might meet clients who have gone through somewhat similar experiences to themselves. While having similar experiences with clients might enable a therapist to empathize with a client at a deeper level, it can also be counterproductive to the therapeutic alliance if countertransference occurs. When this occurs and if a therapist is unable to separate themselves from their client's narratives then therapist may harm the client in the process. Therefore, it is imperative that therapist know what their triggers are and how to catch themselves if they find themselves having a countertransference. If this occurs a therapist should take a step back and examine what is going on within themselves for the sake of their clients and themselves.

What Can Be Done to Maintain the Therapeutic Alliance and Grow as a Therapist?

There are a few things that therapist can do to avoid from over-identifying with their clients. While countertransference is inevitable, being aware of it is essential for effective counselling to take place. One way of doing this is to be aware of the analytic self which is a concept that can be used to enhance a therapist's awareness of their countertransference (Conte, 2009). The analytic self relates to the human psyche and refers to where our capacity for self-awareness exists. It is crucial for therapists to develop the ability to metaphorically separate themselves from themselves to enable them to look at their psyche from an objective point of view and gather the feelings their clients are trying to provoke in them (Conte, 2009). By learning how to do this, therapist not only learn not to personalize things, but it also allows them to recognize physiological signs that the client may perceive as well (e.g., facial expressions, eye contact gestures, etc. Another simpler way of grasping this concept is having the ability to create a different head space when a therapist is present with a client. Example a therapist had introduced another way of looking at things for a client who had to be present at her parent's court hearing by asking her to observe the situation as a detective and not by herself. By doing this the client was able to remain objective throughout the process and was minimally affected. Another example to illustrate this is a lecturer who had given a student another way of remaining focused during the class by asking her to metaphorically put away her troubles in a hypothetical box outside the class. This had enabled the student to pay attention in class because she had chosen a different head space to be at that moment. This is a skill that takes time to build. The first step is to be aware that it exists and start practicing it to see its benefits.

Other than this, it is important for therapist to develop their professional self in understanding how their own feelings, attitudes and relationship with clients are major components in the helping profession and understanding that helping others is a process as well (Urdang, 2010). Developing a professional self includes having an ability to recognize, understand and use the feelings and insights gathered on clients. By developing a professional self, a therapist will be less likely find themselves over-identifying with their clients because there are well aware of the person they are in the therapy room and the role they are playing in the therapeutic setting. Being a therapist is an ongoing journey of building oneself as one goes one and through the process it is important for therapist to engage in the reflection process. To develop a therapeutic alliance a counsellor may look within to find similarities that can help him connect with the client, but the problem arises when a counsellor overidentifies with their clients and becomes uncertain of how to proceed with therapy. When this occurs, it would be helpful for counsellors to look for what is different between themselves and the client in order to help them redirect their focus to the client. Another important step a therapist can take is to be aware of the boundaries they have set for themselves and enforce it while in session to avoid overidentifying with clients.

Moreover, it is crucial that therapist seek continuous supervision throughout their career as a therapist because supervision can help therapist identify their blind spots and as well help them to grow. Supervision is also necessary to ensure that a client's care has not been jeopardized and that they can still be effective helpers to their clients. There are many kinds of supervision that is offered but one kind of supervision that has its origin in the psychoanalytic concepts of transference and countertransference is the concept of parallel process (Sumeral, 1994). When transference occurs, this kind of supervision is carried out by the retelling of the presenting problem and emotions associated to the therapeutic alliance by the counsellor in the supervisory relationship whereas when countertransference occurs the supervisor would respond to the counsellor in the same fashion as the therapist responded to the client (Sumeral, 1994). The re-enacting of the counselling interaction and the supervisory interaction is why it is called the parallel process. Since transference and countertransference are covert behaviour being able to recognize when it happens entails a continual awareness of one's own issues and events that trigger the issues. Though awareness of oneself is the first step, utilizing this awareness can aid in the growth of the counsellor and in turn would help the client as well which is the ultimate goal. The discussion of the parallel process in supervision can heighten a counsellor's awareness of their involvement in the therapeutic and supervisory alliance. Therefore, for this process to be effective the intervention used by supervises using this technique should be simple, tangible and emphasis chiefly on self-awareness issues (Sumeral, 1994).

Importance of Knowing Your Role

20/20: A Vision for the Future of Counseling (2010), came to a consensus of the definition of counselling and defined counselling as a professional relationship that empowers diverse individuals, families, and groups to accomplish mental health, wellness, education, and career goals. However, the American Counselling Association (ACA) (1997) adopted the following definition of professional counselling; 'The application of mental health, psychological, or human development principles, through cognitive, affective, behavioural or systemic intervention strategies, that address wellness, personal growth, or career development, as well as pathology' (as cited in Marini & Stebnicki 2009, p. 16). This definition had created guidelines for the official ACA role of counselling and appears cover a professional that works with the normal population and those with pathology as well. A counsellor helps clients in attaining their optimal level of psychosocial functioning by identifying destructive patterns of coping and equip clients with healthier coping strategies to improve their quality of life.

It is important to remember the definition of what a professional therapist is and does because often times the role of a counsellor can become blurry quickly. Therefore, it is vital that therapist are aware of their roles in the counselling field because clients come from all walks of life and some may bring heart rendering stories that may require you to use your professional judgment to ascertain the best course of action. Thus, it is always important to reflect upon your role first before making any decisions example; I was appointed as a protection assistant at United Nations High Commissioner for Refugees (UNHCR) where my job required me to do a series of things which included interviewing each family member, cross-checking their responses to questions and writing up recommendation reports so that they can be reviewed by another department to be resettled in a 3rd world country. Other times when I was off duty I was asked to mend the front counter where refugees came by to either ask about their status, to inquire about various things or to register for protection with UNHCR. One day as I was mending the front counter, a guy walks up and enquires about insurance for his wife as she was in need of medical assistance. I told him what he needs in order to purchase the insurance and he states that he does not have enough money to purchase the insurance which was RM20. I go to my leader and ask him if I could buy insurance for this guy and immediately without a second thought the leader gives me a blunt no. Despite pleading and coming up with justification to buy this man the insurance the leader just turned around and told me this, ''you can't buy the guy insurance. What about the other 100 people who need it too? This is something that can't be done. I won't allow it'. I was off course devastated as I had to go back to the person and tell them that there was nothing we could do for him. It took me months before I could lay this to rest and I was only able to do so once I examined my role. I was trying to play a role of a well-ware worker when my actual role was an assistant to provide additional help to the team. Often times, being a therapist and coming across many civilians on a day to day basis a therapist is certain to meet people with extraordinary needs which a therapist may be able to provide but since they are in the role of a therapist they should not. It is during this times that therapist need to take a step back and remind themselves of their role as a therapist in order to be an effective helper and also to not face burnout which is a common occurrence in this helping profession.

ENCOUNTERING CLASHES IN CULTURAL VALUES

Explanation

It has been an enduring goal in psychology that therapist are expected to be objective and have unbiased understanding of human beings. Although therapist may have their own values and beliefs towards something, therapists are expected to put aside their values and beliefs in therapist and assume a neutral position (Jackson, Hansen & Cook-Ly, 2013). Therapist are expected to be aware of their client's worldviews so that they would not impose their values on others. However, Gademer (2004), doubts that therapist can put aside their values and contends that both therapist and client's values are something that can't be avoided. However, having value conflicts in therapy has its benefits in therapy and if it is used carefully and ethically it can encourage positive change. Research debates that when a therapist allows clients to come up with their own therapy goals which is termed as liberal individualism is still embedded in value, therapist has imposed their value and treatment goal (Tjeltveit, 1999). Since, therapist have a strong belief in what they deem as positive mental health for clients it is characteristic of having value judgment and therapist should also recognize that being tolerant and having respect for clients' autonomy is values a swell (Jackson, Hansen & Cook-Ly, 2013). Essentially, values lie beneath every definition that therapist constitutes as healthy ways of being and it exists in psychotherapy theories as well. Research has also shown that value convergence and value conversion occurs in therapy and it would be immature to discount the impact that values have on the therapeutic process.

Situations Where Conflicts May Occur

As therapist we are constantly faced with situations that clients bring to us because it is too big for them to figure out what to do on their own. Our role as a therapist is to offer them choices, discuss with them the consequences and support them with the decision they have made. However, sometimes a therapist values and a client can be in conflict especially in cases of abortion where there is pro-choice and pro-life or whether to stay in a marriage or seek for divorce or whether to terminate end of life care or keep the person on a ventilator. All these kinds of situations are hard to deal with but in order to be an effective helper and to allow the client to make an informed decision one must put aside one's own values regarding the situation. It is also important that therapist view the situation from the client's point of view when trying to assist them in making a decision in order to ensure that clients are able to take responsibility for the decision they make. When helping clients make a choice on what sometimes seem like impossible situations it is imperative that therapist assists clients in determining the consequences of their actions because at the end of the day clients have to be able live with the decision they have made.

Ethical Considerations

In looking at issues related to values in therapy to be value neutral it is now being seen as indefensible (Bergin, Payne, & Richards, 1996). However, this raises ethical questions for therapist because values from therapist goes against the core facets of client autonomy and respect of differences that are expressed in the American Psychological Association (APA) (2002) code of ethics. In the APA code of ethics principle D and E addresses therapist values which mostly comes from values and is seen as harmful and steps are taken to ensure that therapist values are kept in check due to fear of ethical concerns of wanting to protect clients right and decreasing unfair influence from therapist beliefs and attitudes. However, there seems to be an argument to Principle A which speak about beneficence and nonmaleficence where it is said to have value judgement of what is seen to be a good outcome compared to a bad one and that it may differ from therapist on what is considered to be a good outcome. This being said the principles drawn up is laden with value issues as well that present ethical concerns. Therefore, a therapist can't avoid having value in the session but they are step that need to be taken to ensure that clients are not harmed and gain the most out of the sessions.

Strategies to Manage Values in Therapy

As therapist are human beings they are expected to have personal feelings about what is deemed as appropriate behaviour ad as professional in the mental health field they are expected to have professional believe about what is surrounds psychological well-being and what outcome are seen as appropriate for clients facing emotional suffering. As such the idea that personal beliefs in therapy pose as an ethical threat can be reduced by differentiating between personal feelings from professional beliefs (Jackson,

Hansen & Cook-Ly, 2013). By differentiating between personal feelings and professional beliefs, therapist can still use values if it is identified as professional ones to facilitate therapy. Other than, client's values can be challenged if therapist find that it would hamper the therapeutic progress and if their view on mental health differs significantly from the therapists Williams and Levitt (2007). As suggested by Strupp (1980) for therapist to share important therapeutic values (professional values) disparate from idiosyncratic value because they are exceptional to the therapist and can be put aside in therapeutic sessions. By doing this a therapist can reduce issues associated to teaching and other ethical concerns with value convergence. Since therapist have a desire to increase client's autonomy, using professional judgment self-disclosure can be used to disclose their professional values in order to discuss differences in values to reduce value convergence. Irrespective of the manner used to manage values, it was found that therapist shared values of individualism such as authenticity, agency and autonomy and worked toward building a client's inner sense of self and their ability to make decisions and be responsible for their own lives (Fisher-Smith, 1999). In terms of therapeutic goals, adjustment might be required to preserve a client's value system. Heilman and Witzum (1997), proposed that therapist take on the value-sensitive approach in therapy by valuing a client's value more than their own. Williams and Levitt (2007), recommended that therapist seek supervision when they feel that their values with the clients vastly differs from theirs to gain a different perspective on the differences. Another way recommended to deal with values in therapy is therapist require training to articulate their values both personal and professional and to understand the importance of values and morality in counselling (Jackson, Hansen & Cook-Ly, 2013). Other recommendations include, getting more training to manage differences in values and gaps that are presented between recommendations and actual practice so that therapist are able to recognize how their own values permeate into therapy and what can be done. It is imperative that therapist understand the sensitive nature of cultural values client bring into therapy and using their professional judgment to figure out what would be the best approach for their clients.

ENCOUNTERING CLASHES IN COMMUNICATION AND THERAPEUTIC STYLES

Explanation on Communication Styles

Therapy is a context where communication plays a vital role in transmitting messages to a listener and there are various ways that the differences in communication styles across races and cultures manifest themselves in the therapeutic alliance (Sue & Sue, 2016). In some cases, difficulties may arise due to different cultural backgrounds or personal experiences one may have. Communication styles often vary vastly between cultures, as such a person who says the same thing to two different individuals who come from different cultures may interpret the message in two totally different ways. A therapist who is a non-native speaker but have native speaking clients or individuals who communicate in languages other than their native language may encounter difficulty in understanding or interpreting certain subtleties or nuances that are easily picked up by native speakers the language. This types of issues can lead to communication breakdown, confusion or conflict in a therapist- client alliance and in some cases may be interpreted as insolence, when it was not even intended in the first place. The implications of being aware of the clashes of communication in therapy are many, for one due to the diversity of culture Malaysian's live in an issue that may be considered a communication problem in one individual from one culture may not be perceived similarly from another individual from another culture. Therefore, it is imperative for therapist to be knowledgeable about the culture they have chosen to work with because having effective communication styles to communicate with different cultures would not only help both parties convey accurate messages to one another, but it would also help therapist build a strong therapeutic alliance which is pivotal for any kind of therapy to take place.

Knowing About the Asian Culture and How They Communicate Using Space, Touch, Tone of Voice and Eye Contact

Hall (1966), has divided space into five sub-sections. First is interpersonal space; different cultures have different agreement about space between individuals in social situations. The differences of communication styles may be evident by how certain cultures use personal space when interacting with one another. Watson (1970), has determined that South America, the Middle East, and Southern Europe as contact cultures whereas Northern Europe, North America and Asia fall under non-contact cultures. In contact cultures where close contract was preferred it was noted that people had a tendency to interact with each other at a close distance, were more directive and utilized more touching and eye contact compared to noncontact cultures Watson (1972). Typically, some cultures like the Western culture prefer to converse at a closer distance as they feels much comfortable doing so whereas other cultures such as the Asian culture may feel uncomfortable conversing at a close proximity as it is seen as an intrusion of personal space. For example, Latin Americans, Africans and Indonesians tend to converse with people much closer as compared to Anglos. A Latin American client may cause a therapist to move back and this behavior may be interpreted as being cold or aloof. In another instance, the therapist may interpret the client's behavior as inappropriate (Sue & Sue, 1977). As such it is important to check in with clients to assess their comfort of the distance between the therapist and themselves. Though touch in therapy has been verified as a powerful nonverbal behavior in therapy seeing that Asians are a non-contact culture, violations of the cultural rule in regard to touch are likely to be deduced similarly to close space as producing aversive consequences. This is especially important to take note for the Muslim culture that do not necessarily welcome touch. So it is pertinent to ask whenever a therapist feels that touch in a particular context may be helpful in conveying a deeper understanding and empathy than verbally expressing could.

Second is olfactory space; different cultures have different ways of utilizing the sense of smell (Hall, 1966). Example the Middle Easterners see olfactory space as a way of sensing another person whereas in Britain, perfumes are used to mask natural smells. It is important to take note of this in the Asian culture as well seeing that the weather in most countries are humid and due to these individuals who live in these countries are likely to perspire more. As such it is important to be aware of one's bodily odor and also the therapeutic space to ensure that clients are able to have a comfortable experience being in therapy. Third is thermal space; the experience of space can be felt through thermal sensations (Hall, 1966) like people who have higher tendencies to blush. In the Asian culture Chinese clients are likely to blush more because of their pale skin so therapist needs to be sensitive in managing this aspect of space as some may be self-conscious of this. Fourth is visual space where space is used to collect and deliver information (Hall, 1966). Though a therapist might not think much of the things they choose to keep in their therapy room it does impact the therapeutic alliance between therapist and clients because everything that is kept in the therapy room is sending a message to clients about the kind of therapist they are seeing, what is important to the therapist and what they can ultimately disclose to their therapist. It is important for therapist to think about the kind of message they are sending their clients and to take time to think about what they place in their therapy room because humans often engage in meaning making and thus, may attach a totally different meaning to what they see in a therapist room. Therefore, it is important that therapist ensure that any symbols that may represent religiosity, photographs, mementos, books, art and whatever else that may be value laden are removed from the therapy room to ensure that the therapy room is neutral and conveys a message to clients that it is safe for them to unload, be themselves and heal from whatever they are struggling with. Lastly, sociofugal and sociopetal space is where different cultures use different ways of arranging their furniture and designing their rooms (Hall, 1966). How furniture's in the therapy room are arranged, where the seats are positioned and where a therapist sits may have certain connotations to clients and implications that can build or rupture their therapeutic alliance between therapist and client. Therefore, a therapist needs to be mindful of the kinds of cultures they are dealing with, so they can adjust to ensure that clients feels safe and comfortable in the therapeutic space.

Other than being aware of the different kind of space in therapy, voice is another important nonverbal-behavior that is able to send many different messages. The usage of voice and verbal style to show and amplify speech differs through cultures. Expressive cultures tend to use louder voices with high speech rates whereas less expressive cultures tend to use softer voices with lower speech rates. Since Asians come from a collectivistic culture and grow up among elders, they typically do not raise their voice and tend to be less expressive in nature. Therefore, a therapist needs to be able to modulate their tone of voice in session and gauge the kind of client that is in front of them. Furthermore, eye contact is also a powerful nonverbal behavior. Different cultures create different rules with regards to eye contact and visual attention because both aggression and connection are behavioral affinities that are vital for stability and maintenance of a group. Eye contact is often used as a nonverbal sign to denote respect and since different cultures have different rules with regards to eye contact, respect using eye contact is conveyed differently in different cultures. Hence, as discussed earlier, Asian cultures are noncontact culture and seeing that the Asians come from a collectivistic culture they tend to view respect differently. As such looking directly at someone whom they are talking to is seen as disrespectful whereas looking away or even looking down is a sign of respect. So it is important for therapist to use caution when using eye contact because to them is may be a sign of disrespect to look another person in the eye but may be more willing to look at the therapist while a therapist are talking because they grew up in a culture that taught them to respect the elderly or people in authority by looking at them while they are spoken to.

Therapeutic Styles and Asian Culture

One facet that is consistent with cultural competence in a therapist is the ability to deliver services that are culturally sensitive (Sue, 1998). Cultural competence is a made up of numerous characteristics or skills and have adequate knowledge and understanding of the cultural groups that therapist work with. Another important component in being a culturally competent therapist is to ensure that the method of delivery of interventions are culturally consistent with what is needed by the individual of that culture, there is increase in credibility of the treatment or therapist applying the treatment modality and treatment is made understandable to ethnic minority clients (Sue, Zane, Nagayama Hall, & Berger, 2009). One way this can be done is to ensure that interventions used are in line with the ethnic language of clients (e.g. translating materials, having a translator or a bilingual therapists presents), ensuring that the interpersonal style used for the intervention is varied or by providing cultural context for interventions used (Andres-Hyman et al., 2006). In order for a therapist to be able to call themselves culturally competent therapist need to be aware of the many components that exists in being culturally competent and put in to practice when conducting sessions.

It is also important to watch the therapeutic styles used when counselling clients of different cultures because some cultures prefer things to be directive (i.e. tell me what to do) whilst other cultures may be open to exploring therapeutic styles which are non-directive in nature. As suggested by Sue and Zane (1987), Asian American clients seem to have the need for gaining immediate benefit from the therapeutic meeting which is helpful for therapist to know in tailoring the approach they use with these kinds of clients to ensure that clients get the most out of the therapy session. In the Chinese culture a lot of time people describe being emotionally disabled due to having their emotions suppressed as it is something that is valued in the culture. This is an important thing for therapist to note when dealing with clients from the Chinese culture as they may expect the therapist to pick up on their indirect cues instead of expressing their feelings directly. This is something that can help the therapist build the therapeutic alliance by understanding that a client's lack of expression might not mean that they are not interested in engaging in a conversation that can potentially help them, but it is because they have grown up in a culture that did not encourage emotional expression that has made them the way they are. In a research carried out by Ng and James (2013) found that Chinese clients appreciated therapists that provided homework, analyzed their issues, spoke about helpful approaches that other clients have utilized, provided guidance through their communications and provided resources. It was also important for Chinese clients to be informed of their understanding of their own responsibility in the therapeutic process. The results found in the research helped delineate Chinese client's preference toward directive approaches is therapy.

MULTICULTURAL COMPETENCE IN A THERAPIST

Explanation

Multiculturalism refers to race, ethnicity and culture whereas diversity refers to dimensions of personal identity and individual differences (Arredondo & Glauner, 1992). The characteristics of cultural competence were acknowledged through the usage of a tripartite model: (1) being aware of one's own personal beliefs, values, biases and attitudes, (2) having awareness and knowledge of the worldview of individuals and groups in diverse cultures and (3) the employment of culturally appropriate intervention skills and strategies (Sue & Sue, 2013). This model takes into account personal identity of differences that exists in humans and the complexities of diversities and shared identity (Arredondo & Glauner, 1992). In order to have multicultural competence a therapist one has to have the knowledge and skills in handling diverse cultures in their practice.

Awareness of Different Aspects That May Impact a Therapy Session

Clocks, Time, and Scheduling Clients

In order to be a multicultural competent or an effective helper in this profession therapist must not only be well versed in their application of skills and have wealth of knowledge in the area of counselling but they must also be mindful of the covert subtleties that exist in creating a conducive therapeutic environment for the therapeutic process to occur. Back when I was a teenager I fell into a deep depression and my parents decided to send me to a therapist to get help. The therapist was mindful of my body language and noticed that I often looked at the clock that was in the sitting area. She decided to move it as she knew it was a distraction. It important to note client's nonverbal behavior in therapy sessions as it is speaks louder than verbal behavior.

Although time is an important social construct that is used in the counselling field; to ensure sessions are kept within time, to ensure the client gains the most out of the session, to schedule sessions a therapist needs to be mindful of the different kinds of times that exists. Hall (1966), came with subdivisions of monochromic time that can have massive implication to the therapeutic alliance between therapists and clients from different cultures. Hall (1966) spoke about appointment times as different cultures have different expectation and practice. 9.00am does not necessarily mean 9.00am exactly as determined by monochromic time. Cultural time adjusts the exact time specified by adding or subtracting time as much as it is culturally understood and agreed upon. Appointment times has huge implications in therapy because not only does it enable therapist to gauge the amount of time they have to work with the client it also is important to ensure that client turn up on the time they set in order for a therapist to set their next appointment. It would be unprofessional if a therapist next client shows up before the previous client leaves the premises. Seeing that in the Asian culture there is still a lot of stigma attached to seeking help for mental health issues having clients meet one another would not be right as this may cause people to talk about the client they saw outside, and this may lead to more issues. Another time that therapist should be aware of is acquaintance time which is usually done in the early stages of therapy (Hall, 1966) to build rapport with the client and this might have considerable implications for therapist as well in terms of their behavior. Other than this, there is discussion time where it has implications in the therapy sessions about who makes decisions about certain things; the therapist or client and who else should be involved in the process (e.g. family and friends). Example in cases of where a client is suicidal it is not always black and white especially if the client is low risk. During this time professional judgment on the therapist part is needed and trust in the client's judgment is needed when making a decision whether to breach confidentiality or to bring in other people. Moreover, there is visiting time to consider where if a therapist makes house call it is only appropriate to allow the client from the culture to determine how long the meeting should last. Lastly, time schedule is an area that is difficult for individuals to gauge who are from different cultural origins and may have different concept of how long things should be. This is especially true for people in the Asian culture as most of them work, housewives with children or students who have to juggle multiple commitments so scheduling sessions may be difficult for them. Since time has huge implications on sessions, therapists should be aware of its existence and ensure that it is practiced accordingly.

Therapeutic Setting

Clients are incredibly sensitive about things and a therapist should take this into account as well. When my parents had sent me to this therapist it so happen that she was my friend's aunt which I have never seen before the session but I knew had lost her brother a year or so ago. So, when I entered therapy her pictures of her brother was placed on the mantel and I could not help but look at it. I felt bad that she had to listen to my troubles when she must have been grieving. Picking up on this she had moved the picture frames to another room and this made me feel better. She was in tuned with what was going on within me and had acted duly to make the therapeutic space more conducive for therapy to proceed. Although this therapist had done her best to accommodate my needs she didn't know I was extremely uncomfortable being in that particular room in the house where my sessions took place because that was the same area where her deceased brother once laid in a coffin and I for one had a lot of experiences with death since young which made me uncomfortable at the time. Looking back as a therapist now I can see how things like this could facilitate a safe environment for the client to talk about their issues or it can hamper their ability to stay focus. Therefore, removing distraction is imminent in creating a conducive therapeutic setting.

Language Proficiency Usage Based on Education and Cultural Background

Since language makes up a huge part of therapy it is important for therapist to gauge what level of language is used with a client. The important thing is to be able to convey messages to the client clearly and ensure they understand what is trying to be communicated to them. Especially, in the Asian culture if a therapist is seeing clients from suburban or urban areas most of the people are educated so they would have high language proficiency and would be able to understand a therapist who communicates using high language proficiency as well. However, it is the opposite for therapist who might see clients from the rural areas. People from the rural areas or people with ow social economic status may have not had proper education and therefore, their language proficiency may be low. Therefore, it is important that therapist assess the clients understanding of the message that is transmitted and based on this assessment a therapist can adjust accordingly to meet the client at where there are at. This would enable the client to receive the most from therapy. It is also important to ease into the way a client communicates so that rapport can be build. Other than that, it is important to use what the client has said instead of adding one's own words when paraphrasing or asking questions as this would likely enable the client to open up and take responsibility for what they are saying. Lastly, in some cultures swearing is acceptable so therapists need to be cautious in using swear words as it may traumatize clients who are not open to that kind of communication and it may also hamper the therapeutic process. Therefore, it is important for therapist to be aware of the usage of language in the therapy session.

Being Open About Disabilities

Therapist should also be open with clients about any disabilities they may have so that any concerns can be addressed openly, and the therapy session can progress smoothly. Example if a therapist with some kind of paralysis were to carry out therapy sessions it would be imperative for the therapist to discuss her disability to allow client to understand the nature of what had happened, and this would allow the client to refocus his attention to the issues that brought him to therapy in the first place. It is important to eliminate distraction in therapy so that the client can get the most out of the therapy session.

Crying in Therapy

Crying refers to shedding tears in response to an emotional state. The production of tears begins with lacrimal system. It is both a secretory system that produces tears and excretory system that drains them. To deal with emotions the limbic system (hypothalamus), which is wired into the autonomic system a part that an individual has no control over goes through via a neurotransmitter called acetylcholine, that has little control over the lacrimal system which is where the tiny molecule from I stimulates tear production (Knight, 2014) To put it simple whenever someone has an emotional reaction to a stimulus it trigger the nervous system which in turn causes the lacrimal system to activate producing tears (Knight, 2014). Since, therapy is an intimate process a lot of what is discovered in therapy sessions may cause clients to cry due to the intensity of emotions that are invoked from talking about certain things with the client. It is hard to decipher what is the best practice of care to give a client when they cry but it is important to know that crying is healing. It is important for therapist to get used to clients crying because it is part of the therapeutic process that enables a client to move through their issues and reach a better understanding of the issues that have brought them into therapy. As long as the function of tears is understood that it has a place in the therapeutic space it is entirely up to a therapist whether to use tissues in a therapeutic setting because the goal is to support the client through their issues. One way to be sure of what to do would be to ask a client what they need. Another was to assess the kind of culture they are from because people from the Asian culture are not openly expressive and may feel embarrassed to cry in front a stranger so therapist needs to give clients assurance that that their tears have a place in therapy.

Reciting Prayers in Therapy

Since therapy is a journey and different things work for different people it is important that therapist ask client their religious affiliation, faith, belief and spirituality to see if it might be a resource that they can tap on. A therapist who is well read about scriptures or is knowledgeable about others religion can use it in therapy if it is something that will help the client. An example of a memorable and powerful use of prayer in therapy was when a Muslim therapist asked the client knowing that she is religious to recite a prayer in the session and the therapist held her hand and respectfully listened to the prayer while it was recited by the Indian client. It was a powerful experience for the client because to have a therapist from a different faith respect her religion and seeing that it helped during the session the client was touched by what had happened in session. Therefore, prayer if used tactfully and in the right situation can impact the client in positive ways.

Managing Dual Relationships

It is undeniable that the ratio of therapist to the community who seek or need mental health services exceeds the number of therapist available to meet the demand. As such therapist who live in suburban or urban and especially rural areas may face challenges such as the client they see might also be their neighbors, friends or people who provide different services. Thought the American Counseling Association (ACA) (2014) code of ethics outlines managing and maintaining boundaries and professional boundaries it is frowned upon when therapist see clients whom they have had A.6a previous relationships with and decide to A.6.b extend counseling boundaries. There is no doubt that the situation is not ideal but due to the shortage of therapist available and the high demand of people seeking out counselling therapist need to make some adjustment to the guidelines given because everyone deserves mental health care and therapist too need to be able to socialize with people. Since this is the reality of the situation therapist need to ensure that certain things are enforced when the therapeutic relationship is extended. Therapist need to ensure that there are boundaries set in place when dual relationship and multiple relationship is present. There are many types of dual relationship that exists such as social, professional, treatment-professional, business, communal, institutional, forensic, supervisory, digital, online or internet and any additional and rare forms of dual relationships adoption of client's children or even referral received from clients to see people they know by the same therapist (Zur, 2015). There is also dual relationship of difference kinds that can be avoidable, unavoidable or mandated; voluntary-avoidable, unavoidable, common-normal, mandated and unexpected (Zur, 2015). Dual relationships can also be concurrent; in a school setting counsellor play both role as teacher and counsellor or in an intuitional setting where lecturers are also counsellors and supervisors (Zur, 2015). Other than this, there is different levels of involvement; low-minimal level, medium level and intense level (Zur, 2015).

According to Zur (2015), things that therapist can take into account when managing dual relationships is in regard to treatment plan; develop a clear treatment plan, consider the clients welfare, effectiveness of treatment, ways to avoid exploitation and bring harm, conflict of interest and impairment of professional judgment. It is also important to act with competence and integrity to minimize any potential risk. Consult with supervisors and legal experts when information is needed on complex cases. Zur (2015) also mentions that it is important that before and during therapy that include dual relationship this are taken into account; being informed of the clinical, ethical, legal, spiritual complications and potential consequences of entering into dual relationships, examine and be aware of your own need, consult with people who have been in the mental health field for long, learn to separate law and ethics from care, integrity and effectiveness and be sure to talk about policies of the risk and benefits of and implement them before session begins. Zur (2015) also outlines the things that therapist need to take into account when it comes to clinical integrity and effectiveness; where therapist need to remember that they are setting examples for clients to emulate, also since we are storied being stories are important part of therapy so therapist need to ensure that stories are told to help clients and not satisfy one's own needs, ensure that no harm is brought to client, explain the nature of the dual relationship, ensure that records are kept throughout therapy sessions, and constantly practice evaluations to ensure the approach used, treatment plan drawn and one's own effectiveness is looked into and be aware that if the dual relationship is not benefiting the client to take remediation steps to ensure the client receives the best care possible. Therapist are required to use their professional judgment when entering into dual or multiple relationship because there are risks involved. Therapist also needs to ensure that whatever decision made to enter a dual relationship is done with caution, ensuring that it would not bring clients harm and it is ethical.

THERAPIST OF COLOUR NEEDING TO PROVE COMPETENCE

What Happens to Therapist of Colour in This Situation?

People who identify with the majority group may overtly or covertly believe that therapist of colour are less capable than therapist from the majority group and this may effect therapist of colour in two ways; they may adopt the belief and stereotypes about themselves and the group they identify themselves from and become victims stereotype threat where therapist may be afraid of confirming a mistaken idea of themselves despite not believing in their own inferiority (Steele, 1997). This tend to happen when therapist have unresolved issues pertaining their racial identities and accept what society at large thinks of them. Due to this therapist of colour may feel the need to prove their competence and capabilities but may look for approval or confirmation from therapist or clients who identify with the majority group.

This has strong implications in the counselling session because therapist may need affirmation from clients and may resign their roles as experts in the session (Sue & Sue, 2016). Therapist of colour may also decline to see clients from majority groups due to feeling uncomfortable in bringing up the racial dynamics that may be present. This situation eventually leads therapist of colour to feel that their competence is threatened and the need to constantly challenge the stereotypes attached to them. This constant need to prove themselves may put them on edge and they may not be effective helpers to clients from the majority group that seek their professional help due to feeling inferior. Therefore, it is important for therapist of colour to know who they are as a person, their racial identity and valid documents to support them in this field so that they can't be shaken by others beliefs of them.

DEALING WITH EXPRESSIONS OF RACIST ATTITUDES/ BELIEFS/BEHAVIORS FROM CLIENTS

How to Manage This Situation Effectively

Therapist are bound to come across expressions in regard to racist attitudes, believes and behaviors from clients. Clients may express this towards the therapist appearance, skin colour, speech or any other characteristics. It is important for therapist to acknowledge differences and investigate the reasons behind the client's reactions as it may affect the therapeutic process. Example clients may call the therapist names that are crude, and this may stir up emotions. However, it is crucial that therapist respond to the client's behavior instead of reacting and do not take what is said personally because it may be a defense mechanism, distraction or even resistance that the client may be facing. Instead of focusing on the issues that brought them into therapy they have chosen to hurl hurtful remarks. Therapist can use this opportunity to circumvent the client's remarks and approach it firmly with facts to substantiate what is said. Other than this, clients from the same race may try to gain the therapist attention by telling stories of their race because indirectly they are either afraid that they might say something offensive or to assess if the therapist is able to understand their experiences. It is important for therapist to be aware of this because it happens covertly, and it is easily missed. It is also important to acknowledge the differences that exists between therapist and clients that are obvious (e.g., gender, age, ethnicity, disabilities) or discovered (e.g., religion, sexual orientation) (Sue & Sue, 2016). Another way to deal with expression of this kind is through self-disclosure if the therapists sees that it would be helpful in as it may aid building stronger therapeutic alliances by reducing worries about differences and increasing feelings of similarity between therapists and client.

RECEIVING AND EXPRESSING RACIAL ANIMOSITY

Importance of Being Aware of Racial Animosity and Circumventing the Situation

Since seeking mental health services in Asian culture still has stigma associated towards it people may use race against therapist for going into the field or clients for seeking help. A lot of psychoeducation that is required to bridge the gap in society about seeking mental health services and clients need to be validated for their effort for coming in for sessions. Since therapy is a journey of self-exploration Asians may view the process as unfitting and may find the need to question the therapist qualification (Sue & Sue, 2016). When this happens, it is good to acknowledge clients concerns and explain to them clearly what therapy is and how it can benefit them. It is also pertinent to discuss any risk that may be involved in therapy and as well as the interventions used. Seeing that there are different views of therapy and mental health practices, several subtleties may exist between racial groups (Sue & Sue, 2016). Example, Muslims in the Asian culture tend to keep therapy as the last resort and tend to value going through the nontraditional counselling or spiritual healing route. Therefore, if a therapist of a different race is not aware of the alternatives that exists in the culture it may impact the therapeutic alliance where the client may view the therapist as someone who would not be able to relate to their problems. This may in turn cause them to question the client's credibility and their trust in the therapist may dwindle which may lead them to constantly test the therapist in different ways to ensure that they can work together. The tests may differ from overt hostility to different forms of resistance (Sue & Sue, 2016). Other than this, therapist of colour may be recipients or perpetrators of racial animosity and the differences may be outlined due to the differences in cultural values and communication styles that may trigger stereotypes that impact both attitudes towards each other (Sue & Sue, 2016). Therefore, it is important to openly speak about it so that the therapeutic process can be salvages and therapeutic alliance can continue to be built.

DEALING WITH THE STAGES OF RACIAL AND CULTURAL IDENTITY OF THERAPISTS AND CLIENTS

Importance of Developing Racial and Cultural Identity

It is important for both therapists and clients to build upon their racial and cultural identity because it creates awareness of one's own race and culture which can impact how one perceives things in their own community and outside the community. The stages of racial and cultural identity development model can provide a structure to assist therapist in understanding their culturally diverse client's attitudes and believes. The attitudes and beliefs that are present are an essential part of forming an individual's identity and are revealed through how a person views themselves, others from the same minority group, other from another minority group and individuals from majority groups (Sue & Sue, 2016). By understanding the stages, therapist can not only build their own racial and cultural identity but can assists clients in understanding the stage they are at and areas that they struggle with. This understanding can help therapist talk to clients about religious beliefs openly and it would aid in more transparency about any issues pertaining to religious beliefs a client may have. Therapist should avoid falling into the trap of who is more oppressed as therapy is not a competition but rather a place for clients to discuss their issues and find alternative ways of coping.

REFERENCES

20/20: A Vision for the Future of Counseling. (2010, March). Consensus definition of counseling. Retrieved from http://www.counseling.org/knowledge-center/20-20-a-vision-for-the-future-of-counseling/consensus-definition-of-counseling.

American Counselling Association. (2014). ACA Code of Ethics. Retrieved from http://www.counseling.org/docs/ethics/2014-aca-code-of-ethics.pdf

American Psychological Association. (2002). Ethical principles of psychologists and code of conduct. *American Psychologist*, 57, 1060–1073. Retrieved from http://apa.org/ethics/code/index.aspx?item=3

Andres-Hyman, R. C., Ortiz, J., Anez, L. M., Paris, M., & Davidson, L. (2006). Culture and clinical practice: Recommendations for working with Puerto Ricans and other Latinas(os) in the United States. *Professional Psychology, Research and Practice*, *37*(6), 694–701. doi:10.1037/0735-7028.37.6.694

Arredondo, P., & Glauner, T. (1992). *Personal dimensions of identity model*. Boston, MA: Empowerment Workshops, Inc.

Bergin, A. E., Payne, R. I., & Richards, P. S. (1996). Values in psychotherapy. In E. Shafranske (Ed.), *Religion and the clinical practice of psychology* (pp. 297–325). Washington, DC: American Psychological Association. doi:10.1037/10199-011

Chapman, R. T. (2006). Internalized racism of the clinician and the treatment dynamic. *Journal of Emotional Abuse*, *6*(2-3), 219–228. doi:10.1300/J135v06n02_13

Conte, C. (2009). *Advanced techniques for counseling and psychotherapy* (pp. 7–8). New York: Sprinter Publishing Company.

Cross, W. E. Jr. (1971). The Negro-to-Black conversion experience. *Black World*, *20*(9), 13–27.

David, L. E., & Gelsomino, J. (1994). An assessment of practitioner cross-racial treatment experiences. *Social Work*, *39*, 116–123. PMID:8310317

Farsimadan, F., Draghi-Lorenz, R., & Ellis, J. (2007). Process and outcome of therapy in ethnically similar and dissimilar therapeutic dyads. *Psychotherapy Research*, *17*(5), 567–575. doi:10.1080/10503300601139996

Fisher-Smith, A. M. (1999). *From value neutrality to value inescapability: A qualitative inquiry into values management in psychotherapy*. Unpublished doctoral dissertation, Brigham Young University, Provo, UT.

Gadamer, H. G. (2004). *Truth and method* (2nd ed.). (J. Weinsheimer & D. G. Marshall, Trans.). New York: Continuum.

Gelso, C. J., & Mohr, J. J. (2001). The working alliance and the transference/countertransference relationship: Their manifestation with racial/ethnic and sexual orientation minority clients 106 and therapists. *Applied & Preventive Psychology*, *10*(1), 51–68. doi:10.1016/S0962-1849(05)80032-0

Hall, E. T. (1966). *The Hidden Dimension*. New York: Anchor Press/Doubleday.

Heilman, S. C., & Witztum, E. (1997). Value-sensitive therapy: Learning from ultra-orthodox patients. *American Journal of Psychotherapy*, *51*(4), 522–541. doi:10.1176/appi.psychotherapy.1997.51.4.522 PMID:9470959

Jackson, A. P., Hansen, J., & Cook-Ly, J. M. (2013). Value conflicts in psychotherapy. *Issues in Religion and Psychotherapy, 35*, 6–15. Retrieved from http://scholarsarchive.byu.edu/irp/vol35/iss1/3

Knight, N. (2014, September 18). Why Do We Cry? The Science of Tears. *The Independent*. Retrieved from http://www.independent.co.uk/life-style/health-and-families/features/why-do-we-cry-the-science-of-tears-9741287.html

Marini, I., & Stebnicki, M. A. (2009). *The professional therapist's desk reference*. New York: Springer.

Ng, C. T. C., & James, S. (2013). "Directive approach" for Chinese clients receiving psychotherapy: Is that really a priority. *Frontiers in Psychology*, *4*(49), 1–13. PMID:23408043

Steele, C. M. (1997). A thereat in the air: How stereotypes shape intellectual identity and performance. *The American Psychologist*, *52*(6), 513–629. doi:10.1037/0003-066X.52.6.613 PMID:9174398

Strupp, H. H. (1980). Humanism and psychotherapy: A personal statement of the therapist's essential values. *Psychotherapy*, *17*(4), 396–400. doi:10.1037/h0085938

Sue, D. W. (2010a). *Microaggressions in everyday life: race gender; and sexual orientation*. Hoboken, NJ: Wiley.

Sue, D. W., & Sue, D. (1977). Barriers to effective cross-cultural counseling. *Journal of Counseling Psychology*, *24*(5), 420–429. doi:10.1037/0022-0167.24.5.420

Sue, D. W., & Sue, D. (2013). *Counseling the culturally diverse: Theory and practice* (6th ed.). New York, NY: John Wiley.

Sue, D. W., & Sue, D. (2016). *Counseling the culturally diverse: Theory and practice* (7th ed.). New York: Wiley.

Sue, S. (1998). In search of cultural competence in psychotherapy and counseling. *The American Psychologist*, *53*(4), 440–118. doi:10.1037/0003-066X.53.4.440 PMID:9572007

Sue, S., & Zane, N. (1987). The role of culture and cultural techniques in psychotherapy: A critique and reformulation. *The American Psychologist*, *42*(1), 35–45. doi:10.1037/0003-066X.42.1.37 PMID:3565913

Sue, S., Zane, N., Nagayama Hall, G. C., & Berger, L. K. (2009). The case for cultural competency in psychotherapeutic interventions. *Annual Review of Psychology*, *60*(1), 525–548. doi:10.1146/annurev.psych.60.110707.163651 PMID:18729724

Sumerel, M. B. (1994). Parallel process in supervision. ERIC Digest. Retrieved from http://eric.ed.gov/?id=ED372347adresinden elde edildi.

Tjeltveit, A. C. (1999). *Ethics and values in psychotherapy*. New York: Routledge. doi:10.4324/9780203360453

Urdang, E. (2010). Awareness of Self: A Critical Tool. *Social Work Education*, *29*(5), 523–538. doi:10.1080/02615470903164950

Watson, O. M. (1970). *Proxemic behaviour. A Cross cultural study*. The Hague, The Netherlands: Mouton.

Watson, O. M. (1972). *Symbolic and Expressive Uses of Space: An Introduction to Proxemic behaviour*. Addison: Wesley Modular.

Williams, D. C., & Levitt, H. M. (2007). A qualitative investigation of eminent therapists' values within psychotherapy: Developing integrative principles for moment-to-moment psychotherapy practice. *Journal of Psychotherapy Integration*, *17*(2), 159–184. doi:10.1037/1053-0479.17.2.159

Zur, O. (2015). Dual relationships, multiple relationships & boundaries in psychotherapy, counseling & mental health. *Zur Institute*. Retrieved from http://www.zurinstitute.com/dualrelationships.html

Chapter 2
Counseling Chinese Communities in Malaysia:
The Challenges and Needs in Mental Health Service Deliverance

Rachel Sing Kiat Ting
Monash University Malaysia, Malaysia

Pei Lynn Foo
Penang Association of Counselling and Psychology, Malaysia

ABSTRACT

This chapter presents the experiences of Chinese in Malaysia (CIM), in the context of mental health services. As the second largest ethnic group in Malaysia, CIM is diverse in its dialectic subculture, education, generation, geography, and degree of assimilation to the mainstream culture. The chapter introduces the ecological characteristics of CIM and how they shape the unique psychological challenges. Though CIM are known for their multilingual ability, strong work ethics, emphasis on education, and family piety, the clashes between tradition and modern values, the marginalized position in the Malaysian political arena, the stereotype of overachiever in education, and the "brain drain" movement of young elite CIM, have all caused a strain in CIM families as well as individuals. Moreover, they face both external and internal barriers in getting quality mental health care. It is therefore imperative to promote a mental health discipline that is open to serve CIM, as well as being sensitive to its cultural and historical backdrop.

INTRODUCTION

In the recent two decades, the discipline of psychology in Asia is arriving at its golden age of development due to waves of globalization, modernization and westernization. Since the publication of the *Handbook of Chinese Psychology* (Bond, 1996), Chinese psychology is deserving much attention in the arena of cross-cultural psychology and cultural psychology. In 2010, there is an updated edition on the Handbook and the chapters expanded from 32 to 40 (Bond, 2010). Many recent empirical researches

DOI: 10.4018/978-1-5225-6073-9.ch002

on the Chinese population have been included in the handbook, which demonstrated that psychological research among this population could confirm, verify and be adapted from certain existing theories from Western psychology. Nevertheless, most of the studies cited in those chapters were based on Chinese populations from Hong Kong and Taiwan, as these regions have a longer history in establishing local psychological disciplines. Overall, there is a scarcity of psychology publications and literatures on Chinese immigrants or diasporas in other regions or societies.

The Chinese people have a long history of migrating overseas. Due to acculturation and assimilation, overseas Chinese espouse multiple identities that add to the richness in manifestation of Chinese personalities. The diverse and multidimensional identities among overseas Chinese can be explored through identity conflict and integration in the experiences of acculturative stress and socio-cultural adaptation, cultural competence mediated by coping strategies, personal and situational factors, social support (i.e. in the context of ethnic communities & host cultures), and the roles and interpersonal relationships within the foundation of the Chinese family (i.e. the concepts of family harmony and filial piety) over time and generations (Ward & Lin, 2010). The voices of Chinese immigrants speak of the evolvement of Chinese culture in new lands, as well as their hybridized identities as overseas Chinese. As a pioneering effort, the authors of this paper endeavor to expound upon the experiences of Chinese in Malaysia (CIM), in the context of mental health services. In comparison to Hong Kong and Taiwan, psychology practice is considered to be in its infancy stage in Malaysia. While academic psychology has existed since the late 1970s, applied psychology disciplines have surfaced only in the past 30 years (Ng, Teoh & Haque, 2003).

The Chinese as the second largest ethnic group in Malaysia with a population of 6,650,000 (23.4%) (Department of Statistics, 2016), is also diverse in its dialectic subculture, education background, generation gap, residential areas, and exposure to the amalgamated mainstream Malaysian culture. The aim of this chapter is to introduce the ecological characteristics of CIM and how they shape the unique needs of mental health among CIM. The objective is to empower mental health practitioners to be culturally sensitive and competent in providing services to the CIM community. Due to their unique migration history and settlement in Malaysia, CIM are known for their multilingual ability, strong work ethics, emphasis on education, and family piety. Their relative absence in the political arena, ethnic identity crisis, mistrust towards governmental system, and lack of solidarity have made them vulnerable to psychological stressors. In recent years, there is a rise in awareness of mental health issues among CIM in the public arena through promotional efforts of NGO services, religious groups, para-counselors, and social media. However, there is still stigma towards mental illness that creates barriers for CIM to seek help, especially among the less Westernized and urbanized populations. Since not all lower class CIM could afford private mental health services and deem such services as priority, many CIM rely mainly on family network or strong relational ties as emotional support. From the practitioners' standpoint, many trained counselors or service providers are not fluent in using Mandarin or other Chinese dialects in providing counseling. Moreover, even when there is an ethnic or language match between the counselors and counselees, the former often found that translation of Western psychological concepts a challenge in the counseling room with CIM, and do not necessarily possess multicultural competency. The uncritical transposition of the Euro-American values embedded in Western psychology also contributes to potential cultural clashes in the counseling room with the more traditional CIM (e.g. assigning labels such as "over-enmeshment" to CIM families). This struggle is quite obvious as Malaysia is an ex-colonized country struggling to find its multiracial-multicultural identity after 60 years of claimed independence from British influence. It is therefore imperative to produce a mental health discipline that is open to serve the CIM population, as well as being sensitive to its cultural and historical backdrop. This chapter will end with practical suggestions for CIM mental health trainers, researchers and practitioners in service delivery, education and policy making.

A BRIEF MIGRATION HISTORY OF CIM

Malaysia has a multi-ethnic naturalized population of about 28.4 million that is made up of three major ethnic groups. The largest ethnic group is the Malays at 68.6%. Those of the Chinese descent make up about 23.4% of the total population (about 6.65 million, which is roughly the size of Hong Kong's population). The Indian ethnic group makes up about 7.0% of the population and the remaining 1.0% consists of the aboriginal people as well as mixed ethnicities (Department of Statistics Malaysia, 2016).

Historically, the Chinese have been settling in Malaya since the days of the Malacca Sultanate, when the Straits of Malacca was a major trading route in the 15th century AD. Many Chinese traders settled and integrated into the Malayan culture since then. The second large wave of Chinese entering Malaysia was after Penang was founded in the late 1700s; many of them were planters, traders and tin miners. The influx of Chinese became more established after the founding of Singapore in the early 1800s, expanding their trade to include manufacturing, banking, and timber trading (Tan, Ho & Tan, 2005).

Due to trading and mining, CIM have been instrumental in the economic development of Malaysia as it is now, especially with regards to commerce and industry. A British administrator in Malaya was quoted as saying,

Under present conditions, the Chinese are the bone and sinew of the Malay states. They are the labourers, the miners, the principal shopkeepers, the capitalists, the holders of the revenue farms, the contributors to almost the whole of the revenue; we cannot do without them (Tan, Ho & Tan, 2005).

Reinforced by the British policy to keep the different ethnic groups in separate sectors, CIM had been seen as leading in business and trading, while Malays dominated the politics and government administration, whereas Indians provided blue-collared manpower (Fu, 2007). As a result, CIM tend to be seen as being on a higher scale with regards to socioeconomic status as compared to other ethnic groups (Fu, 2007). In 1971, the New Economic Policy (NEP) was introduced to eradicate poverty as well as to eliminate racial differences in economic function and geographical location. It was also a vehicle to boost Malay entrepreneurship by encouraging Malays to venture into business. In spite of its controversial implementation, which resulted in decreased Chinese participation in economic activities, the CIM still flourished in business ventures (Fu, 2007).

Traditionally, economic strength of the CIM is very much related to its community leadership. Many community leaders were successful merchant-entrepreneurs or *towkays*. Some of these leaders were conferred formal leadership status, and named *Kapitan Cina* (Chinese Captains) by the Malays. These *Kapitan*s were instrumental in building the Chinese community, in the areas of infrastructure and trading, as they were also appointed to State Councils. Apart from that, "secret societies" were also instrumental in leading the Chinese communities, especially during the early British colonial times. By the end of the 1800s, the Kapitanship was abolished by the British and secret societies were banned. Instead, the secret societies resorted to underground activities that still managed to keep the Chinese economy afloat (Pan, 2006). Influenced by the Confucian work ethics, the early Chinese settlers were known to be very hardworking with strong determination that lasted generations until today, leading to the stereotype of CIM being the most entrepreneurial people. Today, many CIM have ventured into and demonstrated success in various contemporary vocational areas. They also make up the bulk of the population in most urban areas of Malaysia today (Carstens, 2005; Heng, 2006).

UNIQUENESS OF CIM

According to the theory of ecological rationality (Todd & Gigerenzer, 2012; Sundararajan, 2015), human cognition and emotion are shaped by the ecological system we are embedded in. Even among the same Chinese tribe, such as the Yi ethnic minority group, there could be differences in semantic expression of emotions, explanation of suffering, and help-seeking behavior due to different religious practices and beliefs (Ting & Sundararajan, 2017). This theory could explain why CIM are different from other racial groups in Malaysia, as well as Chinese from other countries. We would describe four major environmental factors as having decisive influence on CIM in this section—language, cultural practices, education, and political status.

Language

With regards to language and culture, although most are conversant in the Malay language which is also the national language, each ethnic group in Malaysia still retains most of their original traditions and mother tongue. In addition, most Malaysians are familiar with the English language, which can be traced back to the long history of British colonization. Such multilingual ability is a uniqueness of CIM as compared to the Chinese elsewhere such as Taiwan, Hong Kong, Indonesia and Thailand. Tan (2005) estimated that there were approximately 5,365,875 number of Chinese dialect speakers in 2000, comprising of 94.27% of overall CIM (i.e. 24.45% of the total 2000 Malaysian population)[1] (Department of Statistics, 2001). Though not all CIM could read and write Chinese characters, most of them are fluent in one dialect or more at conversational levels, depending on their education, origin, and exposure. There are also significant differences in the way the Chinese language and dialects are spoken among the CIM. Influenced by the Malay and English languages, the CIM develop their own unique Chinese dialects, such as the Penang Hokkien which is unique and distinct to the northern peninsular region (Ong & Tan, 2017).

Cultural Practice

While most CIM retain their Chinese identity and traditions in their acculturation process, there exist some degrees of differences in the CIM cultural practice compared to those of Mainland China, Taiwan, and Hong Kong. Some traditional festivals celebrated by the Chinese community in Malaysia are no longer widely celebrated in Mainland China after the Chinese Cultural Revolution. This is especially true of certain regional rites and rituals that continue to be celebrated by the CIM. For example, for wedding ceremony in the Cantonese community, elaborated rituals and gift-exchanges are observed between the engaged families. The Chinese New Year, especially the reunion dinner on Chinese New Year eve and the 15th day, are still highly emphasized (Tan, 2005).

More importantly, the ability to preserve their language and cultural practice enable CIM in general to preserve their identity as Chinese, unlike their counterparts in Indonesia and Thailand where national identity precedes ethnic identity. In fact, many CIM still identify themselves as "Chinese," even if they are already acculturated Malaysians for more than a generation (Ang, 2013). For this group of CIM, their healing methods for mental health problems would also strongly tie to the folklore beliefs and practices, such as shamanism or traditional Chinese herbal treatment (*Zhong yao*) (Chang, Tam & Mohd Suki, 2017; Edman & Koon, 2000).

Education

Tan (2000) divided CIM into three major categories based on their education: Chinese-educated, English-educated, and Malay-educated, and he predicted that the second group will disappear as its boundary with the third group becomes gradually blurred with increased shared characteristics. He postulated that the internal diversities of CIM by education have implications on their cultural identities and even political orientation. The mass media they are exposed to also differentiates their level of acculturation and worldviews, with the English-educated CIM more susceptible to Western ideologies (such as democracy), whereas those who are Chinese-educated may know more about the historical facts and cultural values of ancient China. Not surprisingly, the English-educated CIM have remained politically prominent. This difference in educational background would also influence their worldview towards mental illness as well as help-seeking methods.

Socio-Political Status

Given economic strength and recognized leadership, CIM do possess some political influence in the ruling parties as well as the opposition, compared to other ethnic minority groups. Case in point is the state of Penang which has been under the governance of DAP (former opposition party prior to GE14) Chinese chief ministers since 2008 (Banyan, 2013). However, the ethnic Malays still hold the dominant political power in the country and the political involvement of CIM is decreasing (Freedman, 2000). The recent Penang floods debacle in which the plight and appeal for federal aid became political fodder and contention underlines the challenges faced by the minority opposition party (FMT Reporters, 2017).

In terms of inter-racial relationship, CIM seem to prefer to remain within their own race, forming racial cliques at schools and at workplaces. Due to the ethnic-based political structure in Malaysia, ethnocentric sentiments remain entrenched within each ethnic group thus discouraging meaningful inter-racial interaction. As evident in the university students' campaign against having different races to share rooms in hostels (Ng, 1999), which shows that there is still a strong pull towards keeping to one's own racial-ethnic group, leading to a lack of inter-racial understanding. This sociopolitical atmosphere is caused by the oversea immigration trend among CIM since 1980s, and those who remained in the country are faced with psychological insecurity as a racial minority. In fact, rising racial tension can be seen in recent years due to some right-winged ethnic Malay groups' rhetoric on "Ketuanan Melayu" ("Malay Supremacy" in English), and delegation of the ethnic Chinese as "Pendatang" (i.e. immigrants) and second-class citizens which further harmed positive inter-racial relations (Han, 2015).

According to Minkov and Bond (2017), the main predictors of national differences in happiness (i.e. subjective well-being, SWB) are closely connected to "national economic development, democratization, and increasing social tolerance" among different ethnic groups of a nation. Hence, taking the current socio-political challenges faced by the CIM into consideration, it is understandable that in comparison to the other ethnic groups in Malaysia, CIM have been found to have the lowest level of happiness and SWB (Minkov & Bond, 2017).

DIVERSITIES AMONG CIM

Despite much shared experience among the CIM, there exists much diversity among the population. Different scholars also have different taxonomy to differentiate CIM depending on their educational backgrounds, history of immigration and acculturation, language/dialect spoken, and geography of residence. Knowing these subcultures will help counselors better engage with their CIM clients as well as conceptualizing their struggles in a cultural-inclusive perspective.

Cultural Identity

According to Tan (2007), the CIM are broadly categorized into two groups. The first group, constituting 85% of CIM, builds their cultural identity around three pillars: the Chinese-medium schools (currently about 95% of Chinese children study in Chinese schools; there are around 1,300 national and independent Chinese schools across the country), the Chinese newspapers (nine in West Malaysia and eight in East Malaysia) and the Chinese ethnic corporations (including more than 7000 registered cultural heritage, industrial and business associations). They are typically independent business people, whose main concern is political stability for good economic returns. The second group, constituting the remaining 15% of CIM, consists of those who speak mainly English and are non-Chinese educated. Many are Christians, Peranakan, and members of Lion's or Rotary Clubs. This group is often stereotyped by the first group as the "banana" (i.e., yellow skin [Chinese race], white core [pro-Western culture]) (Tan, 2007).

The main difference between the two groups is that the second group does not share the three cultural pillars as part of their identity. Even though some are sending their children to Chinese schools now, this is done more for practical rather than cultural reasons. The two groups differ in their choice of media (English / Malay newspapers vs. Chinese newspapers), which indirectly results in very different perspectives and reactions to sociopolitical events within the country. Inevitably, because of different interests and worldviews, the two groups tend to associate minimally with each another, which further reinforce their prejudice and stereotype of the other party.

Nonetheless, despite their differences in cultural beliefs and identification, Tan (2007) suggested that both groups of CIM ultimately share one mutual concern -- fairness and justice for all people in the country. With general economic stability over generations leading to less hunger for survival, there is also increased interest in ancestral identity among the contemporary CIM (Fu, 2007). However, in recent years, the wealth gap has been increasing among the CIM community, yet not much attention has been paid to the marginalized CIM from lower socio-economic background (FMT Reporters, 2017).

Degree of Assimilation and Acculturation

According to Tan (2000), CIM could be divided into two broad categories — the more assimilated "Peranakan Chinese" and the so-called "Pure Chinese." The former group refers to the Malay-speaking Chinese, including the Baba in Malacca, and Malay-acculturated Chinese from the rural areas of Kelantan and

Terengganu. The origin of this group could be traced back to the 19th century, where interracial marriage occurred between the early Chinese settlers and Malays in those areas. The second group refers broadly to the Chinese who settled in Malaysia in the later stage, and who kept the kinship among themselves. What differentiates them from the first group is that they would never speak Malay among themselves. Their interaction with Malays is more confined to economic exchange (Tan, 2000).

Earlier research on acculturation also showed that those who were able to reach the "integration stage" in the acculturation process tended to have better mental outlook and subjective well-being than those who were stuck in the "marginalized status". Lin and Ting (2014) studied returning oversea Chinese from Southeast Asia to Mainland China during the 1950s, in terms of their re-entry acculturation experience. Many of them experienced cultural shock and disillusionment after returning to China as they lacked language fluency of Mandarin Chinese and still preferred the customs of their original host country (e.g. Thailand, Indonesia, Myanmar). This experience is likely similar to CIM, who although self-identify as "pure Chinese", have already adopted the host country's values and living practices. That is why CIM call themselves as "hua ren" (華人) rather than "Zhong guo ren" (中國人), where the former connotes overseas born Chinese and the latter entails the political nationality as Mainland Chinese.

Nevertheless, there is much variation in the degree of acculturation among CIM and their self-identified status in the society, which manifests as much nuances and complexities in the CIM's identities. For instance, in a preliminary study on psychotherapists in Malaysia (Ng, 2007), when participants were asked whether they would be considered "a member of a social, cultural or ethnic minority" in Malaysia, more Chinese considered themselves as part of the mainstream (60%) than not – a stark contrast with the Indians (about 75% considered themselves a minority), even though both the Chinese and Indians were historically migrants and generally considered the minorities by census. Yet, what makes the CIM very much distinguished from Chinese in other countries is still their hybridized identity shaped by the pluralistic Malaysian culture with the regional social-cultural experience of being Chinese. Bonn and Tam (2015) supported this premise and found that the CIM group carries its own unique cultural values on happiness overlapping with the values from Malays and Mainland Chinese groups respectively.

Dialect Groups

Early Chinese settlers in Malaya were mainly from the Guangdong and Fujian provinces in China. A report by Heng (2006) categorized these settlers into five major dialect groups, with the largest group being the Hokkien (37%), follow by the Hakka (22%), and then the Cantonese (19%), the Teochew (12%) and the Hainanese (4%). The geographical distribution of these groups was not random due to chain migration. The Hokkiens and Teochews mainly settled on the northern and southern coasts, whereas the Hakka and Cantonese settled in the inland regions. In Sarawak, East Malaysia, the Fuzhou and Hakka dialects are more prevalent in most inland and coastal regions, leaving Kuching to be predominantly Hokkien. In Sabah, the Chinese community is largely Hakka, followed by Cantonese and Hokkien (Tan, 2005; Ghazali, 2012). There is also certain bonding within each dialect group due to similar custom, cuisine and heritage.

Geographical Locations

Due to its political backdrop and geographical distance, Chinese in East Malaysia also forms a unique culture and community that is distinctive and different from the Chinese in West Malaysia (Chin, 1981).

Sabah and Sarawak joined Malaysia as a country in 1963, after West Malaysia claimed its independency in 1957. Prior to independence, both were under the ruling of British governors and the Malay Raja (king). Due to the discrepancy in political history, East Malaysians usually do not possess an affiliation with their nationality as strongly as those from West Malaysia ("Civil movement", 2013; "GE 13: Movement", 2013; Rintod, 2013).

The Chinese first came to Sarawak as traders and explorers in the 6th century. Today, they make up 29% of the population of Sarawak and comprise of communities built from the economic migrants of the 19th and early 20th centuries (Hing & Tan, 2000). The first Chinese migrants worked as laborers in the gold mines at Bau or on plantations. Through their clan associations, business acumen (*kongsi)* and work ethics, the Chinese rapidly dominated the commerce sector. There were times of riots with British and Holland colonizers early in the history due to discrimination and oppression. Waves of immigration were agreed upon by the British governor, Charles Brooke, in 1901. Though there was mistrust between the local government and the Chinese immigrants during the communist war in China, the majority of the Chinese abided by the rules of the new Malaysian government, formed in 1963. Today, Chinese are amongst the most prosperous ethnic groups in Sarawak (Chin, 1981).

PSYCHOLOGICAL RESILIENCE OF CIM

After introducing the socio-economic status and ecological system of CIM, this section focuses on the psychological resilience of CIM, as well as resources they inherited from the historical and cultural contexts.

Business Vitality

As illustrated above, CIM has a history of success in entrepreneurship and as a leader in economic development. They have a high visibility in business, both nationwide and internationally. Therefore, though they do not hold much political power, their contribution to the Malaysian economy has been widely acknowledged. This also gave them certain leverage and voice over the mainstream political structures (Gomez, 1999).

Strong Adaptability

CIM has a history of resiliency through immigration and differentiation from China by building a new home and identity in a new land. Within a century, the Chinese have grown into the second largest ethnic group in Malaysia, and its contribution to the nation is undeniable. In spite of all the hardship at the beginning of the 20th century, CIM are able to adapt to the new country and be flexible about their roles in the Malay government.

Family Values

The strong family lineage and concept of filial piety have kept the Chinese families intact. According to the Population and Housing Census 2010 in Malaysia (Department of Statistics Malaysia, 2011), CIM have the lowest divorce rate among all the racial groups. This shows family resilience in facing life challenges, as well as their values of integrity of family as a social unit. Moreover, filial piety is still highly emphasized in the CIM, and it serves as a protective factor for the aging population, as children are expected to take care of the elderly (Simon, Chen, Chang & Dong, 2014). The elder siblings are also expected to take care of the younger siblings. The Confucius hierarchy for the family continues to be passed on through generations. Many researchers have established that the tight networks among blood-tie relationships have served as a buffer against social oppression and marginalization (Ng, Bhugra, Mcmanus & Fennell, 2011; Yeh, Yi, Tsao & Wan, 2013). These networks are even more evident in rural areas, where most of the CIM siblings and relatives stay together in the same neighborhood. In many cases as evidenced in clinical practices, when there is mental illness in the CIM family, all the family members feel obligated to take care of the ill-member, hence decreasing the burden of the social welfare system.

Emphasis on Education

Compared to other ethnic groups, CIM have a reputation of high investment on education for their next generations. Chinese parents usually work very hard to save enough money for their children's post-high school education. In spite of the racial profiling at public education, Chinese parents always try to send their children to foreign countries for better opportunities in education. Private Chinese associations or societies would also sponsor some distinguished students through donations and scholarships. In fact, great pride is bestowed upon young students who excel in academic achievements even at the elementary school levels.

Strong Work Ethics

The strong work ethics among CIM is a continuation of the "survival" mentality since centuries ago, and coined by scholar as high "Confucius dynamism" (Hofstede, 2003). This strong work ethics is not only reflected in the common business sector, but also among mental health professionals in the health care domain as well.

PSYCHOLOGICAL CHALLENGES OF CIM

Despite many strengths and resilience embedded in the CIM community, the clashes between tradition and modern values, the marginalized position in the Malaysian political arena, the stereotype of over-achiever in education, and the "brain drain" movement of young elite CIM, have all caused a strain in CIM families as well as individuals (Sukumaran, 2017). According to the 2015 Malaysia National Health and Morbidity Survey, both CIM adult and children population have seen a significant increasing trend in mental health problems from 1996 to 2015 (Ahmad et al., 2015; Ministry of Health Malaysia, 2015). This section presents more specifically how different age cohorts of CIM face specific external pressures that could add to the mental burden of the individuals. We hope the readers would not generalize or pathologize the problems by stereotyping CIM, but to see their personal responsibilities and solutions in the midst of these social dilemma.

1. Children: Pressures of Achievement (Overachievement/Perfectionism)

In the past decade, the increase of mental health problems among the child and adolescent population in Malaysia has become a significant concern. According to a study comparing data from the Malaysia National Health and Morbidity Survey (NHMS) from 1996, 2006 and 2011, the prevalence of mental health problems among children and adolescents (between the ages of 5 to 15 years) saw an increase of 49.2% across 1996 to 2011. Mental health challenges among preschool aged children (5 to 6 years old) almost doubled in the decade spanning 1996 to 2006 (Ahmad et al., 2015). The latest 2015 Malaysia NHMS highlighted that Malaysian children struggled especially with emotional, conduct, hyperactivity, peer and social problems (Ministry of Health Malaysia, 2015). From the literature reviewed, depression among Chinese children could be associated with family factors, social factors, age and gender, ethnicity and culture, and physical (or body) factors (Zgambo, Kalembo, He & Wang, 2012).

In general, although Ahmad et al. (2015) found that the prevalence of mental health problems among children of Chinese ethnicity was lowest compared to other ethnic groups from 1996 to 2011, mental health problems among CIM children saw an exponential increase of 366.7% from 1996 to 2006. In 2015, the NHMS placed CIM children group second in the prevalence of mental health problems (Ministry of Health Malaysia, 2015). Many CIM children struggle with psychological distress especially pertaining to anxiety, depression and even suicide (Alphonsus, 2012). For the CIM, the pressure to excel and achieve began at a young age, and is invariably closely tied to the Chinese family's interests. Hence, failure to achieve and meet high standards not only reflected poorly on the individual child but impacted the concept of the Chinese family's face, image, pride and integrity. For CIM, such achievement-oriented upbringing and emphasis on family interests served as a double-aged sword for children – especially in the absence of adequate parental and social support, familial and household stability, and positive coping resources – the pressures and stress early in life precipitate significant challenges with mental health adaptability in young children which are unfortunately carried into the later years in life[2] (Alphonsus, 2012; Bernama, 2016; Zgambo, Kalembo, He & Wang, 2012). In fact, research has shown that academic and achievement-oriented stress could actually be carried until the college stage where CIM have been found to have relatively higher levels of stress but lower coping skills in comparison to other ethnic groups (Mazlan, Bahari & Ardillah, 2012).

2. Adolescents: Addiction Problems and Pressures From Authoritarian Parents

As Malaysia goes through the wave of industrialization and modernization under the 2020 vision[3], college students are widely exposed to the most advanced information and technology globally through internet browsing and video gaming. The younger generation has a subcultural of their own with a myriad of cultural exposure that is very different from their parents. The identity crisis of CIM teenagers surfaces in their choice of friendship, dating relationship and career path, as parental authority is still prevalent among CIM (Chen & Liew, 2015). While the traditional CIM parents expect them to be "obedient and filial" children, not many teenagers today can conform to such social norms and expectations. As a matter of fact, in a survey among 2927 secondary schoolers, CIM students were found to have the highest depression rate among all ethnic groups (55%), which is associated with low academic performance and alcoholism (Latiff, Tajik, Ibrahim, Abubakar & Ali, 2016). Similar results were shown in another research in Sarawak, where CIM adolescents had the highest depressive rate among all ethnic groups (Ghazali & Azhar, 2015). Suicidal ideation is also higher in CIM adolescents (7.9%) in comparison to their Malay counterparts according to a survey done in Sabah (Ahmad & Cheong, 2014).

In the counseling room, the therapists might see many CIM teenagers who are having trouble with their parents. Behavioral problems and teenage delinquency are rising as substance abuse becomes prevalent in Malaysia (Singh, Yap, Redpath & Allotey, 2017). According to a survey conducted in Penang (Guan & Rahimi, 2015), self-hurt behavior has also become prevalent for CIM teenagers (56.81%), especially among female students (33.72%). For children who come from families with lack of emotional support (e.g. single parents, absent father figures), their need for mentoring and emotional regulation become the goal of therapy. As mentioned before, many CIM families engage in entrepreneurship and business management, and therefore it is quite common among CIM families for many fathers to be travelling frequently between places while the mothers and grandparents are the housemakers. These "migrant worker" families were quite common in the first and second generation of CIM, and thus created a unique family structure where the grandparent figures became prominent in parenting. The gap between the grandparent generation and the teenager world creates difficulty in mentoring and behavioral monitoring, even though the former could serve as supportive figures for the family. Hence the lack of moral guidance and supervision of parents are quite common in the "high work ethic" CIM families. Many teenage clients in therapy complained that the parents provided only their material needs but neglected their emotional needs. The challenges in working with CIM teenagers would be to reconstruct the family system to make it more flexible and reciprocal using their perceived language of love.

3. Adults: Family Differentiation

As briefly introduced before, though familism is a strong protective factor for CIM against psychological distress, it could also serve as a stressor when the family lacks resources to cope with acculturative and assimilation stress from the mainstream culture. As Malaysia is still a commonwealth country, it is constantly being impacted by globalization and Western values. Though CIM have been persistent in keeping their cultural heritage, the hybridized cultural identity could be clashing with traditional social norms. For example, many CIM adult clients complaint about the enmeshment and interference of their parents in their daily life decisions and not respecting their boundaries and privacy. It is quite common for unmarried adults to still stay with their parents until they get married. Some traditional CIM also value multigenerational living under the same roof (三代同堂) as a sign of prosperity for the family clan. With this kind of living structure, one could imagine the possible conflicts that could occur between in-laws, and those who seek individuation from the family of origin. Studies have identified that post-natal depression and suicide among CIM women could be perpetuated by the unsupportive family system such as lack of support from the husband or due to in-law conflicts (Yusuff, Tang, Binns & Lee, 2014). Having to struggle with the patriarchal family system (e.g. in-law problems) makes CIM married women more vulnerable to mental illness especially depression (Arifin, 2015).

From the first author's clinical practice in the past 10 years, many depressed CIM adults found it suffocating for not being able to be recognized as an "individual," and expected at the same time to be loyal to the family. Issues with authority figures are always a challenge the adult CIM have to work through in the therapy room. Finding their own voice in the traditional Chinese household would be a life-long challenge due to the pressure of being the "perfect child". For example, career choice is often a battle seen in the therapy room when CIM parents insist on the career choice for their young adult children especially sons who carry the family names. More often, the top career choice for their children is the medical profession or computer sciences which could guarantee a secure financial income and white-collar class. However not many CIM students could thrive through competitive programs like medical school, but they are "forced" to honor the parental wish for choosing a career path that is "good for them." This observation is confirmed by several studies which found that parental authority still plays a key factor for individuals of Chinese descent in determining their career goal (Chen & Liew, 2015; Tang, 2002).

Moreover, Mak and Chen (2010) expounded that strong Chinese cultural values pertaining to the maintenance of the family's "face" and interpersonal harmony could inversely contribute to ineffective coping and adaptability. Research have shown that Chinese adults who uphold stronger preference for familial "face" concerns were more likely to report higher levels of psychological distress. The effort invested towards interpersonal dynamics within the family can be psychologically taxing and distressing especially in the event of failure to sustain interpersonal harmony among family members (Mak & Chen, 2010). Hence, CIM who carry strong adherence to the concepts of the Chinese family's face, interests and harmony are more susceptible to sociotropic cognitive vulnerabilities and psychological distress which in turn precipitate challenges with mental health problems.

4. Older Adults: Somatic Complaints and Empty-Nest Syndrome

Many less acculturated CIM older generation still believe in Chinese traditional medicines in interpreting mental problems and healing of ailments. The popular belief in "shen jing shuai ruo" (神经衰弱), translation of neurasthenia, is still pervasive among CIM older adult circles[4]. Older generation CIM would rather equate mental problems such as mood disorder or anxiety disorder as "shen jing shuai ruo" as it is thought to be a "neurological condition" of their mental problems. It serves the function of destigmatizing mental illness, as well as matching the traditional philosophy of mind-body unison (Kleinman, 1982). It has been argued that Westerners conceive depression as an intra-psychic, existential experience, whereas in Chinese and many other non-Western societies, it is most frequently experienced somatically and in terms of interpersonal dysfunction (Chan, 1990; Kleinman, 1982; Watters, 2011). In her dissertation, Ting (2008) showed that Chinese individuals, when using Chinese language, tended to use discourse that was interpersonally focused (e.g., feeling critical of others) in projecting depressive feelings rather than abstract emotional discourse that was intrapersonal (e.g., feeling lonely). The challenges for aging adults then become their inability to express their pain through internal affective language but manifested through somatic and concrete descriptions instead. Their losses and grieves might not be understood by the mental health practitioners or taken seriously by their family members if emotions are being expressed rather indirectly with somatic symptoms (Mak & Chen, 2010; Ting, 2008). The somatization and interpersonal projection of emotional dysfunctions often times do not overlap with Western diagnostic categories for mental disorders (Mak & Chen, 2010).

Another unique phenomenon surfacing in the CIM community is the "international family" constellation, where younger elite CIM migrated to other countries as Permanent Residents in the foreign lands while still carrying Malaysian citizenship. These kinds of global families normally happened in the middle upper class CIM families where the parents encouraged their children to pursue higher education in more developed and immigrant-friendly countries (e.g. Australia, New Zealand, Singapore, Taiwan)[5]. Most of their children continue to stay on in those developed countries for better living and stable subsistence as the Malaysian government provides limited chance or promotion for CIM (Ward & Hewstone, 1985). This trend of re-migration is also known as the "second wave diaspora among CIM" (Ling, 2008; Tan,

2005). However, this creates a vacuum in the CIM community where the aging cohort lacks support from the younger cohort. Many older adults might suffer from empty-nest syndrome with loneliness and depression as their children and grandchildren are not around, which conversely goes against the cultural tenets of filial piety and family ethics (Simon, Chen, Chang & Dong, 2014).

BARRIERS IN RECEIVING MENTAL HEALTH SERVICES

Though CIM displays a relative low rate of mental problems (24.2%), compared to other races in Malaysia, the ratio is still quite high among the CIM community (Krishnaswamy et al., 2012). The ratio of seeking mental health services is quite low for CIM, hence we need to explore further the barriers hindering them from seeking and receiving quality mental health services in Malaysia. Some barriers listed below are internally oriented, but the major barriers lie externally in the scarcity of resources in meeting the heterogeneous needs of CIM.

Shame in Psychopathology

Though there is an increased awareness of mental health among CIM, there is still stigma towards mental illness and seeking help from mental health professionals[6]. The belief of "never air your laundry outside the family" is still prevalent among CIM. They would usually cover up the pathology of individuals within the family through social isolation, in order to avoid "face losing" or "shame". The stigma towards mental illness and the implication of personal and familial failure, weakness and shame invariably result in low help-seeking behavior and service utilization (Hwang, 2006; Mak & Chen, 2010). Therefore, the delay in seeking help often times exacerbates the symptoms of targeted patients, and consequently demands a lot of case management and crisis intervention from mental health professionals. Another reason for treatment delay is due to financial reasons. Besides financial concerns and affordability, some CIM are reluctant to pay a professional fee to seek help from "talk therapy." Many still prefer pro bono or low fee service from non-profit organizations. Those cases that are being seen by the counselors in community usually are chronic, psychotic, low-functioning and severely-ill. Yet they expect a "quick fix" or "magic pill" in one session. The concept of an ongoing treatment plan is still foreign.

Cost-Benefit Concern

Unlike other countries, where mental health services are covered through managed care or insurance plans, most mental health providers in Malaysia are not included in the welfare systems. Hence, the clients have to pay out of their own pockets should they seek private or community psychologists. Governmental clinics or hospitals have very limited positions for clinical or counseling psychologists, and instead largely depend on social workers who might not have the relevant training, background or experience to manage serious mental health cases. Psychiatrists mainly adopt a medical and biological model in approaching the patients. Hence, private counseling centers become the major sources of mental health referral. However, many lower class CIM cannot afford a costly long-term treatment plan. They would rather opt for other forms of treatment, such as traditional herbal medicines for symptom relief (Chang, Tam & Mohd Suki, 2017; Chen, 1981).

Preference for Ethnic Match

From our clinical experiences, if they have a choice, CIM tend to seek private and Chinese-based professionals rather than government agencies catering to a Malay majority. Even within the government setting, where services are more affordable to most people, Chinese clients have been known to ask for Chinese service providers. Reasons for this tendency include language and sociocultural familiarity, and underlying mistrust towards "the others". According to multicultural counseling research in the United States (Sue, 1998), ethnicity match does not predict the efficiency of therapeutic outcome, but would reduce the dropout rate and prolong the length of the treatment among ethnic minority clients. Ironically, due to the stigma of mental illness, seldom would Chinese parents encourage the new generations to pursue a career in the mental health profession, which contributes to the enormous gap between the demand and supply of CIM mental health service delivery.

Lack of Mandarin and Dialect Speaking Practitioners

Though CIM are educated in the Malay and English language, most of their mother tongue are still Chinese dialects (e.g. Cantonese, Hokkien). Research found that interventions conducted in clients' native language were two times more effective (Griner & Smith, 2006). In order to facilitate greater emotional congruence in the counseling room, we need more Mandarin and Chinese dialect speaking mental health professionals who are able to serve the non-Malay and non-English speaking CIM population effectively. With regard to Chinese psychologists in Malaysia, to date it is estimated that up to 56.6% (77 out of 136) of known active clinical psychologists in the country are of Chinese descent[7]. Fortunately, compared to the data collected between 2004-2005 by Ng (2005), the ratio of CIM clinical psychologists has actually increased almost doubly (from 37% to 56.6%). However, the Chinese representation in the registry of the Malaysian Counseling Association is only about 12.7% (907 out of 7157) (Lembaga Kaunselor Malaysia, 2016). With such a limited number of CIM psychologists and counselors serving the whole community of CIM (ratio=1:6758), one could imagine the gap of services in the system.

Lack of Developed Inventories Used for Mental Health Screening and Diagnosis

Most psychological instruments are predominantly in English and normed on Western populations (such as in the United States, United Kingdom or Australia). As such, assessment services in Malaysia are still largely culturally and linguistically biased. The lack of Chinese translated and locally normed tools for intelligence and personality testing have been a dilemma, as many competent CIM researchers and psychologists are English speaking and not fluent in Mandarin. This leaves the Chinese-speaking CIM population underserved and unfairly assessed.

Lack of Multicultural Competence

Not all institutions that train mental health professionals emphasize on multicultural competency training and include it as core coursework. Moreover, the multicultural modules that are adopted by current Malaysian postgraduate programs are often times heavily reliant on the Western model of multicultural diversity; hence, adequate understanding and contextualization of the unique history, challenges and issues of Malaysia's multicultural setting and communities are invariably overlooked in the training of mental health professionals. As counseling is still a young profession, and not many culturally competent senior CIM counselors or therapists are available, the younger generation of mental health professionals often lack supervision and role models, leaving them to stumble their way in gaining more clinical and educational experience (Ching & Ng, 2010; Haque, 2005).

Lack of Regulation on Mental Health Professions

Many of the "counselors" in the Chinese non-profit counseling centers, who have limited training and experiences as para-counselors or volunteers, are not registered with PERKAMA. This could be risky to the clients, especially CIM who are less exposed to the mental health professions. There is a lack of regulatory boards to govern uncertified "therapists" or "psychologists", which leaves the less educated CIM an easy target for scamming or exploitation[8] (The British Psychological Association, 2006).

Lack of Research Funding in the Area of Chinese Psychology in Malaysia

Our feeble effort might be the first formal document in this aspect. Up till date, there is no registered Chinese journal for psychology in Malaysia. There are some local peer-reviewed journals, but the publishing language is mainly in English or Malay. On the other hand, most of the Chinese-speaking NGOs choose to publish their own books and magazines in Mandarin, which could be disseminated to wider readership among the Chinese community. The gap between scholarly work and popular psychology has also hindered the dissemination of appropriate and updated information about mental health to CIM who are fluent in Mandarin only.

Uneven Distribution of Mental Health Services

Most mental health services are concentrated in big cities, such as the Klang valley and Penang (Ng, 2006). There are hardly any counseling services in rural areas or small cities. It is not convenient for people from suburban settings to seek professional counseling. This has become a problem in terms of availability and accessibility of mental health services, especially to those living outside of the city areas, which understandably have lower awareness and greater stigma on mental health issues. In terms of the mental health profession, East Malaysia is still at the infancy stage of development, due to the uneven distribution of resources in governmental sectors. There is limited literature or research conducted in terms of the mental health prevalence and needs among Chinese in East Malaysia. To the authors' knowledge, there is only one clinical psychologist and less than five psychiatrists in the whole Sarawak state; furthermore, most of them reside in big cities. Moreover, most of these mental health professionals are not Chinese and usually would not be conversant in Mandarin or Chinese dialects either. In practice, the mental health professionals working under the government services will rotate to the smaller towns once a month only and would have a very long waitlist of patients which significantly diminishes the quality of care rendered to patients.

Lack of Family Therapists

According to a survey, the mental health profession in Malaysia is dominated by individual-oriented therapists who practice individual therapy (Mohamed & Rahman, 2011; Ng, 2006). Family therapy or other modes of therapy are not as widely practiced due to a lack of training opportunities grounded in the Malaysian context. However, as we have learned, CIM is thickly embedded in familism as well as how mental problems and solutions are perceived and managed. Through the lens of family systems, one could reframe mental illness or psychological struggles in a more dynamic and sensitive language reflected through a multigenerational and familial structure. Aside from the individualistic approach to counseling, mental health practitioners should receive further training in family systems theory or even community psychology (Ching & Ng, 2010), and adopt it to the CIM context. Otherwise, CIM clients would be blinded to their communal resources and be isolated in the therapy room.

SUGGESTIONS FOR FUTURE MENTAL HEALTH DEVELOPMENT

In this section, a blueprint is delineated with the objective and strategy to advance the mental health profession and practice for CIM. The ultimate goals are twofold: First, CIM would be able to access effective and culturally sensitive mental health services; Second, local practitioners will be empowered to take part in discovering a Chinese psychology that is indigenous for CIM. To achieve these goals, the following are some strategies and plans of action in the near future:

1. Indigenizing Research Epistemology and Methodology

While reviewing and researching empirical studies related to CIM, the authors found that ethnicity was seldom a major factor addressed in the literatures. The CIM group was often used as the "comparison group" to the Malay group, and the findings of those papers were also interpreted from the lens of the dominant group where CIM culture was left invisible or not taken seriously. While many anthropologists and sociologists have studied the diversity of CIM in length, Malaysian psychologists are still behind in building a suitable theoretical framework to explain the ethnic differences and uniqueness in our own country. To date, most of the psychological models employed by Malaysian psychologists are either direct translation or importation from developed Western countries. The discipline of psychology practices occur almost exclusively in the Euro–American tradition. There is little awareness of the need to indigenize psychology to fit into the local CIM culture and needs.

International psychologists like Gulerce, Lock and Misra (as cited in Gergen et al., 1996), wondered whether there should be a universally acceptable conception of psychology. These psychologists noted that the journals in their respective countries (i.e., Turkey, New Zealand, and India) seem to differ little from American psychological publications in the methodologies utilized, the issues addressed, or the paradigms adopted. Failure to appreciate cultural particularity tends to result in local phenomena where minority psychologists imitate American models of psychological research (Sundararajan, Misra & Marsella, 2013). In fact, Mohanty (1988) had referred to the replication of Western psychology by Indian psychologists as "Yankee Doodling."

While indigenous psychology may well include non-local wisdom (e.g. scientific methodology), members of the host culture should decide what is to be imported or contextualized in the local culture. Indigenous psychology not only should be built on the collaboration between anthropologists, psychologists, historians, and sociologists, it should also be constructed on relationships of mutual respect and empowerment between the researchers and the lay leaders of local communities. In contrast, mainstream psychology is culturally bound in that it serves and benefits the people in a Western context. It exports the products of psychology to minority cultures through the processes of colonization, commercial exchange, globalization, and westernization. Mainstream psychology's failure to recognize the limitations of Western theories, and the fantasy of creating a universal psychology have not only disempowered the recipients in underdeveloped societies, but also destroyed the shelter built by the traditions of those cultures (Dueck, Ting & Cutiongco, 2007).

It is hoped that indigenous research for CIM would address the social phenomena of CIM, study the psychological concepts espoused by CIM, and develop measurement tools or scales to assess the concepts coherent and pertinent to the CIM community. The mixed method research approach would be best utilized to explore and identify the key factors contributing to mental health issues of CIM and to validate the best treatment approaches. Pedagogical efforts are needed to invest in research topics concerning the wellbeing of CIM, as well as establishing reliable funding agencies to support such efforts. More awareness on the importance of indigenous psychology in the Malaysian mental health field could also promote similar cultural sensitivity towards other ethnic groups as well.

2. Enhancing Multicultural Competency in Training and Education

It is highly recommended that higher education institutions mandate multicultural therapy as core coursework in counseling training programs. For counselors who are providing services to CIM community, it would be imperative to have a clear understanding of CIM culture and subcultures through reading and cultural immersion experiences. Since it is not possible to train multilingual staff, it is more realistic to train multiculturally competent therapists in post-graduate programs. Even if there is an ethnic and language match between the CIM counselors and counselees, there might be values differences due to education background and upbringing (Tan, 2007). For example, a Chinese-educated therapist may not readily empathize with the unique experiences of English-educated Chinese. With multicultural competency, a good counselor will first examine his/her own biases and values toward different groups of CIM. Multicultural competency training would not only include close supervision of intern counselors working with CIM, but also help trainees work through their own cultural stereotypes and counter-transference challenges with various clients.

Besides having cultural sensitivity towards different groups of CIM, a competent counselor would also be trained with therapy skills that are specific to dealing with frequently seen problems among CIM. For example, cognitive-behavior therapy was found to be preferred and effective for Chinese American community (Chen & Davenport, 2005), due to its education and didactic elements. For those CIM clients who prefer a more practical approach and quick fix, a solution-focused approach would be essential. For those CIM clients dealing with family conflicts, therapeutic skills in conducting family sessions would be necessary. Furthermore, knowledge about CIM community resources and traditional wisdom would help the counselors to facilitate referrals for more traditional CIM. As many CIM still practice folk religions (e.g. Taoist) and ancestral worship, counselors also need to have some basic knowledge of these local practices, aside from the common spirituality and religions practiced by CIM.

Another unique socio-political atmosphere for the mental health profession in Malaysia is its "thickness" in religion. Considering the Islamic backdrop in Malaysia, some Islamic psychologists have taken on a leading role in integrating Islamic teaching into psychological practice (Haque & Masuan, 2002). It was found that religious-based therapy serves as a catalyst to recovery from anxiety disorders among religious Malay patients (Razali, Aminah & Khan, 2002). Some CIM mental health practitioners have already started integrating their religious faith into their research and practice, such as mindfulness and meditation for Buddhist therapists, and prayers and scriptures for Christian therapists (Ting & Ng, 2012). Counselors are encouraged to talk to different religious leaders in the CIM community for wider exposure. Academicians could also study the effects of such integrated therapeutic approaches for empirical evidence based therapy.

3. Empowering CIM Community to Take the Lead in Mental Health Service Delivery

It is highly encouraged for the next CIM generation to pursue a career in the mental health profession due to the great need among its own community. In the past, many CIM parents insisted for their children to pursue medicine or law as the symbols of achievement and success, which contributed to the current shortage of CIM mental health professionals. Careers in the mental health field are also associated with the stigma of mental illness. However, there is a turn in the last decade, where greater visibility of psychology and mental health practices among CIM can be seen. The establishment of Chinese counseling centers and associations, coupled with the blossoming of counseling seminars and various continued education courses, have led to a wider acceptance and understanding of counseling and mental health within the Chinese society. More CIM are expressing interest in psychology and counseling courses. These demands further stimulate the expansion of psychology departments in some private institutions in Malaysia (EduAdvisor, 2017).

Many textbooks and literature in counseling/psychology have been translated into Mandarin in Taiwan, Hong Kong and China, and CIM counselors could also benefit from such overseas resources by accessing first-hand knowledge from their counterparts in other countries. There is also more interchange with Taiwan counselors to bridge in such developing skills through intensive training and workshops. Some CIM counselors/therapists have started to publish their own works, as well as contribute to newspaper/journal columns (such as Sinchew Daily and Guangming Daily). Online media exposure such as to radio station interviews could also help to destigmatize the mental health field, as well as promoting the social status of counselors.

In addition, CIM counselors/therapists have a privilege which other racial groups might not have. Ng (2006) found that a substantial number of Chinese therapists (though not all) speak at least one Chinese language/dialect – 70% speak Mandarin, 60% speak Cantonese, 47% speak Hokkien, 16% speak Hakka, and 2% speak Hinoi or Teochew. In addition, most, if not all, CIM therapists are able to speak and write in English and Malay (Ng, 2006). This is an advantage for CIM therapists who can also reach out to non-Chinese clientele, without the need for translators. Unlike other racial groups who are usually monolingual or dual-lingual, multilingual CIM therapists have wider access and flexibility to the general Malaysian population.

4. Building a CIM Friendly Society Through Advocacy and Public Policy

In ensuring quality services not only to CIM but to the general public, we need to continue to ensure the presence of regulatory boards and enforcement of clinical ethics in mental health service delivery. All Malaysian citizens, including CIM, should have equal access to mental health services in the public arena. The counselor registration requirement stipulated by the *Counsellors Act* in Malaysia has a certain positive influence towards the quality control of counselors in Malaysia. The mass media including magazines, television and radio programs very often interview people in the mental health profession, which gives the profession more exposure to the public. This is certainly a reflection of the mental health need in the society, where people are beginning to seek help in this area. The government sectors should also ensure diversity among employed mental health practitioners (e.g. psychiatrists, counselors, psychologists) to serve the diverse CIM population. Many trained CIM clinical psychologists or counselors were actually "drained" to foreign country such as Australia and Singapore as they found current employment in Malaysian governmental sectors not available. Though there is no overt racial oppression and discrimination towards CIM, the implicit racial quota in the government system could be unfair to CIM mental health practitioners. It is urged that all mental health professionals, regardless of ethnic backgrounds, to come together to share resources in the community and promote inter-racial harmony.

Considering the current trend of racial segregation and tight knit CIM community, mental health professionals could utilize community-based services to promote mental health awareness and services to this population. Instead of practicing from an individualistic model, community psychology could help in destigmatizing and demystifying psychotherapy, building a safety net of preventive measures, and decreasing the prevalence of mental illness among CIM. There is also the advantage of mobilizing peer-mentoring groups—such as parenthood groups, adolescent mentoring programs, support groups for family/caretakers of the severely mentally ill, among the CIM community. In rural areas where mental health resources are scarce, the training of lay counselors and peer counselors who come from diverse backgrounds would be a high priority. It is anticipated that local counselors would be able to reach out to the CIM family units in a more culturally appropriate manner than external consultants.

CONCLUSION

Despite the mushrooming number of studies on the mental health of ethnic minorities in the United States over the past three decades (Sue & Sue, 2003), Chinese diaspora remains a novice population to be studied by psychologists and mental health workers. The public slogan of "Satu Malaysia" (One Malaysia) promoted by the Malaysian government with the intention to unite the nationalities, has not been encouraging towards ethnic comparison studies. Emphasizing national identity over ethnic identity is a political strategy that encourages assimilation and reduces tension between multiple races. Yet, if these efforts are not balanced by celebrating diversity under the umbrella of nationality, cultural heritage would be watered down, and the identity of any ethnic group would be compromised. We advocate for a moderate public policy to embrace the diversity within CIM, as well as a mental health field that fosters more peaceful dialogue between CIM and other racial and ethnic groups. Henceforth, this chapter is a feeble attempt to start tackling the complicated mental health issues faced by a heterogeneous group like the CIM. We adopt a psycho-social approach in understanding the diversity and uniqueness of this group, as well as how mental health needs are shaped by the political atmosphere in Malaysia. We address the barriers faced by CIM in getting quality mental health care and services, as well as methods in overcoming these barriers. It is our belief that the mental health profession could promote the welfare of the CIM community by modeling harmony, modesty, justice and peace within and between the mental health professionals.

ACKNOWLEDGMENT

We want to acknowledge the contribution of Dr. Alvin Ng and Dr. Wai Sheng Ng to the initial draft of this paper.

REFERENCES

Ahmad, N., Cheong, S. M., Ibrahim, N., & Rosman, A. (2014). Suicidal ideation among Malaysian adolescents. *Asia-Pacific Journal of Public Health*, *26*(5), 63–69. doi:10.1177/1010539514540746 PMID:25005932

Ahmad, N., MuhdYusoff, F., Ratnasingam, S., Mohamed, F., Nasir, N. H., MohdSallehuddin, S., ... Aris, T. (2015). Trends and factors associated with mental health problems among children and adolescents in Malaysia. *International Journal of Culture and Mental Health*, *8*(2), 125–136. doi:10.1080/17542863.2014.907326 PMID:26000035

Alphonsus, A. (2012, June 18). Chinese youths top suicide list. *Free Malaysia Today*. Retrieved from http://www.freemalaysiatoday.com/category/nation/2012/06/18/chinese-youths-top-suicide-list/

Ang, I. (2014). Beyond Chinese groupism: Chinese Australians between assimilation, multiculturalism and diaspora. *Ethnic and Racial Studies*, *37*(7), 1184–1196. doi:10.1080/01419870.2014.859287

Arifin, M., Roshaidai, S., Cheyne, H., & Maxwell, M. (2015, June). Postnatal depression across cultures: A qualitative study in Malaysia. *Paper presented at NMAHP Research Unit Mini Conference 2015*, Glasgow, Scotland.

Banyan. (2013, April 28). Malaysia's close-fought election: The Penang effect. *The Economist*. Retrieved from https://www.economist.com/blogs/banyan/2013/04/malaysias-close-fought-election

Bernama. (2016, September 12). Mental health of Malaysian students cause of worry: Health Ministry. *The New Straits Times*. Retrieved from https://www.nst.com.my/news/2016/09/172683/mental-health-malaysian-students-cause-worry-health-ministry

Bond, M. H. (Ed.). (2006). *Handbook of Chinese Psychology*. New York: Oxford University Press.

Bond, M. H. (Ed.). (2010). *The Oxford handbook of Chinese psychology*. New York: Oxford University Press. doi:10.1093/oxfordhb/9780199541850.001.0001

Bonn, B., & Tam, C. L. (2015). Imagining a good life in Malaysia and China: Cultural beliefs among Mainland Chinese, Malaysian Chinese, and Malay University students. *Asian Journal of Social Psychology*, *19*(2), 145–153. doi:10.1111/ajsp.12120

Carstens, S. A. (2005). *Histories, cultures, identities: Studies in Malaysian Chinese worlds*. Singapore: Singapore University Press.

Chan, D. W. (1990). The meaning of depression: The Chinese word associations. *Psychologia*, *33*, 191–196.

Chang, M. L., Tam, A., & Mohd Suki, N. (2017). Moderating effect of races towards consumers' feeling of TCM usage. In Handbook of Research on Leveraging Consumer Psychology for Effective Customer Engagement. doi:10.4018/978-1-5225-0746-8.ch020

Chen, L.-S., & Liew, S.-A. (2015, February). Factors influencing career decision making difficulties among graduating students from Malaysian private higher educational institutions. In *Proceedings of the 8th Asia Pacific Business Research Conference*, Kuala Lumpur, Malaysia.

Chen, P. C. Y. (1981). Traditional and modern medicine in Malaysia. *Social Science & Medicine. Part A: Medical Psychology & Medical Sociology*, *7*, 127–136. doi:10.1016/0271-7123(81)90032-8

Chen, S. W. H., & Davenport, D. S. (2005). Cognitive-Behavioral therapy with Chinese American clients: Cautions and modifications. *Psychotherapy (Chicago, Ill.)*, *42*(1), 101–110.

Chin, J. M. (1981). *The Sarawak Chinese*. NY: Oxford University Press.

Ching, M. S., & Ng, K. M. (2010). Counseling in Malaysia: History, current status, and future trends. *Journal of Counseling and Development*, *88*(1), 18–22. doi:10.1002/j.1556-6678.2010.tb00144.x

Civil movement to call for self-government, nationhood for Malaysia's Sarawak. (2013, April 15). *Nationalia Aureli Argemí.* Retrieved from https://www.nationalia.info/new/9822/civil-movement-to-call-for-self-government-nationhood-for-malaysias-sarawak

Department of Statistics, Malaysia. (2001). Population and Housing Census 2000. In *Distribution and Basic Demographic Characteristics Report.* Retrieved from http://www.statistics.gov.my/English/pageDemo.htm

Department of Statistics, Malaysia. (2011). *Population Distribution and Basic Demographic Characteristic Report 2010.* Retrieved from https://www.dosm.gov.my/v1/index.php?r=column/cthemeByCat&cat=117&bul_id=MDMxdHZjWTk1SjFzTzNkRXYzcVZjdz09&menu_id=L0pheU43NWJwRWVSZklWdzQ4TlhUUT09

Department of Statistics, Malaysia. (2016). *Current Population Estimates, Malaysia, 2014 – 2016. Retrieved from* https://web.archive.org/web/20160812014710/ https://www.statistics.gov.my/index.php?r=column%2FcthemeByCat&cat=155&bul_id=OWlxdEVoYlJCS0hUZzJyRUcvZEYxZz09&menu_id=L0pheU43NWJwRWVSZklWdzQ4TlhUUT09

Dueck, A., Ting, S.-K., & Cutiongco, R. (2007). Constantine, Babel, and Yankee Doodling: Whose indigeneity? Whose psychology? *Pastoral Psychology*, *56*(1), 55–72. doi:10.100711089-007-0082-1

Edman, J. L., & Koon, T. Y. (2000). Mental illness beliefs in Malaysia: Ethnic and intergeneration comparisons. *The International Journal of Social Psychiatry*, *46*(2), 101–109. doi:10.1177/002076400004600203 PMID:10950358

EduAdvisor. (2017). *Find and compare psychology degree courses in Malaysia.* Retrieved from https://eduadvisor.my/psychology-degree-institutions/

FMT Reporters. (2017, November 17). Report: Chinese community has the biggest income gap. *Free Malaysia Today.* Retrieved from http://www.freemalaysiatoday.com/category/ nation/2017/11/17/report-chinese-community-has-the-biggest-income-gap/

FMT Reporters. (2017, December 8). MP censures Najib for 'insensitive' remark about Penang floods. *Free Malaysia Today.* Retrieved from http://www.freemalaysiatoday.com/ category/nation/2017/12/08/mp-censures-najib-for-insensitive-remark-about-penang-floods/

Freedman, A. L. (2000). *Political participation and ethnic minorities: Chinese overseas in Malaysia, Indonesia, and the United States*. New York: Routledge.

Fu, C. Q. (2007). *A different Chinese. Petaling Jaya, Malaysia*. Malaysia: Strategic Information and Research Development Centre.

GE13. Movement wants full autonomy for Sarawak. (2013, April 14). *The Star Online.* Retrieved from https://www.thestar.com.my/news/community/2013/04/14/ge13-movement-wants-full-autonomy-for-sarawak/

Gergen, K. J., Gulerce, A., Lock, A., & Misra, G. (1996). Psychological science in cultural context. *The American Psychologist*, *51*(5), 496–503. doi:10.1037/0003-066X.51.5.496

Ghazali, K. (2012, November 2). National identity and minority languages. *UN Chronicle.* Retrieved from https://web.archive.org/web/20121102173228/http://www.un.org/wcm/content/site/chronicle/home/archive/issues2010/un_academic_impact/national_identity_and_minority_languages?ctnscroll_articleContainerList=1_0&ctnlistpagination_articleContainerList=true

Ghazali, S. R., & Azhar, A. (2015). Depressive symptoms, gender, and ethnicity: An exploratory study among cross ethnic adolescents in Sarawak, Malaysia. *Malaysian Journal of Youth Studies*, *13*, 141–152.

Gomez, E. T. (1999). *Chinese Business in Malaysia: Accumulation, Ascendance, Accommodation*. Psychology Press.

Griner, D., & Smith, T. B. (2006). Culturally adapted mental health interventions: A meta-analytic review. *Psychotherapy (Chicago, Ill.)*, *43*(4), 531–548. doi:10.1037/0033-3204.43.4.531 PMID:22122142

Guan, T. E., & Rahimi, C. A. (2015). Prevalence of self-hurt behaviour among Chinese adolescents in Malaysia. *International Journal of Humanities. Arts and Social Sciences*, *1*(2), 108–113.

Han, B. (2015, November 10). Malaysia's Chinese diaspora: The other side of the story. *The Diplomat.* Retrieved from https://thediplomat.com/2015/11/malaysias-chinese-diaspora-the-other-side-of-the-story/

Haque, A. (2005). Mental health concepts and program development in Malaysia. *Journal of Mental Health (Abingdon, England)*, *14*(2), 183–195. doi:10.1080/09638230500059997

Haque, A., & Masuan, K. A. (2002). Religious psychology in Malaysia. *The International Journal for the Psychology of Religion*, *12*(4), 277–289. doi:10.1207/S15327582IJPR1204_05

Heng, P. K. (2006). Patterns of Chinese settlement. In L. Pan (Ed.), *The encyclopedia of the Chinese overseas* (2nd ed.). Singapore: Editions Didier Millet.

Hing, L. K., & Tan, C.-B. (Eds.). (2000). *The Chinese in Malaysia*. New York: Oxford University Press.

Hofstede, G. (2003). *Culture's consequences: comparing values, behaviors, institutions, and organizations across nations* (2nd ed.). CA: Sage Publication.

Hwang, K. K. (2006). Constructive realism and Confucian relationalism: An epistemological strategy for the development of indigenous psychology. In U. Kim, K. Yang, & K. Hwang (Eds.), *Indigenous and cultural psychology: Understanding people in context*. New York: Springer. doi:10.1007/0-387-28662-4_4

Kleinman, A. (1982). Neurasthenia and depression: A study of somatization and culture in China. *Culture, Medicine and Psychiatry*, *6*(2), 117–190. doi:10.1007/BF00051427 PMID:7116909

Krishnaswamy, S., Subramaniam, K., Jemain, A. A., Low, W. Y., Ramachandran, P., Indran, T., & Patel, V. (2012). Common mental disorders in Malaysia: Malaysian mental health survey, 2003–2005. *Asia-Pacific Psychiatry*, *4*(3), 201–209. doi:10.1111/j.1758-5872.2012.00180.x

Latiff, L. A., Tajik, E., Ibrahim, N., Abubakar, A. S., & Ali, S. S. B. A. (2016). Depression and its associated factors among secondary school students in Malaysia. *The Southeast Asian Journal of Tropical Medicine and Public Health*, *47*(1), 131–141. PMID:27086434

Lembaga Kaunselor Malaysia. (2016). *Laporan Tahunan 2016 Lembaga Kaunselor*. Retrieved from https://www.lkm.gov.my/kpwkm/uploads/files/LAPORAN%20TAHUNAN%20 LEMBAGA%20 2016%20%20.pdf

Lin, R. K., & Ting, R. S. K. (2014). Acculturation process of returned overseas Chinese refugees from Southeast Asia: A textual analysis on 10 returned oversea Chinese cases in Zhuba Overseas-Chinese farm, Xiamen. *Hua Ren Yan Jiu Guo Ji Xue Bao*, *6*, 1–26. (in Chinese)

Ling, H. S. (2008). Negotiating Malaysian Chinese ethnic and national identity across borders. Unpublished Master thesis. Retrieved from https://etd.ohiolink.edu/rws_etd/document/get/ohiou1226957088/inline

Mak, W. W. S., & Chen, S. X. (2010). Illness behaviour among the Chinese. In M. H. Bond (Ed.), *The Oxford handbook of Chinese psychology* (pp. 421–439). New York: Oxford University Press.

Mazlan, L. B., Bahari, F., & Ardillah, F. (2012). Stress and coping skills among university students: A preliminary research on ethnicity. *Southeast Asia Psychology Journal*, *1*, 31–37.

Ministry of Health Malaysia. (2015). *National health and morbidity survey 2015 volume II: Non-communicable diseases, risk factors & other health problems*. Retrieved from http://www.iku.gov.my/images/IKU/Document/REPORT/nhmsreport2015vol2.pdf

Minkov, M., & Bond, M. H. (2017). A Genetic component to national differences in happiness. *Journal of Happiness Studies*, *18*(2), 321–340. doi:10.100710902-015-9712-y

Mohamed, Z., & Rahman, A. (2011). Counseling practitioners in Malaysia: Socio-Demographic profile and theoretical approaches in counseling process. *International Journal of Business and Social Science*, *2*(22), 184–188.

Mohanty, C. T. (1988). Under Western eyes: Feminist scholarship and colonial discourses. *Feminist Review*, *30*(1), 65–88. doi:10.1057/fr.1988.42

Mpofu, E., & Conyers, L. M. (2004). A representational theory perspective of minority status and people with disabilities: Implications for rehabilitation education and practice. *Rehabilitation Counseling Bulletin*, *47*(3), 142–151. doi:10.1177/00343552040470030301

Ng, M. N., Bhugra, D., Mcmanus, F., & Fennell, M. (2011). Filial piety as a protective factor for depression in survivors of childhood abuse. *International Review of Psychiatry (Abingdon, England)*, *23*(1), 100–112. doi:10.3109/09540261.2010.544645 PMID:21338305

Ng, L. O. (2007). A brief study into the awareness of the field of clinical psychology among medical and health science professionals in Malaysia. *Malaysian Journal of Health Sciences*, *5*, 23–30.

Ng, L. O. (2008). Clinical psychology update: Challenges for practice and training [Unpublished manuscript].

Ng, L. O., Teoh, H.-J., & Haque, A. (2003). Clinical psychology in Malaysia: A brief overview. *ASEAN Journal of Psychiatry*, *6*, 11–16.

Ng, S. (1999, August 15). Students react to hostel policy. *The Star*. Retrieved April 26, 2004, from http://thestar.com.my/news/storyx1000.asp?file=/1999/8/15/education/15lasaro&sec=

Ng, W. S. (2005). *Psychotherapists in Malaysia: A preliminary study of clinical psychologists.* [Unpublished doctoral Clinical Research Project completion of the Doctor of Psychology].

Ng, W. S. (2007, August). Cultural identity of psychotherapists in Malaysia. *Paper presented at the World Mental Health Congress*, Hong Kong Polytechnic University, Hong Kong.

Ong, K. H., & Tan, J. (2017). Penang Hokkien on life support. *Penang Monthly*. Retrieved from http://penangmonthly.com/article.aspx?pageid=7412&name=penang_hokkien_on_life_support

Pan, L. (Ed.). (2006). *The encyclopedia of the Chinese overseas* (2nd ed.). Singapore: Editions Didier Millet.

Razali, S. M., Aminah, K., & Khan, U. A. (2002). Religious–cultural psychotherapy in the management of anxiety patients. *Transcultural Psychiatry*, *39*(1), 130–136. doi:10.1177/136346150203900106

Rintod, L. (2013, May 30). Working towards reinstating Sarawak's sovereignty. *Free Malaysia Today.* Retrieved from http://www.freemalaysiatoday.com/category/nation/2013/05/30/ working-towards-reinstating-sarawaks-sovereignty/

Simon, M. A., Chen, R., Chang, E., & Dong, X. (2014). The association between filial piety and suicidal ideation: Findings from a community-dwelling Chinese aging population. *The Journals of Gerontology: Series A*, *69*(Suppl. 2), 90–97. doi:10.1093/gerona/glu142 PMID:25378454

Singh, S. K., Yap, K.-H., Reidpath, D. D., & Allotey, P. (2017, August). Binge drinking and associated risk behaviours among youth in three ethnic groups in Malaysia. *Paper presented at 31st annual conference of the European Health Psychology Society*, Padua, Italy, August 29th-September 2.

Sue, S. (1998). In search of cultural competence in psychotherapy and counseling. *The American Psychologist*, *53*(4), 440–448. doi:10.1037/0003-066X.53.4.440 PMID:9572007

Sue, D. W., & Sue, S. (2003). *Counseling the culturally diverse: Theory and practice* (4th ed.). New York: Wiley and Sons.

Sukumaran, T. (2017, May 20). What's causing Malaysia's ethnic Chinese brain drain? *South China Morning Post*. Retrieved from http://www.scmp.com/week-asia/politics/article/2095012/whats-causing-malaysias-ethnic-chinese-brain-drain

Sundararajan, L., Misra, G., & Marsella, A. J. (2013). Indigenous approaches to assessment, diagnosis, and treatment of mental disorders. In F. A. Paniagua & A.-M. Yamada (Eds.), *Handbook of multicultural mental health: Assessment and treatment of diverse populations* (pp. 69–88). London, UK: Elsevier Inc. doi:10.1016/B978-0-12-394420-7.00004-7

Sundararajan, L. (2015). *Understanding Emotion in Chinese Culture:Thinking Through Psychology*. New York: Springer International Publishing. doi:10.1007/978-3-319-18221-6

Tan, C.-B. (2005). Chinese in Malaysia. In M. Ember, C. R. Ember, & I. Skoggard (Eds.), *Encyclopedia of Diasporas: Immigrant and refugee cultures around the world* (pp. 697–706). New York, USA: Springer. doi:10.1007/978-0-387-29904-4_72

Tan, J. (2007, October 28). 马来西亚的华人:一个族群,两种观点 [Malaysian Chinese: One Ethnicity, Two Perspectives]. *Sin Chew Jit Poh* [Sin Chew Forum].

Tan, L. E. (2000). Chinese schools in Malaysia: A case of cultural resilience. In Lee. K. H. & Tan. C. B. (Eds.), The Chinese in Malaysia (pp. 228-254).

Tan, T. J., Ho, W. F., & Tan, J. L. (2005). *The Chinese Malaysian contribution*. Kuala Lumpur: Centre for Malaysian Chinese Studies.

Tang, M. (2002). A comparison of Asian American, Caucasian American and Chinese college students: An initial report. *Journal of Multicultural Counseling and Development*, *30*(2), 124–135. doi:10.1002/j.2161-1912.2002.tb00484.x

The British Psychological Association. (2006). Disciplinary notice: Edward Chan. *The Psychologist*, *19*(10), 619–620.

Ting, S.-K. (2008). *Who am I talking to: The effect of language on bilingual Chinese expression of self-concept and depressive emotion*. Germany: VDM Verlag Dr. Muller.

Ting, R. S. K., & Sundararajan, L. (2017). *Culture, Cognition, and Emotion in China's Religious Ethnic Minorities: Voices of Suffering among the Yi*. Palgrave MacMillan Publication.

Ting, S.-K., & Ng, L. O. (2012). Use of Religious Resources in Psychotherapy from a Tradition-Sensitive Approach: Cases from Chinese in Malaysia. *Pastoral Psychology*, *61*(5-6), 941–957. doi:10.1007/s11089-011-0365-4

Todd, P. M., & Gigerenzer, G. (2012). Ecological rationality: Intelligence in the world. OUP USA. doi:10.1093/acprof:oso/9780195315448.001.0001

Ward, C., & Hewstone, M. (1985). Ethnicity, language and intergroup relations in Malaysia and Singapore: A social psychological analysis. *Journal of Multilingual and Multicultural Development*, *6*(3-4), 271–296. doi:10.1080/01434632.1985.9994207

Ward, C., & Lin, E. (2010). There are homes at the four corners of the seas: acculturation and adaptation of overseas Chinese. In M. H. Bond (Ed.), *The Oxford handbook of Chinese psychology* (pp. 657–677). New York: Oxford University Press. doi:10.1093/oxfordhb/9780199541850.013.0039

Watters, E. (2011). *Crazy Like Us: The Globalization of the American Psyche*. NY: Free Press.

Yeh, K. H., Yi, C., Tsao, W., & Wan, P. (2013). Filial piety in contemporary Chinese societies: A comparative study of Taiwan, Hong Kong, and China. *International Sociology*, *28*(3), 277–296. doi:10.1177/0268580913484345

Yusuff, A. S. M., Tang, L., Binns, C. W., & Lee, A. H. (2014). Prevalence and risk factors for postnatal depression in Sabah, Malaysia: A cohort study. *Women and Birth; Journal of the Australian College of Midwives*, *28*(1), 25–29. doi:10.1016/j.wombi.2014.11.002 PMID:25466643

Zgambo, M., Kalembo, F., He, G., & Wang, H. (2012). Depression among Chinese children and adolescents: A review of the literature. *International Journal of Child, Youth, and Family Studies*, *4*(1), 442–457. doi:10.18357/ijcyfs34.1201211543

KEY TERMS AND DEFINITIONS

Acculturation: The process of social, psychological and identity change resulting from migrating to another culture (i.e. original and host cultures).

Assimilation: The process whereby a minority group gradually adapts to the customs and attitudes of the prevailing culture.

Chinese in Malaysia: Naturalized Malaysians of Chinese descent, mostly descendants of Chinese who arrived in various waves of immigration.

Indigenous Psychology: The scientific study of human behavior and mind that is native, that is not transported from other regions, and that is designed for its people. It involves understanding each culture from its own frame of reference, including its own ecological, historical, philosophical, and religious or spiritual contexts.

Mental Health: A person's condition with regard to their psychological, cognitive, emotional, and social well-being.

Multicultural Competency: The ability to understand, communicate with and effectively interact with people across cultures.

Psychological Challenges: Difficulties or obstacles that affect the individual's mental status.

Resilience: The ability to recover quickly or adjust easily to life difficulties, misfortune or adversities.

ENDNOTES

1 Estimated breakdown of Chinese dialect speakers based on available official data from the 2000 Population and Housing Census of Malaysia.

2 See interview from Kwanghua Newspaper on November 1, 2015 on http://www.kwongwah.com.my/?p=39671

3 Wawasan 2020 was proposed as vision for Malaysia to realize the dream of becoming a developed country.

4 Neurasthenia is a term that denotes a condition with symptoms of fatigue, anxiety, headache, heart palpitations, high blood pressure, neuralgia, and depressed mood, by early neurologist George Miller Beard in 1869. It is currently a diagnosis in the World Health Organization's International Classification of Diseases (and the Chinese Society of Psychiatry's Chinese Classification of Mental Disorders). However, it is no longer included as a diagnosis in the DSM-5 by the American Psychiatric Association.

5 Stanford University's Asia Pacific Brain Drain Project highlighted Malaysia as one of the countries most affected by brain drain. The full report can be accessed at https://cs.stanford.edu/people/eroberts/cs181/projects/2010-11/BrainDrain/Malaysia.html

6 Investigation into the Mental Health Support Needs of International Students with Particular Reference to Chinese and Malaysian Students, September 2011, University of Nottingham.

7 Estimated breakdown based on active clinical psychologists registered under the Malaysian Society of Clinical Psychology (MSCP) as provided by the 2017 MSCP committee.

8 Guang Ming Daily reported on an alleged misrepresentation of an infamous 'psychotherapist' among CIM on 11 November 2009; the alleged 'psychotherapist' also received a formal disciplinary misconduct reprimand from the British Psychological Association for false claims on his qualifications and certification.

Chapter 3
A Case Study of MY Psychology:
Malaysia's First Online Psychoeducational Platform

Chong Shen Hew
MY Psychology, Malaysia

Mu Yi Hor
MY Psychology, Malaysia

Hou Huai Gary Yap
MY Psychology, Malaysia

Tin Fung Chong
MY Psychology, Malaysia

ABSTRACT

MY Psychology is an online educational platform currently based in Malaysia, formed with the intention to spread awareness towards the general public of not only on issues related with mental health and those who suffer under mental illnesses, but also to create a place where psychology as a basic knowledge can be taught and learned. This is in order to correct misunderstandings from the public toward psychology. Operating on the internet requires the company to shift towards a marketing-oriented direction, in the meantime, coping with internal and external challenges in order to strive for greater reach and engagement from the audience.

BACKGROUND HISTORY OF MY PSYCHOLOGY'S FORMATION

A statement made by the Malaysian Psychiatric Association (2013), detailed the shocking rise of mental health problems in children below the age of 15, as the group rose from 13% of the population in the year 1996 to 20% of the population in 2012. Add to that, the recent report made by The Star Online (2017) from a statement by resident consultant psychiatrist in the International Medical University, Dr. Philip George, claiming that the actual numbers of people who had mental health problems might be

DOI: 10.4018/978-1-5225-6073-9.ch003

underreported, maybe due to the stigma often attached to such conditions and the topic in general. As such, a non-conservative estimation of the mentally-ill population would be around 40% of Malaysians (The Star Online, 2017).

To further elaborate upon the role that stigma poses against the advancement of the mental health field in Malaysia, stigma towards mental illness and psychology in general are mostly a result of misunderstandings towards the foundations of the field and of the nature of mental illness in itself. Coupled with a lack of knowledge in the subject matter, this causes such a fear to become widespread not only in real life but also in the virtual realm (online and offline). The deficiency in Malaysia when it comes to the availability of mental health practitioners, according to a recent report made in the NST, stands at 1 psychiatrist for every 200,000 of the total population – much lower than the expected ratio set and recommended by WHO: 1;10,000 (Landau, 2017). The report by the World Health Organization (2011) stated that the mental health expenditures from the local government is only a meagre 0.39% in the total budget allocated to health, and that further expenditures towards mental health hospitals are not even available.

This deficiency, coupled with the fact that mental health problems will be on the rise for the foreseeable future as stress levels in a developing country will potentially be one of the most important risk factors for the population, will inevitably demand a higher level of awareness and knowledge regarding mental health in the general public. So what we have now is a vast range of barriers, from perceived stigma towards the mentally afflicted (Clement et al., 2015), a general uncertainty towards clinical effectiveness among the practitioners themselves (Morriss, 2008), economic issues, and finally a deficiency in trained personnel (Berry & Haddock, 2008), all these varying factors result in a reluctance from those who are currently afflicted with one mental health issue or another that can vastly benefit from psychological interventions are now either unwilling to reach out for help, or are unable to do so from the sheer fact of a lack in sources of help.

One of our main goals in establishing MY Psychology as an online platform is to provide a form of countermeasure towards this issue. Our goal is to provide an outlet of information for general knowledge on common psychological topics, and currently progressing towards the dismantling of stigmatization of mental illness through making interventions and information regarding these interventions available and accessible to the audience. It has been shown by Trefflich, Kalckreuth, Mergl, and Rummel-Kluge (2015) that the levels of internet use in those who are afflicted with mental health issues, including those with severe mental health problems (SMIs), are the same as the general population.

Of course, when MY Psychology was originally formed, we didn't have such lofty aspirations, as our original aim was to provide psychological information towards the general public in digestible and accessible formats. These included, educational videos explaining a psychological concept while incorporating comedy skits, or articles ranging from book and movie reviews, to pieces that highlight a single psychological phenomenon. Our approach gradually shifted since our five-year inception from being a pure content creator to incorporating elements of an online educational platform to better suit the goal that developed further down the line. We aimed to not only provide educational insight into the workings of the psychology field and the mental health faction, but also to dispel psychological misconceptions, as well as to raise awareness towards the predicament of the mentally ill. We are not alone in trying to establish ourselves as online providers of psychological and mental health information in Malaysia as well as abroad, as we have also linked up with multiple similar platforms based in the Canada, Taiwan, as well as the Philippines. But this is still a relatively new path for a field that is previously so grounded in the practice of helping through direct contact, and there are still challenges still ahead of us.

In short, MY Psychology, the first Psychology Educational Platform in Malaysia, operating on the belief that psychological information, including discussions regarding mental health issues, shouldn't just be limited to those who are already in the field, and are only used for academic purposes, as we believe that the permeation and popularization of academic knowledge into everyday knowhow should also be of utmost importance. We believe that as psychology students as well as practitioners of the field, we bear the responsibility to provide psychoeducation to the community. With our motto: "Learn. Share. Apply", MY Psychology has been providing mental health information for online users through multiple approaches such as articles, comics and videos on social media platforms including Facebook and YouTube.

NATURE OF BUSINESS

As a company that originally started from the simple idea of being a hub for all psychologically related content that grew during the process into being one of the leaders in the field in Malaysia, we are what is known as a "startup company", and we commonly refer to ourselves as social entrepreneurs or as a social enterprise (Katila, Chen, & Piezunka, 2012). Seeing as the field of online educational platforms, specifically for psychology, is still a growing need that requires innovative approaches and products in order for it to grow (Katila et al., 2012), we see it as our role to generate this shift in moving psychology from the classroom to the layman on the street, so that psychology can become a common knowledge in the vein of oral healthcare, or nutritional healthcare.

Every member on the team has a different role in the company, though of course, since we are still trying to experiment with our approach towards content creation, our roles are often swapped, and overall every one of our current projects involved every single member and they often required a very hands-on approach to accomplish. We are also currently in the process of recruiting more volunteers, be it in the content creation department, or on the management front, so as to expand our scope of operation.

When it comes to the production of content, we have at the emergence of a wider audience and subscribers, developed an outline of two different formats of products that we will continue to provide through our platform in the near future, in order to fully utilize the strengths of the online platform as an outlet for producing and distributing educational products. They take the shape of a Toolkit vs. First-Aid Kit paradigm. Contents falling into the Toolkit category are more focused on conveying information of everyday psychological/sociological phenomena through an approachable manner. On the other hand. contents in the First-Aid Kit category will be dedicated to information on mental health in general, such as the diagnostic criteria and definition of different types of mental illnesses, and some of the methods used to relieve said illnesses, so that we can create an increase in awareness towards such a commonly stigmatized group of people, as well as the misunderstanding towards mental health and mental illnesses in general that is ingrained in the public.

Both sides of the paradigm are presented using a combination of mediums which include: infographic made from online and offline photo editing programs with a monthly change of themes, articles regularly being uploaded onto our personal web-pages as well as social media sites, or videos focusing on explaining some psychological phenomenon or comedy skits detailing everyday situations where knowledge of some basic psychology can come in handy. But one of our biggest aims that we hope to achieve is the elimination of the perception that psychology is a pseudoscience and to increase the awareness of the availability of help for those who faced mental health problems. One of our newest addition to our provided services is the Messenger Bot, which enables anyone with access to our Facebook page to directly inquire for help. In it are directories to our published content that is readily available on our website, as well as a growing list of contacts of mental institutes and healthcare centres in Malaysia, categorized according to each respective state. We are currently inviting more centres to join our efforts.

CURRENT PROJECTS AND FUTURE PROSPECTS

In addition to expanding the database for the Messenger Bot to include more centres and mental health hospitals in Malaysia, we also plan to extend beyond Malaysia and taking our project into Southeast Asia, and then internationally, in the near future. This is of course a very long running project, and we are constantly upgrading the efficiency of our Messenger Bot, so that it would be able to respond to a wider array of questions, as well as provide faster and more accurate responses. On the content creation front, we have already semi-transitioned into a platform, and although the majority of the content we posted daily on to our website as well as our Facebook page is still produced by us, we have also opened the possibility of being part of our team via a registration page on our webpage, allowing users to write articles, and once filtered and approved by our editors, be able to publish it under our brand.

Currently, our newest product is the production of a video series comprising of short videos between one to three minute that attempt to provide a basic outline of either comparisons between differing concepts that lay people usually misunderstood (psychologists vs psychiatrists), or a simple introduction towards a complicated subject matter (i.e. legitimacy of LGBTQ). We plan to release these videos in seasonal formats, with each season taking on topics with a different nature (i.e. first season is comparisons, second season focusing on debating, etc.). This format of videos will be much easier to produce than our older videos, which involved complicated procedures of shooting on location, as well as the addition of skits. In the future, we aim to establish a stable production line for our videos, so that we can be able to produce these videos on a weekly basis.

The other project that we are currently involved in is the production of a monthly web magazines. Currently we have produced two such magazines, and we think that this is an interesting and beautiful way to present our articles as well as entertainment, such as quizzes or infographics, to our audience. Besides that, we would be able to provide more content towards our patrons on our Patreon page, providing them with a summary of each month's best articles. For this, we hope that we would be able to form a team of writers who will be directly responsible for the production of such a magazine.

CURRENT CHALLENGES

The challenges of establishing and running an online psychology educational platform ranged greatly, from internal maintenance of our motivation and company efficiency to external outreach in our attempts to reach our targeted audience and the market. This includes the concerns we have with regards to technological challenges, optimizing the outreach of our content with a limited budget, consistent content creation process as well as handling the new challenges of our messenger bot. These will be discussed accordingly in the following paragraphs.

Audience and Market Needs

The survival of an educational platform is closely related to whether it is serving the need and solving a problem faced by the community. In other words, it is about whether the existence of the platform itself is celebrated and welcomed by the community, or else the platform will just end up providing content with no response or engagement from the receiving end. To further elaborate upon this: multiple factors need to be considered, including mental health literacy and awareness among the community and the motivation behind help-seeking behaviors.

As noted before, stigma and discrimination are always recognized as one of the most significant barriers to mental health seeking behaviours as well as social inclusion of that particular individual (Corrigan & Wassel, 2008). The stigma towards mental illness is not only limited to the Western context, but also to the Asian context including Malaysia (Ng, 1997). The manifestation of the stigma in a Malaysian context not only brings adverse impact to various important aspects of the lives of the affected population, in terms of their wellbeing and their employment rates, it will also influence the perception of their families in seeing them as disabled and shameful besides avoiding the disclosure in order to protect the family from 'losing face' (Chang & Horrocks, 2006).

All these negative consequences stemming from stigmatization will limit available support given to the affected population. With this, an online psychology educational platform might have its place of being an alternative option in filling up the gap via providing accurate information about mental disorders and giving directions for getting the right help. To MY Psychology, our audiences can be broadly divided into two groups: the in-group and the out-group. In-group here is referred to psychology students, psychology graduates and professionals who are already familiar with the field, and this group will have a strong interest or even a career related to psychology. They have a higher tendency and motivation to know more about psychology and also to gather as much mental health information as possible. As such, they are easier audience to be targeted for our online psychology learning platform.

In contrast, the out-group refers to the general population, including those who have mental disorders who are 'outside' of the field or who has never heard about psychology except through popular myths such as psychology being "mind-reading" or "mind-control" tactics. This population may have lower awareness and are thus less likely to realize the importance of understanding about psychology and mental health. It is reasonable to anticipate a larger degree of difficulty in targeting and attracting them to learn psychology online. The efforts of generating interest amongst them, converting their online behaviour to click on psychology platforms and the latter phase of directing them to the right help is definitely way more challenging than the in-group.

As such, the approach of running an online psychology platform needs to be even more proactive in reaching out to the community. Based on our trial-and-errors, here are a few criteria that needed to be considered for content creators. First, the content itself needs to be educational in nature so that the audience can at least learn something from viewing the content such as knowing about the fact that "Depression is not just sadness". Second, the content needs to be entertaining because it has to provide a pleasurable learning experience for the audience. Third, the content has to be short and precise, also known as "bite-size content". Keep in mind that the targeted audiences are not professionals in the field which indicates that their initial passions and interests are less connected to the nature of the content, so explaining the content from its history to theories would be a redundant and unproductive effort. The content itself needs to be short, easy to understand and relatable to them so that the engagement level can be further elevated.

Current Technological Concerns

The challenges of connecting psychology and mental health information to the public are undoubtedly bounded within social media marketing methods and techniques. The most common online social media platform is Facebook. However, the trickiest part of posting content on Facebook is the number of followers on our page doesn't guarantee the exposure and audience outreach of published contents, meaning that not everyone in the 100k audience population will have received every single update of our newly published posts. In fact, the organic reach which is defined as "the number of people who saw your page posts not due to paid advertising" depends much more on the interaction of various factors including adherence to Facebook's algorithm, the peak period of the contents being posted, audiences' reactions towards the post or photos.

According to the Social@Ogily's report analysis of more than 100 brand pages of various products and industries, there was a concerning decline in average organic reach from 12.05% in October 2013 to 6.15% in February 2014 (Manson, 2014). The biggest decline was found in the month of December, during the period when Facebook's company revealed a major change in algorithm. Regardless of our respective Facebook page sizes and our number of followers, organic reach has shown persistent decline over time, indicating that gaining organic reach from audiences has become more and more difficult.

With that, paid advertising becomes another option to increase the exposure of published contents. Facebook fans will be able to see the content and circulate it on their own Facebook timelines if the content itself is interesting enough. According to Neisen (2012), having a friend's endorsement towards a published content can probably generate higher recall from the advertising campaign. Relating this back to the context of our platform MY Psychology, it is unavoidable that we have to employ both strategies: the organic reach and paid reach in order to increase and maintain the exposure of our contents. Paid advertising campaign has undoubtedly achieved its effectiveness by influencing audiences' online behaviour such as increasing buying behaviour on company's product (Comscore, 2012). However, with the limited budget and the lack of income from our platform, it makes the effort of targeting audiences even harder and a more detailed plan has to be structured out in advertising our contents.

Content Creation Process

With the evolution of Facebook into a platform which publishes and broadcasts contents for the community, the editorial model has become more prominent in publishing about recent news and events with the hope of gaining fan engagement (Malson, 2014). This informs the need of becoming more selective in publishing related contents to generate more engagement and discussion among the fan community. For instance, MY Psychology has adopted some recent news such as school bullying and stigma in job employment as a theme of discussion and also daily canvas pictures that deliver a more holistic approach in discussing about such matters.

This is also related to posting frequencies on our Facebook page, in which posting too little or too often will ultimately kill page engagement. Posting at two extremes is not encouraged and hence more careful choices and considerations have to be taken into consideration to publish quality content less frequently but comes with greater potential in good story-telling methods such as psychology short videos with catchy titles and illustrative themes of mental illness. There is no best method for all pages, but it depends on the data of the page. We have to study and analyze the data about users' engagement and reactions including likes, comments and share towards certain post at certain period of time informs the "do" and "don't" in planning and designing future posts. Relating back to the content of MY Psychology, we have found that our audiences are not fond of articles relating to psychological research but show more engagement when it comes to debunking popular myths, telling the differences between two confusing topics such as "Obsessive-Compulsive Disorder versus Perfectionism" and also funny videos related to Psychological concepts and myths.

To run MY Psychology, basic knowledge about psychology and keeping ourselves updated to recent news are insufficient. The information of the fans in our Facebook page is very important because it allows us to identify their behavioural information including their motivation of liking and following our page, their reactions towards certain posts, their highest or last engagement with the content as well as their profile and our audience demographic information. Taking cultural background and language into account, these data can become the variables that serve as cues in informing the direction of our platform, whether the platform is publishing potential viral content such as psychology puns and jokes to generate the "wow" effect that attract audiences who jump on merely for similar contents or the platform is attracting a more people who truly want to know more about psychology. The key challenge that always remains on our platform is to publish content that speaks about the core values of MY Psychology and optimize the content outreach at its best among the community of different ethnicities and background.

To improve our targeting functionality, the analysis of the community on our platform along with Social Customer Relationship Management (CRM) is greatly needed to derive an effective communication model such as one-to-one or one-to-many with the audiences in order to narrow down the focus and customize their experience. For instance, we are serving various kinds of contents for our audiences such as publishing daily pictures of bite-size psychology information, monthly articles and psychology-related videos for audiences who are actively engaging with those contents. Also, we post questions such as asking for their opinions on certain topics of interest or even controversy, which can generate engaging discussions, while increasing more chances for audiences to interact with one another so that they can feel the uniqueness of the experience gained from our platform. Trial and error of posting contents in different layout and designs allows us to compare and contrast the effectiveness of the post. Being aware of the limitations allows us to harness the potential of future posts in deriving greater audiences' engagement and reactions.

Bot Creation and Business Connections

Facebook Messenger Bot is undoubtedly one of the most welcomed user features in the coming years as it has been shown that messaging apps have surprisingly surpassed the social networks (Ballve, 2015). The present efforts in integrating business model into the Facebook Messenger Bot is anticipated and the birth of Chatbot which is a software embedded in Messenger Bot with artificial intelligence that can communicate and establish highly personalized conversations with users is well celebrated because it establishes a firm digital presence and friendly approach to the users who are familiar with messaging apps.

Compared to the traditional strategy of utilizing email strategies and websites, the content delivered in Messenger Bot has higher read rates with up to 90% with greater user retention because the message received by users from the Chatbot generates a similar feeling as personal messages sent by their social circles through mobile devices and apps.

With the vision of increasing the mental health awareness against the mental health stigma whereby people are still reluctant to open up for help, Messenger Bot establishes a safer environment which allows users to communicate with the chatbot in a more personalized way, just like how they send and receive message with their friends without needing to post it online on personal Facebook timelines or in a Facebook group. Messenger Bot can also be seen as a way to overcome the algorithm in the social media especially Facebook page in which we don't have full control of the exposure of our published contents.

MY Psychology has soft-launched its bot platform in early July this year (2017) with the hope of being a directory in connecting the users to psychological help. By doing so, our team has extracted the contact details of the local government hospitals into the chatbot which allows the users to contact and check the available centres at their fingertips. We have also contacted private centers and community organizations that provide mental health services as an alternative to centres in government sectors for our users. With this, we hope to increase the act of getting mental help among the community and connect them to the right services at the right time.

The key challenges of executing the Chatbot are that the initial purpose is to connect users to the local mental health services in Malaysia. However, it isn't yet ready for use by those living in countries especially in the Southeast Asian region where mental health stigma is still prevalent and there is a lack of legislation bodies in regulating the services. The next goal of our team then is not only aiming to establish a more complete directory of mental health services in Malaysia, but also open a new door to international audiences so that they can have access to this service as well.

Sustainability and Future Direction

One of the key challenges which is consistently faced by MY Psychology is the company's long-term sustainability due to us providing free online psychology contents regularly which does not generate profit in return because there is no product that can be sold other than providing information. Hence, getting funding for MY Psychology would be limited compared to other startups which may come with a business model that can drive profit from the users. Sponsorship could come from companies that wish to advertise or increase brand awareness on the platform. Prior to attracting that sponsorship, the number of followers and the statistics in term of audiences' engagement are undoubtedly the key factors that inform the potential optimized outreach of the company's exposure and the engagement itself is embedded within the strategy of designing and publishing contents on a regular basis.

In order to publish content on a regular basis to promote and maintain the audience engagement, manpower in the content creation process is very important and that brings us to the recruitment and management of workload levels that requires detailed planning and production line. Recently, MY Psychology has started to expand its team and recruit a few key members to take respective roles according to their interests and ability. More and more challenges ahead are anticipated.

The future of MY Psychology is uncertain, as always as it is. Being one of the leading platforms in providing bite-size information in Malaysia where the level of mental health literacy and awareness among the community is still very low definitely invites many unforeseen challenges. Yet, it is believed that it has at least taken the initiative in the hopes of advancing the field of mental health in the country.

POTENTIAL SOLUTIONS

Integrative Platform

As stated above, to achieve self-sustainability, we have to seek for funding and or sponsorships due to the non-profitable nature of our products and provided services, and several such attempts has been implemented. We have set up our own Patreon page in order to gain financial support from the public. Patreon is a membership platform that provides business tools for creators to run a subscription-based service, as well as ways for artists to build relationships and provide exclusive experiences and contents to their subscribers, or "patrons." It is popular among Youtube videographers, webcomic artists, writers, podcasters, musicians, and other categories of creators who regularly posted their creations online. It allows artists to receive funding directly from their fans, or patrons, on a recurring basis or per work of art. Despite the slow progress and growth, we have a few patrons who are subscribing to our platform now. The money collected from patrons can be used to pay our writers who contributed articles and designers who compiled them and produce our first issue of the psychology magazine. Hence, MY Psychology would want to use this method to gather funds from our audiences and use them to grow and expand the platform.

MY Psychology's plan is to create a psychology community in which we can connect psychology graduates, students, professionals and the public community en large. By integrating the resources and connecting people from various walks of life, we can easily deliver bite-sized psychology knowledge from credible sources to the public, increase mental health awareness and tackle social stigma towards mental illness. MY psychology has currently been in connection with more than 20 psychological centers in Malaysia and are partners with more than 10 similar psychology online platforms from different countries such as Singapore, Taiwan, Philippines, Canada, and Malaysia. In the journey of promoting psychology and mental health, MY Psychology hope to form an alliance, a community and a closed connection with all the related parties.

Due to the fact that the core members of MY Psychology have their limitations, not only limited time but also are financially insufficient. Without the support from the communities and the public, we would not be able to sustain the platform. For instance, the video series we have been creating as stated before, have achieved quite the success, but because of limited manpower, we are only able to produce one video every two weeks. In order to deliver correct information and credible knowledge from reliable sources to our audience, a much larger quantity of effort is needed. To achieve sustainability, we have to achieve the goal of being able to recruit volunteers first, through the creation of a system, a "psychology content factory", to put it simply. By recruiting talented writers and content creators, we can consistently produce bite-sized psychology infographic, videos, articles, comic and podcast for our audiences as well as controlling the "quality" of the content to make sure each piece of content originated from reliable and credible sources.

Products and Services

MY Psych has several services and products that possess huge potentials in creating job and internship opportunities for Psychology graduates and interns. In order to advance the mental health field, we need to retain the talents in the field, and to provide opportunities for them. MY Psych's current two projects, Bot messenger and Psychology E-magazine, requires a lot of manpower and we are planning use this opportunity to mass recruit psychology students and graduates as volunteers to make these plans achievable. The common problem for psychology students after graduation is not being able to find psychology related jobs and internship opportunities; by promoting these two projects, we can provide these opportunities to the psychology graduates and in turn let them contribute their knowledge and talent back to the society as well as helping them to achieve a better job prospect or academic advancement.

Through this process of hiring psychology students/graduates as writers for our magazine; we gain profit from the public by selling our magazine, and in turn we can use the profit to hire more psychology graduates/ students and to improve the quality of the contents which can later be contributed back to the public once again, in the hopes of creating a positive cycle that can advance the field of psychology in Malaysia.

Media Attention: Offline Connections

Having media attention on our platform can give us the edge we need to grow for years to come if we use it correctly. Publicity will raise the awareness of our platform and we can use that new-found awareness to grow the events attendance and spread our messages. Having major sources provide coverage of our platform speaks volume for our page credibility, as well as lending the mental health cause a big boost in visibility and attention. Because of this, MY Psychology will continue to pursue further into online marketing.

One such way to gain the necessary attention towards our platform is through the organization of a series of workshops and seminars, as it not only fosters a culture of spreading psychology knowledge but also improve the relationship among the mental health professionals from all over the world. To do this require intensive cooperation between us and the universities. In addition, such a relationship can also improve the welfare of psychology students. For instance, MY Psychology can compile various information of psychology courses from several universities for our audiences who might be interested in pursuing psychology. We might be able to gain exclusive "scholarship", "internship", "financial support" opportunities for our audiences. In addition, MY Psychology can also promote any workshops, seminars or talks that organized by the universities. In other words, My Psychology acts as the integrative platform that provides various psychology information for the students or non-students who are interested in psychology.

Such offline activities have the added advantage to connect with our audiences physically and provide face-to-face interactions with the public. Also, MY Psychology can recruit talented people who are interested to become volunteers through these offline campaigns and events. During these offline campaigns, we can invite the public audience to follow our online platform and get the most updated news. By doing this not only increase our exposure in the public, but also attract media attention and perhaps sponsorship.

MY PSYCHOLOGY'S CURRENT IMPACT

The public conception of psychology in Southeast Asia is heavily clouded by myths. The media often portrays psychology in a constant negative light, and the permeation of notions such as 'if you study psychology, you will become crazy' or 'you won't be able to find a job if you study psychology' are common. These myths are harmful and halt the progress that we are trying to gain when it comes to the advancement of the field as a whole, because widespread misconceptions stop the public from truly understanding the core of psychology.

One of the ways in which we achieve the goal of clarification is through creating a structured and easily understood outline of psychoeducation, we hope to create the proper expectations and atmosphere for the public in order to clarify what we as psychology students actually studied. The monthly psychological project offers us a chance to focus and zero in on specific mental illnesses, giving the audience an overview towards these afflictions, and their respective treatment methods. As of today, we have already completed two such monthly projects: a month on depression, and the other on anxiety disorders.

The impact might not seem significant at this point of time but we truly believe that change occurs gradually, and we hope that by influencing others, the change that we hope for can happen, as more and more join in on our efforts. What we truly wanted to achieve is the dismantling of stigmatizations so that people won't hesitate to learn psychology, and that the afflicted won't be afraid to seek for help.

The other achievement of ours is that we have slowly expanded beyond the confines of education and have now stationed ourselves as a middle point between the public and the professional. We have, since our inception, been receiving messages seeking for help when it comes to depression, a trouble in grieving or even suicidal notions through our inbox. We have to clarify with each of them since it is beyond our capabilities and qualifications to provide professional help, but it is hard to just turn our back on these people and draw a clear line.

This is where the Messenger Bot comes into play, as it has the potential to become a constant source of information when our audience came for guidance or seek for help, through its automatic feedback towards help seekers, and as a constant presence, they are able to inquire upon such subjects even when we are not available. We had recently gathered and prepared a long list of emergency hotlines, and upon request, the bot will provide instant replies containing contacts that they can reach to. This is still a task in progress and we hope to cover a wider range of help in the near future.

We also managed to generate an interest in learning more about psychology through our recent video series. Videos, in our opinion, can be an effective medium to share information if used correctly. The contents mainly involve around introducing the right meaning of psychology terms and breaking psychology myths. If you are familiar with YouTube education related channels, when you think of minutes science, you will remember 'AsapScience.' When you think of physics, you will remember 'Veritasium.' There are a lot of channels working now in creating educational videos and gaining a huge wave of support but most of them are from western countries. The successful online education model can be learnt and duplicated, but of course, there are cultural differences between different countries and we should not generalize between these two audiences, and should actively strive for a balance in order to cater to our specific audience.

We are nowhere near the top education channels at this moment, but we hope to introduce the possibility of making education videos in Southeast Asia. When one channel had successfully proven that educational videos could work, others would quickly follow. As of today, while we are writing this, we had two successful videos reaching more than 100k views on Facebook. Shortly after that, we have already received a few invitations to collaborate and produce similar contents. We have also inspired and share our tips to a few psychology graduates and professions to start their own social media page. The online psychoeducation will have a bigger impact to the public if there are more creators joining into this wave, adding depth and variety to the scene and community. We foresee a healthy competition between each group and also a growth in motivation to foster organic growth of the field.

FUTURE RECOMMENDATIONS

First of all, we must repeat that we are not professionals when it comes to online psychoeducation. Our findings are mostly based upon our own experiences, as well as through a painstaking process of trial and error. Nevertheless, we took care to research into every possible outcome as much as we can. Hence, what we shared in this case study is solely for the purpose of sharing our experiences to those who wished to join in the effort in advancing the field of online psychoeducation. We hope these would help future content creators and educators, to create a clearer direction, and to act as a paving stone for those who choose such a path.

Know Your Psychology Knowledge

Identify your own level of knowledge on psychology to avoid sharing wrong information. Often there are pages sharing "*psychology says*" without solid research or further readings. Share the right information and along the way, try to explore further into other areas of psychology knowledge. Be ambitious, but be careful when sharing knowledge. You may encounter people who will inform you that your research findings are outdated, and update you on the latest finding in this field.

Know Your IT Skills

The fastest way for an information to go viral is with the aid of a right platform and creative designs. Graphic design is a skill worth enhancing. Creating creative infographics with bite size psychology knowledge can be a good starting point. With the aid of free graphic design platforms online, simple graphic designs can be generated with no hassle. Other than presenting these in picture forms, a more engaging method would be to present information in video forms. Do note that editing a one minute video consumes much more time and would be harder to execute without proper training. There are pros and cons to this but you can always find the style that suits you the most.

Know Your Platform Well

Upon spending all that time on your infographic and videos, you would want to be sure it can reach optimum audience. One main difference between online education and offline education is that you can gather feedback accurately. You can observe the number of viewers and reaction to the video. These two information serves as feedback. Study your audiences well to know the kind of content you should generate. For example, content with bigger font for old age audiences and colorful infographics to attract younger audiences. Also observe when to post these contents as time is a crucial factor.

Study Your Time

At macro level, to raising public awareness on the importance of psychology requires consistent commitment and a long period of time. To change a stereotype or raise awareness is different from teaching. Sometimes, scientifically proven data and/or statistical data may not be enough to convince people. Convincing requires ample time, detailed explanation and sometimes aid of recent events to educate the public. For example, when an influential figure (such as an idol) committed suicide due to depression, then it would be a good time to share knowledge about depression. Not only does the creation of true impact requires a long time, sometimes it requires good timing too.

Personally, how much time are we willing to invest in this? It is important to do a quick check before executing any project. To simplify; are you willing to commit full time to online psychoeducation? If you are, then you are able to create consistent content and subsequently, content which probably consumes a lot of your time. If you able to commit only a few hours per day or per week, then you may want to consider projects which fits in with your available time. It is often easy to get too ambitious, only to realize later on that we are not in the capacity to complete what was started.

Settle With Right Expectations

In comparison to traditional platforms, one of downsides of online education is the lack of positive reward you obtain. Not just in the form of monetary compensation, but also in terms of observing the effects of our effort. To illustrate, we may feel a sense of pride knowing we helped an elderly cross the road, but we may not be able to tell if we have successfully encouraged three patients with mental health problems to seek for help. Despite the powerful impact of our contribution to the society, it can be relatively hard to notice. Raw data shown on the paper will never show the direct effect we have made. So, set your expectations straight. We cannot change the minds of thousands who assumes depression will only affect those who have weak mentalities, but we may be able to save a depressed individual from committing suicide.

Currently, the awareness level towards psychology in Southeast Asia is far behind in comparison with other countries, therefore presenting us with a large barrier to overcome. But at the same time, we are lucky because we now have better tools and platforms to help us achieve our goals. Through online platforms, we are able to easily reach and influence more people. However, it also has the power to mislead if we are not careful enough. Unethical creators can abuse the power of social media and online platforms, spreading misleading information as long as it shows good results and lead to monetary gains.

To paraphrase the cliché sayings of Uncle Ben, if you have the obligation to do the right thing, and if it is within your power to do so, then you are required to be responsible for any such actions. In short, we hope that we have successfully provided steps as to how to start your journey in this field. So, shall we begin?

REFERENCES

Ballve. (2015). Messaging apps are overtaking social networks to become the dominant platforms on phones. *Business Insider*. Retrieved from http://www.businessinsider.com/messaging-apps-have-completely-overtaken-social-networks-to-become-the-dominant-platforms-on-phones-2015-4/?IR=T&r=MY

Berry, K., & Haddock, G. (2008). The implementation of the NICE guidelines for schizophrenia: Barriers to the implementation of psychological interventions and recommendations for the future. *Psychology and Psychotherapy: Theory, Research and Practice*, *81*(4), 419–436. doi:10.1348/147608308X329540 PMID:18652741

Chang, K. H., & Horrocks, S. (2006). Lived experiences of family caregivers of mentally ill relatives. *Journal of Advanced Nursing*, *53*(4), 435–443. doi:10.1111/j.1365-2648.2006.03732.x PMID:16448486

Clement, S., Schauman, O., Graham, T., Maggioni, F., Evans-Lacko, S., Bezborodovs, N., ... Thornicroft, G. (2015). What is the impact of mental health-related stigma on help-seeking? A systematic review of quantitative and qualitative studies. *Psychological Medicine*, *45*(1), 11–27. doi:10.1017/S0033291714000129 PMID:24569086

ComScore. (2012). *The Power of Like 2*. Retrieved from http://www.comscore.com/Insights/Presentations_and_Whitepapers/2012/The_Power_of_Like_2_How_Social_Marketing_Works

Corrigan, P. W., & Wassel, A. (2008). Understanding and influencing the stigma of mental illness. *Journal of Psychosocial Nursing and Mental Health Services*, *46*(1), 42–48. doi:10.3928/02793695-20080101-04 PMID:18251351

Cummings, E. J. (2009). Trends in mental health googling. *The Psychiatrist*, *33*(11), 437–437.

Katila, R., Chen, E. L., & Piezunka, H. (2012). All the right moves: How entrepreneurial firms compete effectively. *Strategic Entrepreneurship Journal*, *6*(2), 116–132. doi:10.1002ej.1130

Landau, E. (2017, July 1). Malaysia needs 3,000 registered psychiatrists to meet WHO recommendation: Lee. *New Straits Times Online*. Retrieved from https://www.nst.com.my/news/nation/2017/07/253500/malaysia-needs-3000-registered-psychiatrists-meet-who-recommendation-lee

Malaysian Psychiatric Association. (2013). *Mental health: With compassion we can help them cope*. Retrieved from https://www.psychiatry-malaysia.org/article.php?aid=1757

Manson, M. (2014, March 6). *Analysis of 100 Facebook Pages conducted by Social@Ogilvy [Digital image]*. Retrieved November 18, 2017, from https://social.ogilvy.com/facebook-zero-considering-life-after-the-demise-of-organic-reach/

Manson, M. (2014). *Facebook zero: Considering life after the demise of organic reach*. Retrieved from https://social.ogilvy.com/facebook-zero-considering-life-after-the- demise-of-organic-reach/

Ng, C. H. (1997). The stigma of mental illness in Asian cultures. *The Australian and New Zealand Journal of Psychiatry*, *31*(3), 382–390. doi:10.3109/00048679709073848 PMID:9226084

Nielsen. (2012, April). Global Trust in Advertising and Brand Messages. Retrieved from http://www.nielsen.com/content/dam/corporate/us/en/reports-downloads/2012-Reports/global-trust-inadvertising-2012.pdf

The Star Online. (2017). *Depression: 40% of Malaysians will suffer from mental health issues in their lifetime*. Retrieved from https://www.thestar.com.my/news /nation /2017/04/02/malaysians-will-suffer-from-mental-health-issues-in-their-lifetime/

Trefflich, F., Kalckreuth, S., Mergl, R., & Rummel-Kluge, C. (2015). Psychiatric patients' internet use corresponds to the internet use of the general public. *Psychiatry Research*, *226*(1), 136–141. doi:10.1016/j.psychres.2014.12.037 PMID:25623020

World Health Organization. (2011). Malaysia. Retrieved from http://www.who.int/mental_health/evidence/atlas/profiles/mys_mh_profile.pdf

Chapter 4
Revised Reality Therapy:
A New Intervention to Help Boost Self-Esteem in Malaysian Secondary Schools

Joo Hou Ng
University of Exeter, UK

Aaron Page
University of Exeter, UK

ABSTRACT

This chapter proposes an intervention – revised reality therapy – that has been developed to help school guidance counsellors treat low self-esteem in Malaysian secondary schools. Revised reality therapy has been developed using literature from a range of fields, including: choice theory, reality therapy, social identity approach, and first-hand experience in Malaysian secondary schools. The proposed intervention uses a simple, easy to use method which - for the convenience of school guidance counsellors and laypeople alike – has been presented as a six-step process. The theoretical background, implementation, and validity of revised reality therapy will be presented in this chapter. Future directions and limitations are also discussed.

INTRODUCTION

Imagine you are a student who attends a secondary school, you have just received important academic results and you rush home to share the results with your family. After sharing your results, you ask your family what they think. "The results are not good enough" is the reply you receive. How do you feel in this situation? Ashamed, disappointed, embarrassed, like you have let your family down? In Malaysian society, being below average is unacceptable. Most Malaysian students strive to achieve outstanding academic results. However, in the real world, it is impossible for everyone to achieve outstanding results. Consequently, many people fall short of their expectations, and often think "I'm not good enough". This form of negative self-evaluation is formally known as low self-esteem.

DOI: 10.4018/978-1-5225-6073-9.ch004

Self-esteem is broadly defined as a person's subjective evaluation of their worth as an individual (See, e.g., Donnellan, Trzesniewski, & Robins, 2011). In contrast to what many people think, low self-esteem is not a reflection of a person's ability, and it certainly is not a representation of how a person is evaluated by others. Instead, low self-esteem is a negative pattern of thoughts, characterized by a person's subjective perception that they are inadequate in many facets of life (Sorensen, 2018).

For many years, psychologists have recognized that self-esteem is an important aspect of mental-health and is relevant for many important life outcomes. For example, high self-esteem predicts happiness, better job performance and academic achievement (Baumeister, Campbell, Krueger, & Vohs, 2003; Judge & Bono, 2001; Marsh & Craven, 2006). In contrast, low self-esteem predicts antisocial behavior, delinquency, anxiety and depression (Donnellan, Trzesniewski, Robins, Moffitt, & Caspi, 2005; Sowislo & Orth, 2013; Steiger, Allemand, Robins, & Fend, 2014; Trzesniewski, Donnellan, Moffitt, Robins, Poulton, & Caspi, 2006). So, on the basis of the literature discussed, you may now - as the authors of this present chapter did before you – ponder the following question, surely Malaysian schools have effective interventions to help students overcome low self-esteem?

Evidence suggests this may not be the case. In recent years, Malaysian secondary schools have been teetering on the edge of a 'self-esteem crisis'. Nationally the number of Malaysian students suffering from low self-esteem has risen from ten-percent to twenty-percent, meaning that low self-esteem currently affects one-in-five Malaysian students (The Sun Daily, 2016; Yaacob, Juhari, Talib, & Uba, 2009). Given that low self-esteem is a strong predictor of many detrimental life outcomes (e.g., depression, delinquency, antisocial behavior etc.), the looming 'self-esteem crisis' represents a serious problem for Malaysian students.

Currently, within context of the Malaysian education system, 'school guidance counsellors' play a crucial role in helping students with low self-esteem. For many students, school guidance counsellors provide an essential, valuable service that – to a certain extent – helps treat low self-esteem. However, a school guidance counsellor's ability to help treat low self-esteem has been hindered by a number of barriers, such as: (1) a lack of support from school faculty, who prioritize academic grades and teaching; (2) a lack of cooperation from the parents of students; (3) being assigned admin tasks, such as photocopying and delivering reports; (4) being responsible for roughly five-hundred students; and finally (5) the incompatibility of Western interventions in Malaysian schools (Low, Kok & Lee, 2013; Othman & Abdullah, 2015). In short, many barriers impede a school guidance counsellor's ability to help Malaysian students suffering from low self-esteem.

It is beyond the scope of the present chapter to address all the barriers listed. In truth, a textbook chapter can have little influence on the culture of schools, parenting styles and the workload of school guidance counsellors. However, in line with previous literature, this chapter acknowledges that there is a need for a Malaysian compatible intervention to help boost self-esteem (Othman & Abdullah, 2015).

So, the aim of the current chapter is to introduce a new, innovative intervention that has been developed in the context of Malaysian Secondary Schools. On the basis of literature on choice theory and reality therapy (Glasser, 1998; Wubbolding, 2015), social identity approach (e.g., Haslam, 2001), and first-hand experience in Malaysian secondary schools, this chapter will propose a simple 'step-by-step' intervention to help boost the self-esteem of Malaysian secondary school students.

For the benefit of those who are unfamiliar with the theories mentioned, a brief laypersons introduction to the key principles of choice theory and reality therapy, and social identity approach will be presented. In the following sections, each of the theories will be mentioned in isolation, then the overall framework for the new intervention will be presented.

Choice Theory

Choice theory, developed by William Glasser, is a theoretical explanation of human behavior and mental health. Critically, this theory can help explain the origins of low self-esteem. The cornerstone principle of choice theory is the assumption that human behavior is a choice, and these choices are driven by basic needs. According to Glasser (1998), humans have five genetically encoded needs: survival, belonging, power, independence, and enjoyment.

The need of survival, the most basic of human needs, is the physiological requirement to stay alive. Belonging reflects a feeling of connectedness with family and friends. The need of power is the drive to experience success and self-worth. Independence is the need for a sense of autonomy and free-will. Finally, enjoyment is the desire to feel pleasure and have fun. Each person has a specific set of needs they perceive as important, in choice theory this is called a person's 'quality world' (Glasser, 2000). Each person's 'quality world' differs depending on many contextual factors – for example, a student may desire power and autonomy, whereas a retired businessperson may desire enjoyment and belonging. When the external world does not satisfy a person's 'quality world' they experience psychological imbalance (i.e., unhappiness), and ultimately, this leads to mental health problems (e.g., low self-esteem). To resolve this discrepancy, a person should be "motivated" to make a behavioral change to influence the external world, thus restoring psychological balance.

For example, in the context of Malaysian schools, a student who has the basic need of belonging may, as a result, value friendships with other students. However, this student may experience low self-esteem if their friendships are jeopardized (i.e., their external world is not fulfilling their needs). To resolve this, choice theory posits that a behavioral change needs to occur, such as seeking friendship from other sources, to help the student fulfil their needs. Ultimately, this should help the student experience an increase in self-esteem.

In short, choice theory offers a theoretical basis to help understand what causes a person to venture into the mental state of low self-esteem (i.e., a person's 'needs' not being satisfied by the external world), and offers a means for improving self-esteem (i.e., by altering behaviors to change the external world). Building on the theoretical foundations of choice theory, Wubbolding (1988) conceived a therapeutic approach – named reality therapy – that has been widely used by therapists in western cultures to treat low self-esteem. This therapeutic approach, described below, shall form the crux of the new revised intervention.

Reality Therapy

Reality therapy is based upon the principles of choice theory. Thus, reality therapy postulates that mental health problems are the product of a person being unable to satisfy the basic needs they value. The process of reality therapy involves establishing non-coercive and non-judgmental relationships, encouraging the client to take responsibility for behavior, and implementing behavior change to satisfy the basic needs a client values.

In contrast to many therapeutic approaches, reality therapy is surprisingly easy to understand. In the late 1980's, Robert Wubbolding (1988) developed the acronym WDEP to summarize the series of interventions that make up reality therapy. The W represents the process whereby the therapist establishes what basic needs the client 'Wants'. The D is a process in which the therapist explores what the client is 'Doing' to meet their needs. The E reflects a period of 'Evaluation' where the therapist assists the client in evaluating their commitment to change. The final intervention is P, this is where the therapist and client develop a 'Plan' to help the client meet their 'Wants'. So, reality therapy provides the client with a plan, as well as creating a satisfying client-counsellor relationship, that – in many cases – leads to an increase in self-esteem.

In sum, reality therapy is a useful theoretical approach for treating individuals who suffer from low self-esteem. Using principles from choice theory, school guidance counsellors can establish the basic needs a student desires (i.e., 'Wants'), and subsequently, can use this information to elicit behavioral change to help meet the student's desires, which consequently promotes the student's self-esteem. However, from the perspective of a social psychologist, reality therapy lacks a solid theory-driven approach to help school guidance counsellors build effective relationships with clients. Currently, the directions given to counsellors (e.g., "structure the relationship") are limited, ambiguous, and lack a theoretical basis. In response to this issue, this chapter will now review social identity approach, a pioneering theory from the field of social psychology that can help therapists build effective counsellor-client relationships.

Social Identity Approach

Social identity theory (Tajfel & Turner, 1979) and self-categorization theory (Turner, 1985; Turner, Hogg, Oakes, Reicher, & Wetherell, 1987) are together known as social identity approach. According to social identity approach, behavior is driven by both individual thoughts, feelings, and actions (i.e., as "I" in terms of personal identity) and through a sense of social identity (i.e., as "we" in terms of group membership). Scholars argue that social identity forms the basis of all group-based behavior. Indeed, when an individual classifies a co-present other as sharing their social identity (e.g., 'we both belong to this group') several transformations occur. Initially, there is a process of cognitive transformation, this is where an individual assumes they and the co-present other share the same beliefs and values (Haslam, Oakes, Reynolds, & Turner, 1999; Haslam & Reicher, 2012; Turner, Oakes, Haslam, & McGarty, 1994). Subsequently, a process called 'relational transformation' occurs, whereby the collective feeling of "us" leads to an improvement in social relations. Indeed, experimental research has shown that shared social identity facilitates trust, respect, communication, and comfort between individuals (Greenaway, Wright, Willingham, Reynolds, & Haslam, 2015; Novelli, Drury, & Reicher, 2010; Renger & Simon, 2011; Tyler & Blader, 2000).

Therefore, it is clear to see, social identity approach serves as an effective theoretical framework for building the counsellor-client relationship. Initially, a client may view the client-counsellor relationship as "me and you"; however, using social identity approach, the counsellor can create a shared sense of social identity, making the client view the client-counsellor relationship as "us". Ultimately, the collective sense of "us" improves social relations, and thus, should help with the application of a therapeutic intervention.

The Intervention: Revised Reality Therapy

Given that current western-developed interventions for boosting self-esteem are proving to be ineffective in the Malaysian context (Othman & Abdullah, 2015), and the number of Malaysian students suffering from low self-esteem is set to increase, this chapter will propose a new innovative, easy-to-use intervention based on the principles of reality therapy and social identity approach.

The intervention, revised reality therapy, has been developed using the experiences of a Malaysian school guidance counsellor - who used the principles of social identity theory and reality therapy to help Malaysian students who suffer from low self-esteem. The intervention can be simplified into six "steps". The six steps are as follows: 1) establish shared social identity, 2) build mutual trust, 3) awareness of "total behavior", 4) WDEP formulation, 5) implement plan and support, and finally 6) persevere and seek help. The proposed intervention is summarized in Figure 1.

Moving forward, this chapter shall now discuss each stage of revised reality therapy. To help visualize the application of revised reality therapy, each stage will refer to the field notes of a Malaysian guidance counsellor[1], called JN, who used this revised reality therapy to help students suffering from low self-esteem.

Step 1: Establish Shared Social Identity

A critical component of any counselling process is the creation and maintenance of a non-threatening counsellor-client relationship (e.g., Wubbolding, 2015). Revised reality therapy is no exception to this rule; however, in contrast to other counselling approaches, it provides an empirically supported, theoretical framework to help counsellors form an effective counsellor-client relationship.

On the basis of social identity approach, revised reality therapy suggests that a shared sense of identity between a counsellor and client is the key determinant for an effective counselling relationship. A shared sense of social identity occurs when one perceives a co-present other (i.e., counsellor) as an ingroup member (i.e., "we both belong to the same social group"). For example, a shared sense of social identity would occur if the counsellor stated that they support the same football team as the client – thus making the client think "we are both supporters of this football team". Alternatively, a counsellor may wish to activate the salience of a wider social group, stating that they both like sports – making the client think "we are both interested in sports". This perception of shared social identity should facilitate a feeling of similarity, communication, trust, respect, and comfort between the client and counsellor (Greenaway et al., 2015; Hogg & Hardie, 1991; Novelli et al., 2010; Renger & Simon, 2011; Tyler & Blader, 2000). In

Figure 1. An intervention to help improve self-esteem in Malaysian secondary schools: revised reality therapy

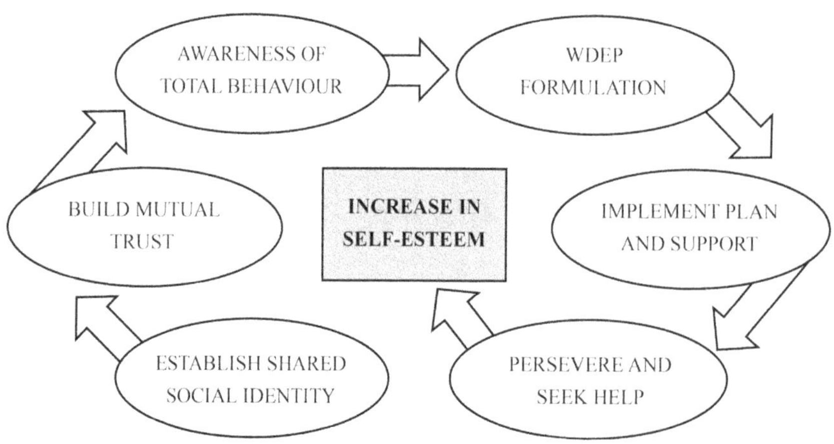

addition, this 'facilitating effect' can be strengthened by the counsellor making themselves more representative of the 'ingroup' they share with the client (e.g., Hogg & Hains, 1996). In summary, when a client perceives a counsellor as "belonging to my social group" a psychological process occurs which, ultimately, facilitates the formation of an effective counsellor-client relationship.

Moving on from the psychological processes that help form an effective counsellor-client relationship, it is also important to consider how a counsellor can create this feeling of shared identity. First, the counsellor must establish a social identity (i.e., social group membership) they share with the client. Second, the counsellor should choose how they wish to express this shared social identity – this could be done using physical cues (i.e., wearing the shirt of a sports team both the counsellor and client support), telling the client verbally that they are both members of the same group, or alternatively, the counsellor could inform the client they have shared experience of the same event (i.e., the counsellor could say they suffered from the affliction that is currently harming the client) (e.g., Drury, Cocking, & Reicher, 2009; Levine, Prosser, Evans & Reicher, 2005). As discussed, creating a sense of shared identity (i.e., "we both belong to the same social group") should help facilitate the counsellor-client relationship.

To help illustrate the application of Step 1 (i.e., establish shared social identity) this chapter will refer to the personal experience of a Malaysian school guidance counsellor, JN, who applied social identity approach to help establish a relationship with 12 boys who suffered from low self-esteem. The boys were referred to the counsellor after they received bad grades in a Malay language exam, which subsequently contributed to the boys experiencing low self-esteem. At the start of the revised reality theory session, JN (i.e., the counsellor) established a shared sense of social identity by referring to a shared experience:

JN[2]: In my experience, when I was once a high school student, I was forced to learn many different subjects that I disliked. When I studied in the last class during my Sixth Form, I was being teased at getting bad grades. The feeling of being teased was not a good feeling.

One of the 12 boys: Really? Is this true?

JN: Yes. I felt really bad, especially when my teachers compared me with other students from the front classes, without truly understand me first. It was really unfair.

JN retrospectively noted: All 12 boys stared with disbelief. I managed to capture the boys' attention and interest.

After JN established a shared sense of social identity, all 12 boys showed a willingness to cooperate and communicate – thus strengthening the counsellor-client relationship. Ultimately, establishing a shared social identity allowed JN to effectively implement revised reality therapy.

Step 2: Build Mutual Trust

Mutual trust is a crucial component of revised reality therapy. Here, 'mutual trust' is defined as the feeling of confidence a client has when in the presence of a counsellor, and vice-versa (Covey, 2006). Building on this definition, 'mutual trust' reflects a social context in which the counsellor has faith in their client's ability to learn and develop, and the client has confidence in the counsellor's ability to implement revised reality therapy. Often, when a client suffers from low self-esteem they are demotivated, for example, a client with low self-esteem may say "what's the point in trying to change. I will always be a failure". By creating this feeling of mutual trust, the counsellor motivates the client to improve, and ultimately, this facilitates the application of revised reality therapy.

To help build mutual trust, this chapter has developed a framework for building mutual trust (See Figure 2). Specifically, this framework shows how mutual trust can be achieved by focusing on four areas: 1) express care and encouragement; 2) express confidence in the client's ability to improve; 3) use vulnerability to connect; and 4) apply connecting habits (i.e., listening, supporting, encouraging, negotiating, respecting, accepting, and trusting) and avoid controlling habits (i.e., blaming, criticizing, complaining, nagging, rewarding to control, threatening, and punishing) for the duration of the counselling session (Glasser, 2000).

To help illustrate the application of Step 2 (i.e., build mutual trust) this chapter will refer to the experience of a school guidance counsellor, JN, who used the framework discussed to build mutual trust with a student suffering from low self-esteem. The student, referred to as G, suffered from low self-esteem. Initially, JN attempted to build mutual trust with G by expressing care and encouragement.

G: (quiet, kept his head down, staring on the desk)

JN: (with a smile) Hi, what do you want to talk about?

G: (kept his head down, quiet).

The silence went about 10 minutes. Then JN dismissed G.

JN: (requested to meet G's class monitor).

G's class monitor: G is very quiet in class, plays badminton during Physical Education, likes to draw comics, and plays online computer games with a few other boys.

Figure 2. Framework for building mutual trust

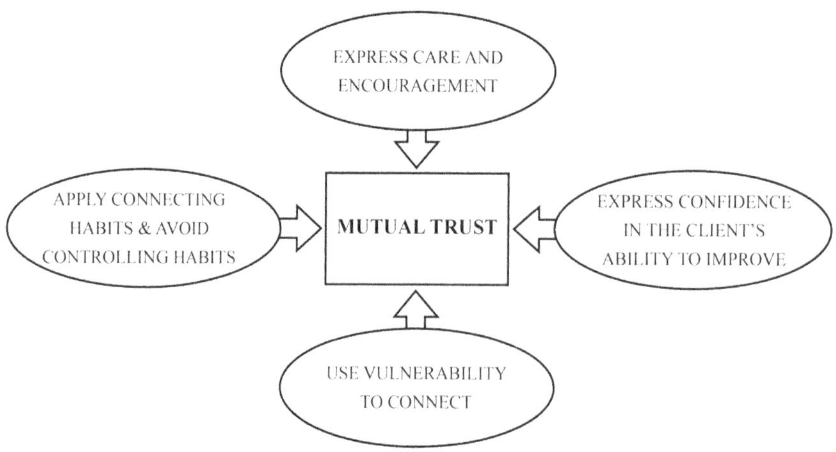

JN: (thanked the class monitor) I really hope to help G to improve in his studies.

G's class monitor: I will pass that message to G.

One week later, JN met G for a second session. JN, aware that G previously showed mistrust and was demotivated to engage in the counselling process, continued to build mutual trust by expressing confidence in G's ability to improve:

JN: I want to know you better. I need to communicate with you, to know your thoughts. I have met your class monitor, and he said that you like to draw. Can you draw something for me?

G: (took the pencil and paper and wrote in Chinese) I don't want to be in here.

JN: Do you know why you are in this room with me?

G: (wrote on the paper) I am stupid.

JN: I don't think you are stupid. Let me ask you a question. If a person gets sick, where will that person go?

G: (wrote on the paper) Doctor.

JN: If the doctor cannot help that person, because that person's sickness is very bad, no cure at all, what will that person become?

G: (wrote on the paper) Die.

JN: So, if the doctor thinks that person is very sick, and no cure, that doctor will send that person back and let that person die. On the other hand, if the doctor thinks that person is able to recover from the sickness, the doctor will continue to give treatment to that person. Am I correct?

G: (nodded head softly)

JN: The school sends you here, to meet me, in my room. This means you are able to recover, to bounce back from your failures in your academic subjects. If the school thinks you cannot be helped, then the school will send you home. You get my point?

G: (looked up for the first time): You think I can be helped?

JN: Don't worry. I believe that you can be helped, and I am here to help you.

Using the framework outlined in step two (See Figure 2) JN was able to communicate with G, expressing that he believed G had the potential to improve. This marked the start of G trusting JN. What follows next is JN's attempt to further develop mutual trust, JN did this by expressing shared vulnerabilities with G:

G: I always procrastinate, especially on the homework that I find difficult. I am very bad, but you still believe that I can improve. I don't think I can improve.

JN: I sense that you are very brave to be honest with me on this.

G: Brave?

JN: Yes, it takes courage to admit one's weaknesses. Look, I procrastinate in marking these exercise books too, as I dislike marking essays.

G: Teacher, you procrastinate too?

JN: Yes, I think a lot of us procrastinate, especially on the tasks that we dislike.

G: So, teacher, you won't mark? Because in the end, I won't do those homework.

JN: In the end, I still have to mark those essays, as this is my responsibility. It's a matter of choice.

Finally, one can see that JN continuously - throughout the counselling sessions noted - used connecting habits (i.e., listening, supporting, encouraging, negotiating, respecting, accepting, and trusting) and simultaneously avoided controlling habits (i.e., blaming, criticizing, complaining, nagging, rewarding to control, threatening, and punishing) while counselling G.

In short, Step 2 can be achieved by referring to the building mutual trust framework, which posits that mutual trust can be achieved by focusing on four areas: 1) express care and encouragement; 2) express confidence in the client's ability to improve; 3) use shared vulnerability to connect; and finally, 4) apply connecting habits and avoid controlling habits for the duration of the counselling session. Ultimately, establishing this sense of mutual trust motivates the client to believe they can improve, and thus, facilitates the application of revised reality therapy.

Step 3: Awareness of Total Behavior

The principle of total behavior – which assumes all forms of behavior can be controlled by an individual – is crucial for the application of revised reality therapy. The principle of 'total behavior' states that behavior has four inseparable components: actions, thoughts, emotions, and physiology. Of these components, a person has direct control over the first two, actions and thoughts. For example, if a person performs an action (e.g., sits down and admires a picturesque view) and has positive thoughts (e.g., "what a beautiful day"), this will have an indirect influence on emotions (e.g., feeling of happiness, acceptance, pleasure), and naturally, the action itself will influence physiology (e.g., the persons heart rate will reduce) (Wubbolding, 2015). Thus, using the principle of total behavior, logic posits that one of the most direct ways of changing emotions (i.e., low self-esteem) is to change actions.

Typically, a person who suffers from low self-esteem does not appreciate the power of actions. For example, a student suffering from low self-esteem may not realize that changing their actions (i.e., revising effectively, preparing well for exams) can lead to a boost in self-esteem. Understanding this principle is vital to revised reality therapy. So, a counsellor must teach the client 'total behavior'. To do this, revised reality theory advises the use of an analogy. In what follows, four analogies will be presented, each varying in complexity:

- **The Car Analogy:** Glasser (2005) presented the car analogy as a method for describing total behavior to clients. Here, the front wheels of the car represent actions and thoughts; whereas, the back wheels represent emotions and physiology. The steering wheel reflects what a person 'Wants' from their external world. Thus, if a person wishes to turn the steering wheel (achieve their Wants), the front wheels (i.e., actions and thoughts) will need to turn first, and then finally, the back wheels (i.e., emotions and physiology) will follow the front wheels. In short, to achieve a person's wants, a person must first change the 'direction' of their actions and thoughts (i.e., the front wheels), and then emotions and physiology will follow (i.e., the back wheels). This analogy is a useful tool to help clients understand 'total behavior'. However, some people may struggle to understand this analogy - particularly young Malaysian students who don't understand the mechanisms of a car – so a counsellor may opt for an alternative analogy.
- **The Suitcase Analogy:** Developed by Wubbolding (2015b), this analogy describes total behavior using a suitcase. The handle of the suitcase reflects actions, and the suitcase itself contains thoughts, emotions, and physiology. So, when a person lifts the suitcase via its handle (i.e., actions) all components of behavior are lifted off the ground too. In short, actions (i.e., the handle of the suitcase) impact all aspects of behavior (i.e., the contents of the suitcase). This example is simpler than the car analogy, and a counsellor may even choose to use a real suitcase to demonstrate how lifting the suitcase via its handle (i.e., actions) will influence thoughts, emotions, and physiology (i.e., the contents of the suitcase).
- **The Captain America Analogy:** Developed by Ng and Jegathesan (in press), this analogy uses a scene from 'Captain America: The First Avenger' to describe total behavior. Initially, the counsellor should play the 'flag pole scene' from the film. In this scene, a sergeant says to his soldiers "that flag means you were only at the half way point. The first man to bring it to me gets a ride home with Agent Carter [...] nobody has got that flag in 17 years". In response, all the soldiers, except for Captain America, try and climb up the pole. In what follows, Captain America's behavior can be described in terms of total behavior – Captain America used thoughts (i.e., there must be a way) and actions (i.e., stood still, analyzed the problem, then lowered down the pole using a joint at the base of the pole) to achieve his goal (i.e., to get the flag), and subsequently, experienced a change in emotions (i.e., feeling confident and happy). This analogy has three benefits: (1) it uses a video to describe total behavior, meaning the effectiveness of the analogy isn't dependent on the clients ability to imagine; (2) Captain America is a role model for many young adolescents, meaning this analogy should be more engaging than the ones discussed so far; and finally (3) its shows how two different actions created two opposing emotional outcomes, Captain America felt confident and happy, whereas the other soldiers – who didn't use their thoughts and actions with tact – felt annoyed and disappointed.
- **The Bread Analogy:** Developed by Ng and Jegathesan (in press), this analogy uses a piece of bread to describe total behavior. Initially, the counsellor would pass the client a piece of bread and say, "please feel free to eat the bread". Then, the counsellor would use the way the student went about eating the bread to describe total behavior. Initially, the client uses thoughts (i.e., deciding how to eat the bread, or deciding not to eat the bread) and actions (i.e., eating the bread, or not),

and consequently, the client will experience changes in physiology (i.e., their mouth is full, or their mouth is empty) and emotions (i.e., now they are happier because they feel less hungry, or they feel nothing as they did not eat the bread). Thus, the counsellor can use this analogy to demonstrate how different actions (i.e., eating the bread) can elicit different emotions. Further still, a counsellor may choose to use sweets or chocolate as an alternative to bread.

It is imperative that the counsellor teaches the client about the principles of total behavior. This can be done using the analogies discussed: the car analogy, the suitcase analogy, the Captain America analogy, or alternatively, the bread analogy. Once the client understands total behavior, they will realize that changing their actions is an effective way of improving self-esteem. As previously mentioned, knowledge of the importance of actions is vital for the application of the next stage of reality therapy – where client and counsellor will complete WDEP formulation.

Step 4: WDEP Formulation

WDEP formulation is a key step in revised reality therapy. As previously discussed, low self-esteem is caused by the external world failing to satisfy a person's desires. WDEP formulation aims to resolve this discrepancy by creating a plan to help clients change their behaviors and actions, which ultimately should lead clients to achieve their desires and experience an increase in self-esteem (Wubbolding, 2015).

WDEP formation is a four-stage process: first, a counsellor establishes what client 'Wants' from their external world; second, a counsellor reviews what the client is currently 'Doing' to help them fulfil their wants; third, the counsellor 'Evaluates' what is hindering and helping the client in their attempts to achieve what they 'Want'; and finally, fourth, the counsellor helps the client create a 'Plan' to change the client's behavior and actions, which ultimately, should lead the client to get what they 'Want' from the external world. In short, WDEP formation leaves the client with an achievable 'Plan' which, if followed, should help boost self-esteem.

Traditionally, counsellors would complete WDEP formation verbally. However, revised reality therapy recommends the use of a specialized WDEP Form (See Appendix, Figure 3). Specifically, the WDEP Form is a one-page document containing boxes corresponding to the four-stages of the WDEP process. The counsellor and client work through the WDEP Form together, following the steps of WDEP formulation. The WDEP Form has two key benefits over the traditional verbal approach: (1) it acts as an effective method for carrying out WDEP formulation, and (2) it can be used as a record of the WDEP process in future counselling sessions.

To help illustrate the application of Step 4 (i.e., WDEP formulation) this chapter will refer to a Malaysian guidance counsellor, JN, conducting WDEP formulation with a student. The student, called H, was bullied extensively after failing several school subjects (English, Malay language, Mathematics, and Science), and as a result, developed low self-esteem. What follows is JN conducting WDEP formulation with H:

JN: (took out H's WDEP form) So, from this form, I notice that you are very clear of your 'Wants' (H had noted: obtain an O-Level certificate and then get a good job), and you have listed down all your 'Doing' to achieve your 'Wants'. Can we discuss more on the 'Evaluations' section?

H: Okay.

JN: In evaluating what you are currently 'Doing', classes in school and tuition classes help you to achieve your 'Wants'. Am I correct?

H: Yes.

JN: So, what is not helping? What is hindering you in achieving your 'Wants'?

H: I don't know.

JN: Hmm, do you revise at home?

H: A bit.

JN: Why only a bit.

H: I don't know.

JN: So, what happens at home? Is it that, you have seven siblings, right? Are they too noisy that you cannot revise at home? Or, you need to take care of them, and hence you cannot revise?

H: My mum will take care of them. They are noisy, but I can study upstairs.

JN: I am hearing that at home, you can study upstairs, but you only study a bit.

H: Yes.

JN: Do you mind telling me why?

H: I am scared and sad at home. I cannot study.

JN: Can you tell me more?

H: Dad argues with mum because of not enough money. Then he will beat her. I hear all their arguments and do nothing. I can only do nothing.

JN: How often does this happen?

H: Every night, after dad comes back from work.

With reference to the example above, JN established what H 'Wants' (i.e., to get good academic grades), what H is doing to achieve these 'Wants' (i.e., being attentive in class, attending tuition classes, and attempting to revise at home), and crucially, JN helped 'Evaluate' the factors that are hindering H's attempts to achieve his 'Wants' (i.e., family dysfunction at home). In what follows, JN suggested a 'Plan' to help H achieve his goals:

JN: Looking at your family's situation, what actually do you really 'Want'?

H: To get the O-Level certificate, get a job, and help provide for my family.

JN: Good. So, we will first focus on getting the O-Level certificate. Attending classes in school and tuition classes after school, is helping you towards achieving this goal. Staying at home every night is hindering your attempts to achieve this goal, because you cannot study at home. And looking at your trial exams grades, you really need to have extra revision, so that you can pass these subjects and get the certificate. Am I correct?

H: Yes.

JN: So, I am thinking, if you stay with one of your friends, do you think you can do more revision?

H: I have never thought of this, but I think I can.

JN: Is it okay for you to temporarily be away from your current house, with your parents' permission, get help from a friend on your studies, and focus more on your grades?

H: Yes. I would love to. I mean, I love my family, but I dislike my parents arguing, if you get what I mean.

Here, JN used WDEP formulation to help create a 'Plan' that will eventually boost H's self-esteem. In short, JN helped clarify H's 'Wants' (i.e., to get good grades), and ultimately, this led to the creation of a 'Plan' to help H achieve these 'Wants' (i.e., stay with a friend so H can revise). So, it is clear to see, WDEP formulation is a useful process which – when followed properly – provides the client with a 'Plan' to help boost self-esteem.

Step 5: Implement Plan and Support

Following on from WDEP formulation, the counsellor must help the client implement the proposed 'Plan'. To do this, revised reality therapy emphasizes the importance of the counsellor executing two steps: (1) stress the importance of the client raising any issues experienced during the implementation of the 'Plan'; and (2) regardless of the client's progress, arrange regular progress meetings. Thus, it is clear to see, this step requires the client to take on a degree of responsibility – as the client is now responsible for raising any issues experienced. Should the client raise any issues during this period, the counsellor should review the proposed 'Plan' and establish solutions to any problems raised.

To help illustrate the application of Step 5 (i.e., implement plan and support), let's refer to the example used in Step 4. Now, JN has met with H one-week after the implementation of the 'Plan' created during WDEP formation (i.e., H had been staying in his friend's house for a week). Below is a conversation between JN and H:

H: Teacher, I realized one problem when staying in my friend's house. My friend's house has iPad and internet access. I spent quite an amount of time watching YouTube video clips. It was really enjoyable at first. But after that, I started to feel guilty.

JN: Do share more about you feeling guilty.

H: I mean, I know I should study.

JN: I am glad that you have this awareness. I believe that you know that you need to take responsibility in all your actions, and all your actions will lead to specific consequences. So, with you spending time on iPad and not revision, are you aware of the consequences?

H: Yes.

JN: So, I sense that you have identified spending time on iPad as hindering you to achieve your goal in getting your O-Level certificate, am I correct?

H: Yes.

JN: So, what is your 'Plan' to overcome this?

H: Self-control?

JN: Yup. Have you heard of delayed gratification?

H: Erm, nope.

JN: Delayed gratification, for example, revise a certain amount of topic, or complete a certain amount of pages on past-year exam questions, only then you can use the iPad to watch YouTube video clips for a certain amount of time.

H: That sounds like a good idea.

JN: Remember, life is a process of learning. As we are aware of actions that are hindering us to achieve our goals, we stop, reflect, and change. We always learn from our past mistakes. The main point is constant improvement.

H: Thank you teacher.

JN: All the best to you.

This step sees a gradual shift occur in the counselling process, where the client takes responsibility for raising issues experienced during the implementation of the 'Plan'. When presented with any problems, the counsellor should support the client, and offer solutions to help the client execute their 'Plan'. This step should not be viewed as a linear process, as the counsellor may need to provide support to their client on many occasions. Therefore, this step should be an ongoing process until the client has become confident enough to seek help from other sources.

Step 6: Persevere and Seek Help

A growing theme in the latter steps of revised reality therapy is the client taking on more responsibility. Indeed, Step 5 saw the client take control of raising any issues they encounter during the implementation of the 'Plan' created in WDEP formation. The final step builds on this, with the client being responsible for 'seeking help from others' and 'persevering'.

The process of 'seeking help from others' reflects an important stage of revised reality therapy, as the client is now empowered to make behavioral changes that will help them achieve their 'Wants'. At this stage the client knows the principles of WDEP formation, meaning they should be able to identity individuals who can help them achieve their goals. For example, again referring to the experiences of the counsellor JN, emphasizing the importance of 'seeking help from others' made a client – whose 'Wants' concerned academic achievement - actively approach a math teacher for help with revision.

In addition, the counsellor must also stress the importance of 'perseverance'. Here, revised reality therapy defines perseverance as: continuing to implement the 'Plan' despite experiencing trouble or delay in achieving what the client 'Wants' from the external world. In many contexts, particularly in Malaysian secondary schools, achieving 'Wants' (e.g., achieving good academic grades) takes time. Thus, perseverance with the revised reality therapy is crucial.

Ultimately, 'perseverance' and 'seeking help from others' helps the client achieve what they 'Want' from the external world, and this will lead the client to experience an increase in self-esteem.

REVISED REALITY THERAPY: DOES IT WORK?

Thus far, this chapter has presented the theoretical basis and application of revised reality therapy. But, now you may ask one important question, is revised reality therapy going to be effective in boosting self-esteem in Malaysian schools?

As previously discussed, revised reality therapy is based upon reality therapy. To date, a body of empirical evidence has shown that reality therapy is a useful intervention for improving self-esteem. Indeed, a meta-analysis found that individuals who received reality therapy experienced an increase in self-esteem, which led the authors to conclude reality therapy is "effective for improving self-esteem" (Kim & Hwang, 2006, p.29). Furthermore, several studies have found consistent results, noting increases in self-esteem after individuals received reality therapy (e.g., Jusoh, Mahmud, & Ishak, 2008; Loyd, 2005). However, due to the changes made to the application of reality theory, the present chapter cannot generalize these findings to the new intervention – revised reality therapy.

To date, only one item of research has explored the effectiveness of revised reality therapy. The study, a long-term qualitative study conducted by Ng (2015), followed seven Malaysian Chinese students who received revised reality therapy. Initially, all students had failed in their academic studies, and as a result, developed low self-esteem. In response to this, all seven students were given revised reality therapy. After receiving revised reality therapy, all seven students made changes in their actions, and as a result, achieved what they wanted from their academic studies and reported an increase in self-esteem.

Together, then, literature suggests that revised reality therapy could be a useful tool for improving Malaysian students' self-esteem. However, in truth, only one qualitative research study has been conducted on revised reality therapy. So, as is often the case in academia, now psychologists and counsellors must take steps towards empirically validating the use of revised reality therapy for boosting self-esteem.

CONCLUSION

This chapter has proposed a new, innovative intervention that could help boost self-esteem. Revised reality therapy improves on its predecessor (i.e., reality therapy) in 3 crucial ways: 1) it uses contemporary social psychological theory to help counsellors build effective counsellor-client relationships; 2) it has been presented in a 'easy-to-use' six-step format; and finally, 3) it has been created and applied in the Malaysian context. In short, revised reality therapy could be a useful intervention for boosting self-esteem in Malaysian secondary schools.

Putting the proposed intervention aside, the focus of this chapter now turns to policy makers in Malaysia. All school guidance counsellors must be given a mandatory, validated, easy-to-use intervention to help improve self-esteem in Malaysian secondary schools; and such an intervention now exists – revised reality therapy. It is important to note that there is no 'silver bullet' to eradicate low self-esteem in Malaysian schools. However, the authors of the present chapter believe that revised reality theory, together with alternative interventions (e.g., Cognitive Behavioral Therapy), can be used by school guidance counsellors to help treat Malaysian students suffering from low self-esteem, and consequently, help Malaysian schools avoid an impending 'self-esteem crisis'. However – as mentioned earlier - before this intervention is used across Malaysia, empirical research should validate the proposed intervention. Only then can revised reality therapy be used to boost students' self-esteem across Malaysia.

In conclusion, this chapter has proposed a new intervention – revised reality therapy – that could be used to assist Malaysian students who suffer from low self-esteem. Unlike other interventions, revised reality therapy combines theory and practice to deliver a six-step therapeutic approach that can be applied to all Malaysian secondary schools. Now, counsellors have a tool that has been developed in the Malaysian context and could serve as an effective intervention to help treat low self-esteem. So, while you reflect on what this chapter has proposed, let's turn to Winston Churchill, former British Prime Minister, to summarize this chapter's efforts to address low self-esteem in Malaysian secondary schools "Now this is not the end. It is not even the beginning of the end. But it is, perhaps, the end of the beginning".

ACKNOWLEDGMENT

First, the authors would like to thank the editors, Prof. Anasuya Jegathevi Jegathesan and Dr. Siti Salina Abdullah, thank you for the opportunity to contribute to this book. In addition, the authors would also like to thank Dr. Ch'ng Xin Ying and Aaron Koh Boon Winn, who contributed to the proof reading of this chapter.

REFERENCES

Baumeister, R. F., Campbell, J. D., Krueger, J. I., & Vohs, K. D. (2003). Does high self-esteem cause better performance, interpersonal success, happiness, or healthier lifestyles? *Psychological Science in the Public Interest*, *4*(1), 1–44. doi:10.1111/1529-1006.01431 PMID:26151640

Covey, S. M. R. (2006). *The Speed of Trust: The one thing that changes everything*. London: Simon & Schuster UK Ltd.

Donnellan, M. B., Trzesniewski, K. H., & Robins, R. W. (2011). Self-esteem: Enduring issues and controversies. In T. Chamorro-Premuzic, S. von Stumm, & A. Furnham (Eds.), *The Wiley-Blackwell handbook of individual differences* (pp. 718–746). Chichester, UK: Wiley-Blackwell.

Donnellan, M. B., Trzesniewski, K. H., Robins, R. W., Moffitt, T. E., & Caspi, A. (2005). Low self-esteem is related to aggression, antisocial behavior, and delinquency. *Psychological Science*, *16*(4), 328–335. doi:10.1111/j.0956-7976.2005.01535.x PMID:15828981

Drury, J., Cocking, C., & Reicher, S. (2009). Everyone for themselves? A comparative study of crowd solidarity among emergency survivors. *British Journal of Social Psychology*, *48*(3), 487–506. doi:10.1348/014466608X357893 PMID:18789185

Glasser, W. (1998). *Choice theory: a new psychology of personal freedom*. New York: Harper Perennial.

Glasser, W. (2000). *Every student can succeed*. Chula Vista: Black Forest Press.

Glasser, W. (2005). *How the brain works chart*. Tempe: The William Glasser Institute.

Greenaway, K. H., Wright, R. G., Willingham, J., Reynolds, K. J., & Haslam, S. A. (2015). Shared identity is key to effective communication. *Personality and Social Psychology Bulletin*, *41*(2), 171–182. doi:10.1177/0146167214559709 PMID:25416042

Haslam, S. A. (2001). *Psychology in organizations: The social identity approach*. London: Sage.

Haslam, S. A., Oakes, P. J., Reynolds, K. J., & Turner, J. C. (1999). Social identity salience and the emergence of stereotype consensus. *Personality and Social Psychology Bulletin*, *25*(7), 809–818. doi:10.1177/0146167299025007004

Haslam, S. A., & Reicher, S. D. (2012). When prisoners take over the prison a social psychology of resistance. *Personality and Social Psychology Review*, *16*(2), 154–179. doi:10.1177/1088868311419864 PMID:21885855

Hogg, M. A., & Hains, S. C. (1996). Intergroup Relations and Group Solidarity. *Journal of Personality and Social Psychology*, *70*(2), 295–309. doi:10.1037/0022-3514.70.2.295

Hogg, M. A., & Hardie, E. A. (1991). Social Attraction, Personal Attraction, and Self-Categorization-, A Field Study. *Personality and Social Psychology Bulletin*, *17*(2), 175–180. doi:10.1177/014616729101700209

Judge, T. A., & Bono, J. E. (2001). Relationship of core self-evaluations traits—self-esteem, generalized self-efficacy, locus of control, and emotional stability—with job satisfaction and job performance: A meta-analysis. *The Journal of Applied Psychology*, *86*(1), 80–92. doi:10.1037/0021-9010.86.1.80 PMID:11302235

Jusoh, A. J., Mahmud, Z., & Ishak, N. M. (2008). The patterns of reality therapy usage among Malaysian counselors. *International Journal of Reality Therapy*, *28*, 5–14.

Kim, R. I., & Hwang, M. (2006). A meta-analysis of reality therapy and choice theory group programs for self-esteem and locus of control in Korea. *International Journal of Choice Theory*, *1*, 25–30.

Levine, M., Prosser, A., Evans, D., & Reicher, S. (2005). Identity and emergency intervention: How social group membership and inclusiveness of group boundaries shape helping behavior. *Personality and Social Psychology Bulletin*, *31*(4), 443–453. doi:10.1177/0146167204271651 PMID:15743980

Low, S. K., Kok, J. K., & Lee, M. N. (2013). A holistic approach to school-based counselling and guidance services in Malaysia. *School Psychology International*, *34*(2), 190–201. doi:10.1177/0143034312453398

Loyd, B. D. (2005). The Effects of Reality Therapy/Choice Theory Principles on High School Students' Perception of Needs Satisfaction And Behavioral Change. *International Journal of Reality Therapy*, *25*, 5–9.

Marsh, H. W., & Craven, R. G. (2006). Reciprocal effects of self-concept and performance from a multidimensional perspective: Beyond seductive pleasure and unidimensional perspectives. *Perspectives on Psychological Science*, *1*(2), 133–163. doi:10.1111/j.1745-6916.2006.00010.x PMID:26151468

Ng, J. H. (2015). *Lived Experiences of Chinese Adolescents Who From Failing In Their Academic Studies Journey into Passing Grades*. unpublished master's thesis, HELP University.

Ng, J. H., & Jegathesan, A. J. (in press). Malaysian Chinese youths: Learning CTRT is fun and impactful! *International Journal of Choice Theory and Reality Therapy.*

Novelli, D., Drury, J., & Reicher, S. (2010). Come together: Two studies concerning the impact of group relations on personal space. *British Journal of Social Psychology*, *49*(2), 223–236. doi:10.1348/014466609X449377 PMID:19523278

Othman, A., & Abdullah, S. S. (2015). Counselling in Malaysia: Trends and Practice with the Malays. *International Journal of Business and Applied Social Science*, *1*, 1–10.

Renger, D., & Simon, B. (2011). Social recognition as an equal: The role of equality-based respect in group life. *European Journal of Social Psychology*, *41*(4), 501–507. doi:10.1002/ejsp.814

Sorensen, M. (2018). What is Low Self-Esteem? *The Self-Esteem Institute.* Retrieved from http://getesteem.com/about/

Sowislo, J. F., & Orth, U. (2013). Does low self-esteem predict depression and anxiety? A meta-analysis of longitudinal studies. *Psychological Bulletin*, *139*(1), 213–240. doi:10.1037/a0028931 PMID:22730921

Steiger, A. E., Allemand, M., Robins, R. W., & Fend, H. A. (2014). Low and decreasing self-esteem during adolescence predict adult depression two decades later. *Journal of Personality and Social Psychology*, *106*(2), 325–338. doi:10.1037/a0035133 PMID:24467425

Tajfel, H., & Turner, J. C. (1979). An integrative theory of intergroup conflict. In W. G. Austin & S. Worchel (Eds.), *The social psychology of intergroup relations* (pp. 33–47). Monterey: Brooks/Cole.

The Sun Daily. (2016). *Mental health of Malaysian students worrisome*. Retrieved from http://www.thesundaily.my/news/1967970

Trzesniewski, K. H., Donnellan, M. B., Moffitt, T. E., Robins, R. W., Poulton, R., & Caspi, A. (2006). Low self-esteem during adolescence predicts poor health, criminal behavior, and limited economic prospects during adulthood. *Developmental Psychology*, *42*(2), 381–390. doi:10.1037/0012-1649.42.2.381 PMID:16569175

Turner, J. C. (1985). Social categorization and the self-concept: A cognitive theory of group behaviour. In E. J. Lawler (Ed.), *Advances in group processes*. Greenwich, US: JAI Press.

Turner, J. C., Hogg, M. A., Oakes, P. J., Reicher, S. D., & Wetherell, M. S. (1987). *Rediscovering the social group: A self-categorization theory*. Cambridge, US: Basil Blackwell.

Turner, J. C., Oakes, P. J., Haslam, S. A., & McGarty, C. (1994). Self and collective: Cognition and social context. *Personality and Social Psychology Bulletin*, *20*(5), 454–463. doi:10.1177/0146167294205002

Tyler, T. R., & Blader, S. L. (2000). *Cooperation in groups: Procedural justice, social identity, and behavioral engagement*. New York: Psychology Press.

Wubbolding, R. E. (1988). *Using reality therapy*. New York: Harper & Row.

Wubbolding, R. E. (2015). The voice of William Glasser: Accessing the continuing evolution of reality therapy. *Journal of Mental Health Counseling*, *37*(3), 189–205. doi:10.17744/mehc.37.3.01

Wubbolding, R. E. (2015b). *Reality therapy training manual. 16th revision*. Cincinnati: Center for Reality Therapy.

Yaacob, S. N., Juhari, R., Talib, M. A., & Uba, I. (2009). Loneliness, stress, self-esteem and depression among Malaysian adolescents. *Jurnal Kemanusiaan*, *7*, 85–95.

ENDNOTES

1. Trained in Choice Theory Reality Therapy (*William Glasser International*), and a registered counsellor in Malaysia since 2015.
2. The dialogues reported in the current chapter are directly translated from Mandarin into English.

APPENDIX

WDEP Form

Figure 3. WDPE form

<table>
<tr><td rowspan="5">Wants</td><td rowspan="5" colspan="2"></td><td>Love & Belonging</td></tr>
<tr><td>Power (achievement)</td></tr>
<tr><td>Survival</td></tr>
<tr><td>Freedom</td></tr>
<tr><td>Fun</td></tr>
<tr><td>Doing</td><td colspan="3"></td></tr>
<tr><td>Evaluation</td><td>What is helping?</td><td colspan="2">What is hindering?</td></tr>
<tr><td>Plan</td><td colspan="3"></td></tr>
</table>

Chapter 5
Filial Play Therapy Process of a Malaysian Parent

Diana-Lea Baranovich
University of Malaya, Malaysia

Cheng Chue Han
University of Malaya, Malaysia

ABSTRACT

In Malaysia, some parents leave the duties of child rearing to their domestic helpers. This can cause much trauma to a preschool child who has been raised by his domestic helper if the domestic helper leaves the family. The domestic helper was the primary caregiver of the child; hence, when the domestic helper leaves, the child feels that his "mother" has abandoned him. This in turn cause the child to respond via very negative acting out behaviors. This chapter presents a case study using filial play therapy as a therapeutic intervention for a pre-school child and his mother after the domestic helper left the family. This therapeutic process enhanced the bonding between the child and his mother. As a result of better bonding, the child's negative behaviors subsided.

INTRODUCTION

Great emphasis has been placed on the importance of being a multicultural counseling in the new millennium. A multicultural aware counselor is, in the context of psychotherapies, a type of therapy which takes into account both racial and ethnic diversities of the client, further taking into consideration their sexual orientation, spirituality, ability and any disabilities, social class and economics, and the potential for any cultural bias by the practitioner. The American Psychological Association (2017) defines multicultural counseling as counseling patients while taking into consideration their cultural believes and how that may affect their treatment. Multicultural counseling is especially important to Malaysian mental health practitioners because Malaysia is a multicultural country that comprises mostly of three main races: Malays (who account for more than 50% of the population), Chinese (who comprise of roughly 25% of the population), and Indians (around 10% of the population). Other ethnic groups do exist within the country as well such as people from Indigenous tribes and those of Eurasian decent (WorldAtlas, 2017).

DOI: 10.4018/978-1-5225-6073-9.ch005

One aspect of human development is universal is the attachment and bonding process between infants and children and their primary caregiver. As John Bowlby stated, "The bond that a child develops to the person who cares for his in his early years is the foundation for his future relationships. (Bowlby, 1979)

However, there are times when secure attachment between an infant and his mother is not created due to a myriad of reasons. One such reason here in Malaysia is when the mother, consciously or unconsciously relinquishes caregiver of the child to their live-in domestic helper. This in turn creates a situation whereby the domestic helper becomes the "mother" figure in the child's life and the birth mother becomes a secondary caregiver. Such a family dynamic becomes detrimental to the child when the caregiver leaves the family during the child's pre-school years. The child feels abandoned. This often leads to oppositional behaviors in the child. At this point not only is grief therapy needed for the child, but attachment therapy for the mother and child.

One form of child – parent attachment therapy that has proven to be successful in several countries with diverse populations is filial play therapy.

In 1964, Bernard Guerney formally introduced filial therapy to help children who experience behavioral and emotional issues. In filial therapy, parents are trained to be therapeutic agents by the therapist and have to engage in twice- weekly 20 minutes of non-directive play with the target child. Filial therapy has been tested as an effective method across various cultures, family structures, and presenting issues. Filial therapy is coined as the golden therapy by Cornett and Bratton (2015) simply for the reason that it has yielded an abundance of valuable and long lasting benefits for parents and children. From the psychological perspective, filial therapy is a therapy that emphasizes the connection between parent and child in term of emotion, behavior, and understanding. The tool of the filial therapy is playing. Play and children is a crucial combination. The child needs to play to help the growth and develop in a healthy situation. Children also use play to find solutions to problems. Play can be healing too in some cases that involve emotion and behavior issue. In addition, as an adult parent will understand how a child views the world by watching and joining in their play. Filial therapy also enhances parents parenting skill. Parents have the opportunity to learn special skills for the play sessions which these skills might be transferred to daily life practice. The main skills are structuring skills, emphatics skills, imaginative play skills, and limit setting skills. One might say that filial therapy will give benefit to both child and parent.

The effectiveness of filial therapy with a variety of populations was supported by researches, such as those with Hispanic parents (Sangganjanavanich, Cook, & Rangel-Gomez, 2010), African American parents (Solis, Meyers, & Varjas, 2004), Iranian single parents (Alivandi Vafa & Khaidzir Hj. Ismail, 2009), Jamaican parents (Edwards, Ladner, & White, 2007), foster children (Cornett & Bratton, 2014), married couples (Bavin-Hoffman, Jennings, & Landreth, 1996), and incarcerated fathers (Landreth & Lobaugh, 1998). With so much international success of the use of filial play therapy with families throughout the world, it is hypothesized that child-centered filial play therapy will be beneficial to children and families of Malaysia.

A one-shot single case study was recently conducted in Malaysia as a pilot study to gather information of the child – center filial play therapy experience with a Chinese- Malaysian five- year old boy and his mother and compare the experience to other filial therapy studies throughout the world.

Research Objectives

There were three research objectives explored in this study.

1. To explore the outcomes of using child-centered filial therapy as a counseling intervention with a five-year old boy experiencing behavior issues due to insecure attachment.
2. To explore and describe the experiences of the parent in the process of filial intervention.
3. To compare the outcome with the outcomes of other studies throughout the world.

Research Questions

1. Does child-centered filial play therapy help enhance the parent-child bonding and pro-social behavior of the five-year old boy.
2. What are the mother's experiences of the child-centered filial play therapy process.
3. How do the findings of this study compare to overseas studies.

LITERATURE REVIEW: FILIAL THERAPY IN INTERNATIONAL CONTEXT

Oftentimes, in therapy there is hesitation to adopt "Western" modalities in the "Eastern" setting as the questions of appropriateness and responsibility to be culturally sensitive needs to be addressed. In this section, the cultural sensitive issue of filial therapy in the Eastern context will be discussed to enhance the understanding of applying filial therapy in Malaysia.

Filial therapist is facilitative and educative in nature. He or she plays the role to educate and guide the learning process for parents instead of being viewed as expert and distant. This may be a more acceptable therapeutic intervention for families in Asia that generally have a collectivistic culture. The group learning in filial therapy also enables parents to feel supported by other parents and they received empowerment from each other (Sangganjanavanich et al., 2010). Although filial therapy was started from the Western setting, the nature of the therapy is collectivist and systemic. Hence, the practice of filial therapy in Malaysia is appropriate based on the collectivistic value shared amongst Malaysians.

Indeed, parenting training programs are not uncommon in Malaysia. The National Population and Family Development Board (NPFDB) under the ministry of Women, Family, and Community Development is the main government agency providing parenting education. In 1993, NPFDB first introduced the parenting module to develop happy families through parenting education. Later in 2008, to present, NPFDB had launched the KASIH Module that covers from pre-parenthood, fatherhood, parenting of young children, parenting of adolescents, to adolescent development (Ministry of Women, Family and Community Development, 2017). Furthermore, several other counseling center, private agencies, and NGOs have also been active in providing parenting training programs; for example: Focus on the Family Malaysia, Agape Counselling Center Malaysia, and Malaysian Pediatric Association (MPA). Thus, attending parenting training program is not strange amongst Malaysian parents.

Additionally, filial therapy is not problem-focused intervention to address children's behavioral problems, rather it emphasizes on building the relationship. The importance of family and kin-relationship is a universal phenomenon that is cross-cultural. The foundation of a good relationship is essential to mend any kind of problems and challenges in a family. Hence, filial therapy is meant for parents who want to enter their child's world and make a connection regardless of their races, cultures, religious believe and socioeconomic status. By focusing on building relationships rather than "problem fixing" we can attempt to avoid labeling the child as "problematic".

The existing research on cross-cultural filial therapy included populations of Chinese from Canada (Yuen, 1997), Chinese parents (Chau & Landreth, 1997), Indian parents (Raman & Singhal, 2015), and Korean parents (Lee, 2003). The results of these studies have been consistently positive which lead to the assumption of the current study – which most likely may yield positive results on the family in Malaysia. Guo (2005) even mentioned that filial therapy will be an assuring and practical treatment modality in China because it helps Chinese parents to be more sensitive and understanding towards their children. He reviewed filial therapy researches that involved ethnic groups and concluded that filial therapy is a culturally sensitive and effective treatment.

To date, there is no formal research being done at the context of Malaysia on filial therapy to the best knowledge of the researcher. It is highly expected that the parents and children will benefit from filial therapy given its past strong evidences across cultures and types of populations. Hence, the focus of the current study is targeted on the parent who is going to walk through the filial therapy process and reap the benefits from it.

METHODOLOGY

A single case study was chosen, as the research methodology is consistent with the focus and objectives of this study. A case study is an in-depth description and analysis of a bounded system (Merriam, 2009 p.40). The bounded system in this study refers to the journey of a parent going through the process of filial therapy. The phenomenon of how a parent is responding to filial therapy is also the central tenet and unit of analysis in the study. Thus, the case study is deemed to be the most relevant research methodology for the study due to the epistemological assumption that the experiences are rooted in context (Merriam, 2009). The proposed study employs a laser focus on the case within a bounded system in order to obtain thick and meaningful data of the phenomenon that is studied in this research.

Filial therapy is at its infancy stage in Malaysia, the exploratory nature of the research is most suitable to be approached through individual case basis. The thick description allows other researchers and practitioners to relate and inspire their current practice. Shields (2007) puts forth the following argument in favor of qualitative case studies:

The strength of qualitative approaches is that they account for and include differences – ideologically, epistemologically, methodologically – and most importantly, humanly. They do not attempt to eliminate what cannot be discounted. They do not simplify what cannot be simplified. Thus, it is precisely because case study includes paradoxes and acknowledges that there are no simple answers, that it can and should qualify as the gold standard (p. 13).

Participant Selection

The participants chosen for this study were a five- year old boy, and only child, and his mother, who is the primary caregiver. The boy and his mother were recommended for the study by a neighbor of the principal investigator. The child was well behaved for the first four and a half years of his life until the domestic helper, who was his primary caregiver, resigned and went back to her country of origin. At the time of the study, eight months had past and the child's behavior continued to be very oppositional. The participants met the criteria, which included a neuro-typical, pre-school child who was experiencing behavior issues and insecure attachment with his mother. Both the mother and child were interviewed separately and both the mother and son reported that because the mom works so much the child was raised by the family's domestic helper. On Sundays, the child is usually left with his maternal grandmother while his mother ran household errands and visited friends. The presenting behavior problems were throwing temper tantrums when he doesn't get his way, not following directions at school, talking back to the teacher and stealing from other classmates. The child's father is an international businessman and often travels overseas. Furthermore, at the time of this study neither the child nor the other family members were suffering any illnesses or had any special needs that would serve to be an extraneous variable to the study.

Before the start of the study it was recommended that the child engage in three months of grief therapy with a qualified child psychologist or counselor before beginning filial play therapy sessions as attachment therapy.

The child chooses the activity – there is no teaching or learning. The play is conducted on the same days at the same times and in the same space. The parent stays totally involved with he child. The only guideline is safety.

Data Collection Process

The mother carried out a total of 20 filial play sessions over a period of 10 weeks. Once every two weeks the researcher observed an entire play session and took notes on the interaction. The observation was followed by a one-hour consultation. During the consultation, the therapist provided constructive feed back to the parent. Skills that needed more practice were gone over and the parent could use this time to ask any questions. The child's behavior in general was also discussed.

Coding was used during each filial session that was observed. Also, the parent wrote process notes after each session. These notes consisted of what activities were played, what toys and materials were used and the mother's feelings about the interaction dynamics between herself and the child. Furthermore, the mother kept a diary about her daily interactions with and observations of her son's behavior, reports from the pre-school, and observations of her son playing with friends either at the house or on playgrounds. The purpose of these diary reflections is to track his behavior and whether or not there was improvement or setbacks throughout the 10-week period.

Pre-Session Training

The Filial Therapist conducted one, two– hour psycho-educational consultations to educate the child's mother on attachment theory and the importance of bonding. This was followed by five, one-hour training sessions over a period of three weeks to teach the mother the theory and techniques of Child – Centered Filial Play Therapy.

FINDINGS

Both the mother and child were very consistent throughout the filial play therapy training and sessions. The mother, for her part, seemed very dedicated to the process and following through correctly. During the first five sessions the mom had the most difficulties with not labeling toys and tacking. The child very much enjoyed the sessions and had difficulties stopping the sessions after 20 minutes. During the first consultation session, the filial therapist practiced tracking and referring to toys as this, that, these or those. Overall the child was well – behaved during sessions; however, it was reported that his behavior otherwise remained the same.

During sessions six through 10, the mother felt much more competent in implementing the techniques. The mother reported that she found herself speaking more positively to the child outside of the sessions and the child began to show some progress in his oppositional behaviors. During the consultation after the tenth session, the mother began to inquire how she could change aspects of her parenting to help her child. She reported that she is beginning to feel differently toward her son, less impatient and irritated with him. The mother chose on her own to not go out on weekends and spend more time with her child. The teacher reported that the child was less disruptive in class. He had not stolen anything in the past two weeks; however, he still had a tendency to not stay focused and follow directions.

During sessions 11 through 15, the mother was very confident in her ability to implement the techniques during the sessions. It was noted that the child appeared to take an interest in participating in the mother's activities such as helping her cook dinner by putting the carrots in the pot and setting the table for dinner. It was also reported that his temper tantrums subsided. The mother also added in 10-minute story times each night before the child went to bed. The mother also commented that she was enjoying playing at a child's level. The teachers reported that overall there was noticeable improvement with peer relationships; however, focus and attention is still lacking.

During sessions 16 through 20, the mother continued to incorporate techniques of child-centered filial play therapy. It was observed she was able to incorporate these methods more effortlessly and comfortably. The child chose to engage in watercolor painting during these four sessions. This is a new activity for the child. He experienced watercolor paints in his art class at school and really enjoyed this activity. His mother bought a set of watercolor paints for him. During the filial session that was observed, the child was imitating his teacher and teaching his mother how to properly use watercolors, such as rinsing the brush before using a different color. The child was very proud of himself. The consultation session was spent discussing ways to continue the process and make recommendations. The mother was keen on continuing the scheduled play sessions. The mother also commented on how her son had begun wanting to engage in more activities with his mother outside of special time, such as going to the park and the grocery store.

In referring to the research questions outlined for this study, based on observations of the filial play therapy sessions of the mother and child we can say that filial play therapy appears to have helped in promoting a bond between the child and his mother – a finding that matches those found from previous researches conducted. The mother also seemed to open up and enjoy the filial play therapy sessions and noted the positive changes she observed in her child. As noted by the mother. the child appeared to be less oppositional and teachers noted that acts of physical aggression displayed towards other children seemed to have declined. The mother also reported that her child was less domineering during play dates. In the past he would have a tendency to boss his friends around by saying what toys would be played with and how. The child is now being less domineering and allowing his friends to lead in games and activities. This is an indication of filial play therapy's ability to promote pro-social behavior.

Similar to previous studies conducted, the findings from this research indicate that filial play therapy is a therapy technique that is cross-cultural. While results of this study cannot be generalized across the

Malaysian population, the results would indicate that this therapy technique would find success with other children living in Malaysia, or Asian countries; such as the findings mentioned in the literature review where this technique was conducted on Asian populations that included Chinese, Indian and Korean (Yuen, 1997; Chau & Landreth, 1997; Raman & Singhal, 2015; and Lee, 2003).

Significance of the Findings

Based on the findings of this case study, the child – centered filial play therapy process helped the mother to feel more comfortable around her child. Hence, a more bonded relationship began to developed. This, in-turn, motivated the mother to spend more time with her child in addition to the sessions. As a result of an enhanced bond between the mother and child, the child's behaviors began to improve. In reference to this study, it cannot be said that the filial play therapy sessions alone enhanced the bonding between the mother and child, which in-turn helped the child's behavior; however, it can be said that the filial therapy sessions served to be a catalyst for the bonding process. As the mother began to feel comfortable relating to her child at his level, she herself began to feel more comfortable being with her child, which motivated her to spend even more quality time with her son. As a result of this quality time, the child began to feel more secure; hence his social behavior began to improve.

This single case study serves to promote awareness about filial play therapy to parents, counselors, psychologist and other mental health providers. Furthermore, it serves as a spring board for more in-depth empirical studies on filial play therapy.

CONCLUSION

One of the most important elements in Filial therapy is that the parent focuses exclusively on the child during the play period, and the sessions are led by the child. This situation may help the child exhibit his/her self-confidence in conducting the play. Another reason is that the filial play decreases the negative parent-child interaction and develops positive and harmonious parent-child interactions. Overall, filial therapy is one of the best therapeutic therapy techniques that can assist in helping children and their families overcome psychological issues.

Filial therapy is a form of therapy that works for various family cultures, structures and presenting issues. Over the course of five decades the literature and research on the topic has come out in support of the effectiveness of therapy in helping to enhance bonds and reduce occurrences of behavioral issues in children. The outcomes of the studies have resulted the expansion of filial therapy to various types of families. It is common to have outcome-oriented studies to test the efficacy of a therapy modality and thus process oriented researches may be overlooked. The importance of process study is to enhance the understanding of practitioner and researcher in the implementation of filial therapy. It is strongly believed that the Malaysian families will benefit from filial therapy as well as families in other Asian countries. Filial therapy is at its infancy stage in Malaysia, a case study enables researchers to obtain rich and thick data for exploratory purpose. Future studies stemming from this proposal will broaden the field of practical implementation of filial therapy.

REFERENCES

Alivandi Vafa & Ismail. (2009). Reaching Out to Single Parent Children through Filial Therapy. *Online Submission, 6*(2), 1–12. Retrieved from https://manowar.tamucc.edu/login?url=http://search.ebscohost.com/login.aspx?direct=true&db=eric&AN=ED504968&site=eds-live&scope=site&scope=cite

American Psychological Dictionary. (2017). Washington, DC: American Psychological Association.

Bavin-hoffman, R., Jennings, G., & Landreth, G. (1996). Filial Therapy: Parental Perceptions of the Process. *International Journal of Play Therapy*, *5*(5), 45–58. doi:10.1037/h0089109

Bowlby, J. (1979). *Seperation and anxiety*. London, UK: Routledge Classics.

Chau, I. Y., & Landreth, G. L. (1997). Filial therapy with Chinese parents: Effects on parental empathic interactions, parental acceptance of child and parental stress. *International Journal of Play Therapy*, *6*(2), 75–92. doi:10.1037/h0089409

Cornett, N., & Bratton, S. C. (2014). Examining the impact of child parent relationship therapy (CPRT) on family functioning. *Journal of Marital and Family Therapy*, *40*(3), 302–318. doi:10.1111/jmft.12014 PMID:24749890

Cornett, N., & Bratton, S. C. (2015). A Golden Intervention : 50 Years of Research on Filial Therapy. *International Journal of Play Therapy*, *24*(3), 119–133. doi:10.1037/a0039088

Edwards, N. A., Ladner, J., & White, J. (2007). Perceived effectiveness of filial therapy for a Jamaican mother: A qualitative case study. *International Journal of Play Therapy*, *16*(1), 36–53. doi:10.1037/1555-6824.16.1.36

Guo, Y. (2005a). Emotional Problems in Mainland China. *Journal of Child and Adolescent Psychiatric Nursing*, *18*(4), 171–180. doi:10.1111/j.1744-6171.2005.00028.x PMID:16236099

Guo, Y. (2005b). Filial Therapy for Children's Behavioral and Emotional Problems in Mainland China. *JCAPN Journal of Child and Adolescent Psychiatric Nursing JCAP Journal of Child and Adolescent Psychiatric Nursing*, *18*(4), 171–180. doi:10.1111/j.1744-6171.2005.00028.x PMID:16236099

Landreth, G. L., & Lobaugh, A. F. (1998). Filial therapy with incarcerated fathers: Effects on parental acceptance of child, parental stress, and child adjustmend. *Journal of Counseling and Development*, *76*(2), 157–165. doi:10.1002/j.1556-6676.1998.tb02388.x

Lee, M.-K., & Landreth, G. L. (2003). Filial therapy with immigrant Korean parents in the United States. *International Journal of Play Therapy*, *12*(2), 67–85. doi:10.1037/h0088879

Merriam, S. B. (2009). *Qualitative Research: A guide to design and interpretation*. San Francisco: Jossey-Bass.

Ministry of Women, Family, and Community Development. (2017). *KASIH package module*. Retrieved from http://www.lppkn.gov.my/index.php/en/family-development-services/168-pk0003.html

Raman, V., & Singhal, M. (2015). Play therapy with children: Its relevance and utility in the Indian context. *Journal of Indian Association for Child & Adolescent Mental Health*, *11*(2), 121–157.

Sangganjanavanich, V. F., Cook, K., & Rangel-Gomez, M. (2010). Filial therapy with monolingual Spanish-speaking mothers: A phenomenological study. *The Family Journal (Alexandria, Va.)*, *18*(2), 195–201. doi:10.1177/1066480710364320

Shields, C. M. (2007). *Can case studies achieve the "gold standard"? Or when methodology meets politics.* Paper presented at the Annual Meeting of the American Educational Research Association, Chicago, IL.

Solis, C. M., Meyers, J., & Varjas, K. M. (2004). A qualitative case study of the process and impact of filial therapy with an African American parent. *International Journal of Play Therapy*, *13*(2), 99–118. doi:10.1037/h0088892

World Atlas. (2017). *People of Malaysia*. Retrieved from, http://www.worldatlas.com/articles/ethnic-groups-of-malaysia.html

Yuen, T. C.-M. (1997). Filial therapy with immigrant Chinese parents in Canada. *Dissertation Abstracts International. A, The Humanities and Social Sciences*. Retrieved from http://search.ebscohost.com/login.aspx?direct=true&db=psyh&AN=1997-95017-304&site=ehost-live

Chapter 6
The Experience of Volunteers and Frontline Workers in Marginalized Communities Across Southeast Asia

Chuah Siew Mooi
HELP University, Malaysia

Ann Nicole Nunis
HELP University, Malaysia

ABSTRACT

This chapter focuses on the experience of volunteers and frontline workers who serve in marginalized communities across Southeast Asia. More frontline workers and volunteers are taking the initiative to support marginalized communities in the region. With the rise of human rights violations towards marginalized communities in the past decade, frontline workers and volunteers face unique experiences in working with these communities, ranging from stigma and discrimination to unaddressed levels of burnout. Based on the authors' experiences working with these communities and the summary of the interviews with fellow frontline workers, the experience of working with marginalized communities, particularly those affected by HIV/AIDS and refugees, are elaborated in this chapter. Current challenges as well as recommendations are highlighted to ensure that the frontline workers and volunteers are supported throughout their vital work towards society.

INTRODUCTION

In community service, frontline workers serve as the first point of contact and avenue of support for clients. Even though they are usually associated with healthcare workers and supporting physicians in a medical setting, the roles are changing to fit the current needs of the communities in the environment they live. Now, frontline workers are divided into a several categories – administrative support, community outreach or public health, physician-related care as well as mental health (Ross, Svajlenka,

DOI: 10.4018/978-1-5225-6073-9.ch006

& Wiliams, 2014; IntraHealth, 2016). However, the increased spread of social and health issues has encouraged organizations to create a new form of workforce which is the volunteer sector. Currently, millions of volunteers are engaging with communities on the ground to deliver healthcare, education and social protection services in areas with limited access to health and government support (Bansal, 2012).

Volunteers and primary frontline workers are currently recognized as vital components in the area of community service. Volunteerism and community work has been cited as the society's Third Sector which contributes to the growth of the nation. It is recognized as an important agent of democracy due to the diverse backgrounds of its volunteers and workers that transcends borders (United Nations Volunteers, 2015).Local support is a huge contribution to get communities involved in managing social issues and strengthening public health programs. With the reduction of international funding, grassroots NGOs and campaigns have included more volunteers as part of their workforce (Bansal, 2012).

It is acknowledged that volunteers and non- medical frontline workers contribute to increased organizational efficiency by handling the 'human' aspect of the work such as administrative duties, connecting with community leaders, and managing networks between communities (Randle & Dolnicar, 2012). Most of them are posted in areas impacted by poverty, famine, or war whereas others do focus on urbanized communities which have less visible issues such as child abuse, gender-based violence, and discrimination. This is based on the Millennium Developmental Goals (MDGs), a declaration signed by a total of 189 countries to eradicate poverty across the globe (Brassard, Sherraden, & Lough, 2010; MDG Achievement Fund, 2017). There are a total of eight goals in the declaration as of the year 2015 – the eradication of extreme poverty and hunger; universal primary education for all; gender equality and women empowerment; the reduction of child mortality rate; the improvement of maternal health; the work to combat HIV, AIDS, malaria and other diseases; environment sustainability and; the development of a global partnership (Jung, 2010; United Nations Development Programme, 2017).

However, frontline workers and volunteers aren't just labels or figures in an annual report. They are people. They are human beings with emotions and lives that have been enriched by the work that they do to serve those who are less fortunate. As both frontline workers and volunteers based in Malaysia, we were given the opportunity to experience what it was like to be on the ground with a few of the marginalized communities. Based on our combined experiences as well as interviews with our fellow colleagues in our line of work, this chapter highlights the characteristics and challenges that frontline workers and volunteers experience as they work with marginalized communities in Southeast Asia.

SOUTHEAST ASIA

Southeast Asia is a region well-known for its melting pot of cultures and diversity. With a population of roughly 600 million as of 2010, Southeast Asia is considered as one of the least populated regions in Asia with rapid urbanization and growing equality between genders and social statuses (Jones, 2013; CARE, 2014). Despite its smaller visibility in global politics, economics, and global health as compared to India and China, the region is currently undergoing rapid expansion, thanks to financial support from China (Hashim et al., 2012). Therefore, it is no surprise to know that the economic growth of Southeast Asia is a source of admiration and envy for other regions (Patel, 2017). However, seeing this region through rose-tinted glasses is deemed unwise by many. Since development has accelerated across the region in the past decades, this gives way to a raised awareness of the social issues that have plagued its citizens such as child abuse and racial violence that has displaced countless people to different areas.

The past few decades have witnessed this region being under scrutiny for various number of human rights violations. On November 2016 in Malaysia, Maria Chin Abdullah was detained under the draconian laws of the Sedition Act and the Security Offenses Special Measures Act for leading the Bersih protest – a peaceful call for electoral reform and transparency (Patel, 2017). Discrimination towards transgenders and men who have sex in men (MSM) in Malaysia is legalized in which any cross-dressing activities or anal sex can result in prosecution by the law. In Myanmar itself, the world witnessed the massacre of the Rohingya community in the northern Rakhine state which amounted to crimes against humanity (Patel, 2017). It is estimated that roughly 500,000 Rohingya refugees flee the affected state into neighbouring countries and the numbers continue to increase to this day (UNHCR, 2017). The callous response from the Myanmar government drew in a lot of flak from whistleblowers and human rights organizations globally (Patel, 2017). The region of the Philippines is also currently under the spotlight due to the drug war that was declared by the government since 2016. A total of 12,000 deaths were reported to date with the majority coming from urban poor areas (Human Rights Watch, 2017). This had caused a huge amount of backlash on an international scale, with several sources citing that the actions of the new Philippines government are equivalent to crimes against humanity as well (Patel, 2017).

Despite the current political environment which has spurred various human rights violations, non-governmental organizations (NGOs) in the Philippines, Malaysia, Cambodia, Vietnam and Indonesia have strived to address the issues related to poverty, education, gender equality, maternal health and transmittable diseases (Jung, 2010). Since the declaration of Millennium Developmental Goals (MDGs) in the year 2000, the Southeast Asian region has seen a spike on best practices in order to fulfil the goals based on the declaration. Jung (2010) noted that the local organizations did not have the capacity to engage in partnerships with larger and more established international NGOs. Yet, that did not stop them from initiating strategic partnerships with other local NGOs by dispersing information with each other, creating coalitions with NGOs that have similar values, attending conferences together and using the partnership as a catalyst for advocacy work (Jung, 2010). Examples of such coalitions include the Joint Action Group (JAG) for Gender Equality in Malaysia, Child Rights Coalition Asia (CRC Asia) in the Philippines, and the ISEAN-Hivos program in the region.

With the increase of awareness towards critical social issues in the region, volunteerism is needed now more than ever, especially participation from the local communities. Local volunteerism has benefitted the government and the communities by acting as a bridge between these two stakeholders (United Nations Volunteers, 2015). However, social work has been largely spearheaded by frontline workers for many years in Southeast Asia. This includes health workers, social workers, mental health professionals and other service providers to the community. Recently, the concept of a more formal involvement of volunteers is starting to develop in certain Southeast Asian countries such as Cambodia (Bansal, 2012). As people are more receptive to the idea of living cooperatively with marginalized communities, they are more willing to assist with community development and report to have an increased engagement with members of the communities (CARE, 2014).

WORKING WITH MARGINALIZED COMMUNITIES

In this section, we will describe the experiences and challenges faced when volunteers and frontline workers serve in marginalized and vulnerable communities across the region. Marginalized and/or vulnerable communities are comprised of groups of people which have limited access to resources and are exposed to high levels of violence due to their identity in the community. This includes groups such as sex workers, sexual minorities (LGBTQs), people living with HIV (PLHIV), people with disabilities and female migrants (rural women who moved into urban areas) (CARE, 2014).

Frontline workers and volunteers working in marginalized and vulnerable communities are usually comprised of healthcare professionals, social workers, and outreach workers. Due to the fluid nature of community service as stated in the previous section, frontline workers and volunteers are expected to wear different 'hats' in order to fill up the most needed roles. In order to provide a more holistic care, mental health practitioners are heavily involved with the mental wellbeing of the marginalized communities. Most practitioners also serve as frontline workers in which they are the first to respond to the needs of the members from the community. Based on our professional experience from working with LGBTQs, people living with HIV (PLHIV) and refugees, this section is divided into two parts – the experience of working with these communities and the experience of managing volunteers within the communities. This section is also a culmination of our observations of other frontline workers and volunteers working with two of the most marginalized and vulnerable communities in the region – key populations affected by HIV/AIDS and refugees.

Key Populations Affected by HIV and AIDS

There are roughly 1.7 million people living with HIV in Southeast Asia (ASEAN, 2016). Between the years 2010 to 2015, deaths related to AIDS have been declining across the region with the exception of Indonesia. However, the region has yet to achieve the 90-90-90 goal set by UNAIDS to eradicate AIDS by 2030 (Pendse, Gupta, Yu, & Sarkar, 2016). The term 'key affected population' is coined to describe "those who are most likely to be exposed to HIV or to transmit it, and whose engagement is critical to a successful response" (UNICEF, 2012, p. 11). Many of them are also vulnerable due to barriers in accessing healthcare services related to sexual health and HIV (UNICEF, 2012; AVERT, 2017). Most countries categorize key affected populations to include men-who-have-sex-with-men (MSM), people who inject drugs (PWID), sex workers, transgenders, women and children.

Currently, the growing epidemic and prevalence in the region is focused on two populations – men who have sex with men (MSM) and transgender (ASEAN, 2016). Although people who inject drugs (PWID) have the highest HIV prevalence among the other key affected populations, countries such as Indonesia, Myanmar, Thailand, and Malaysia have introduced harm reduction strategies which significantly impacted prevalence rates in this population (ASEAN, 2016). However, it is reported that the epidemic is still growing among men who have sex with men (MSM), transgender and people who inject drugs (PWID) as not many of them are aware of their own HIV status, thus preventing effective interventions to curb further infections (ASEAN, 2016).

However, not all is hope is lost. One of the greatest success stories on the region's efforts to manage the HIV epidemic was the consistent drop in HIV prevalence among female sex workers (FSW) (ASEAN, 2016). The consistent efforts in educating the population and providing contraceptives as well as free screening has paid off in the past couple of years (ASEAN, 2016). As for mother-to-child transmission of HIV, Thailand was the first country to fully eliminate it together with Syphilis in the region which is a testament of the effective collaboration between the government and community organizations in eliminating the epidemic (Sidibe & Singh, 2016).

In the public health industry, frontline workers and volunteers face interesting times as they reach out to the most vulnerable communities affected by the HIV/AIDS epidemic. One of them is the shift of the main mode of transmission of the disease. Recent years have revealed that sexual transmission has overtaken intravenous drug usage as the main mode of transmission for HIV. For example, in Malaysia and Thailand, roughly 90% of new HIV+ cases are caused by sexual transmission itself (AVERT, 2017). Since sex is more readily available as compared to intravenous drugs, it comes as no surprise that condom distribution alone would not be sufficient in preventing the spread of HIV. Thus, the focus has shifted to safer sex education, prevention through early detection particularly within the key affected populations.

Key Populations Affected by Migration and Persecution

Migration has always existed across the world but not since World War II has the world experienced the mass migration and displacement of people as it is at the current moment. Across the Asia and Pacific regions, there are 7.7 million people of concerns to the United Nations High Commissioner for Refugees (UNHCR) (UNHCR, 2017). This includes 3.5 million refugees, 1.9 million displaced persons and 1.4 million stateless persons. Currently, the majority of these numbers are made of individuals from Afghanistan and Myanmar. In Southeast Asia, a vast number of refugees live in urban city centres thus gaining the term urban refugees (Jones, 2017). This means that refugees in urban areas live their daily lives side by side with citizens and foreign nationals in apartments, markets, restaurants and public transportation, often blending into the crowd but for one major compromising factor; the lack of legal and valid identification documents. This makes them vulnerable to arrest, detention and even deportation.

Despite the vast numbers across Asia, there remains a vague stance by governments toward the growing refugee crisis. Under the Association of Southeast Asian Nations (ASEAN), refugees fall into the categorical definition of irregular migration, a title that includes economic and political migrants (Pitsuwan & Paramenwaran, 2015). Despite the ASEAN Head of States adopting the ASEAN Human Rights Declaration in 2012, which posits that an individual has the right to seek and receive asylum in another State in accordance with the laws of the respective State and signed international treaties, ASEAN members have failed to place asylum seeker issues as an urgent topic for discussion (Taylor, 2017). This is in the face of boats of asylum seekers being left adrift in the seas in (BBC, 2015) and mass migrant graves found north of the Malaysia-Thailand border in 2015 pointing to the human trafficking of peoples fleeing persecution (The Guardian, 2015). Thus it falls to organisations such as the UNHCR and other NGOs to fill the gaps of protection and living needs that go unmet by host counties in Southeast Asia (Jones, 2017).

The lack of legal status that most refugees living in Southeast Asia face compounds the ability of refugees to earn a living whilst awaiting a long term durable outcome. Refugees frequently work in informal work areas in what the United Nations High Commissioner of Refugees has classified as 3D jobs – dirty, dangerous, difficult (United Nations High Commissioner for Refugees, 2016). Working in these fields further compromises the safety of refugees, in particular female refugees who are frequently sexually harassed and exploited by their employers (Buscher & Heller, 2010). Yet, day to day, refugees work within their communities to help one another survive. This includes assisting community members in day to day activities including providing translation for community members unable to speak the local language, providing help in child care, assisting one another in the learning of a new language or in basic reading and writing.

Futhermore, the experiences of loss, violence, torture coupled with postmigration experiences of detention, discrimination and further economic hardships can lead an individual to experience stress and hopelessness which can further lead to suicide ideation and attempts (Vijayakumar, 2016). The combination of stress and trauma experienced throughout the journey of a refugee can also lead to the development of unhealthy coping habits such as alcohol and drug misuse, trafficking and domestic violence. Issues of pre-migration torture and trauma, intergenerational conflict, and adjustment difficulties in countries of resettlement including the exposure to substance are contributing factors of alcohol and other drug disorders (Posselt, Proctor, Galletly, de Crespigny, 2014). The experience of being a refugee can further increase poor living environment including poverty, homelessness, and criminal victimization (McCloskey, Southwick, 1996).

Profile of the Frontline Workers and Volunteers

The demographics of frontline workers and volunteers who choose to work with marginalized communities come from a variety of backgrounds. For example, due to the nature of refugee work where an individual's life is uprooted and placed in environment with little to no control over access to basic needs, frontline workers typically have some skill or training in legal, protection, or health backgrounds. Some are also equipped with background training in psychological support in order to provide immediate psychological support in situations of crisis or for ongoing treatment support of more serious mental health issues such as schizophrenia. All individuals who work with this population are usually trained on the country adopted policy framework in working with refugees and asylum seekers, the country and region wide issues as well as ethical boundaries and challenges that may arise in dealing with a population who typically have constricted mobility and access to basic needs.

A majority of the frontline workers dealing with the HIV and AIDS epidemic are from the healthcare or NGO industry. This includes doctors, nurses and anyone involved in direct care of the clients. Social workers, outreach workers and volunteers handle the pre-test procedures and post-diagnosis support such as peer counselling, group support, and social welfare. Depending on the country of service, frontline workers and volunteers who work directly with blood may require to undergo a series of medical tests to ensure that their HIV, TB and Hepatitis C status remains negative due to healthcare policies. However, this does not indicate that PLHIVs aren't allowed to contribute their efforts within the community as there are other categories of the workforce that do not require direct blood contact such as outreach work for pre- and post-diagnosis assistance. Everyone who works with key populations affected by HIV/AIDS are well versed with the medical information related to this disease as well as the policies practiced by their country of service which have a direct impact on the clients.

Frontline workers and volunteers working with marginalized communities tend to be familiar with providing service to a diverse range of clientele from various sociodemographic backgrounds. One example are individuals who identify themselves with more than two communities. A male client who has sex with men and also identifies as a person who injects drugs (PWID), carries a different level of risk as compared to a client who is a female sex worker. When these communities overlap, it is common to see frontline workers and volunteer cater to their needs by focusing on the differences while at the same time, addressing similarities among the communities such as the need for safer sex education. This can be further compounded if this client holds a refugee status which can complicate access to medical care and drug rehabilitation. In cases like this, it would be hard to focus on one aspect of the needs but rather would need the intervention of more than one organisation in order to provide sufficient assistance in meeting medical, protection and safety needs.

In the case of working with marginalized communities such as LGBTQs, most of the frontline workers and volunteers are from the key affected populations itself, especially those who are working outside of direct healthcare such as outreach workers, volunteers, case workers and social workers. Although there are no statements or legislations that prevent people from other communities to join this workforce, it is common to note the inclusive nature of the frontline workers and volunteers depending on the nature of the population that they serve in. For example, majority of the frontline workers and volunteers of NGOs that focus on HIV/AIDS prevention among the community of men who have sex with men (MSM) come from the same community itself. This is applicable to other populations as well such as transgenders, sex workers, people who inject drugs (PWID), and women or children affected by HIV/AIDS. However, the community is accepting towards help received from frontline workers and volunteers who have different statuses or identities as long as non-judgmental values are demonstrated in their line of work.

Usually, frontline workers and volunteers do not focus on HIV/AIDS prevention and post-diagnosis support alone. They also deal with other social issues that concurrently affect the population they serve in. LGBTQ issues and HIV/AIDS are usually associated with each other due to the fact that the two key populations affected by HIV/AIDS, namely men who have sex with men (MSM) and transgender (TG), are part of the LGBTQ umbrella. Issues on gender equality and domestic abuse are also highlighted within women and children who live with HIV. As for frontline workers and volunteers serving people who inject drugs (PWID), not only do they emphasize on harm reduction strategies such as needle exchange programs, they also cover on issues related to sexual transmission, HIV/AIDS prevention and drug rehabilitation.

In the case of refugees and asylum seekers, frontline workers and volunteers typically have to work towards assisting refugees to meet most of their basic needs. This is a population that typically arrives with little to no identification. Therefore, gaining identification through refugee community based organisations or through the UNHCR is one of the first priorities. However, frontline workers and volunteers can typically only assist with the registering of asylum seekers pending a refugee status determination process under the UNHCR. Further, refugees typically arrive with health concerns that may have existed prior to migration or that have been sustained during their journey. This includes beriberi, hypertension, and other infectious diseases such as tuberculosis, and chronic intestinal parasites. This coupled with violence, separation from family and other mental health impacts they may have experienced during the journey would mean that frontline workers and volunteers would need to work swiftly in addressing these issues so that it does not worsen over time. Thus, frontline workers and volunteers would have to work in not only preventing further health, protection and mental health issues but also in mitigating these factors from worsening through outreach, mobile clinics, community based interventions and psychoeducation.

It would seem that frontline workers and volunteers working with these communities are like utility knives – they have the equipped skills to handle specific issues when it is required of them. Most of them approach their clients in a holistic manner by addressing the need for support on psychological wellbeing as well as the clients' healthcare, protection and basic living needs. The diverse nature and culture of each of the key populations itself trains frontline workers and volunteers to adapt to many situations that require their attention due to the overlapping social issues that this community experiences on a constant basis. Despite the various background and statuses, those who work at the frontlines strive to provide the best quality of service for marginalized communities.

The Experience of Frontline Workers and Volunteers Working With Key Populations

Combating stigma and discrimination towards this community seems to be one of the goals for most frontline workers and volunteers in Southeast Asia. There are a several valid reasons for doing so. For one, there are legal repercussions identifying oneself as either a gay/bisexual man or a transgender with countries such as Malaysia, prohibiting actions associated with this community such as sexual practices and physical appearances. Likewise, providing services and support to refugees, particularly in countries that do not legally recognize refugees, can endanger an individual's safety as they may be liable to having their business or organisation shut down, fined or individuals held in remand for assisting a group of persons who are considered undocumented or illegal. When faced with such severe repercussions, it is common for individuals from these communities to delay seeking assistance or to conceal urgent medical or psychological issues. A person who has recently been diagnosed with HIV or who may have the beginnings of a contractible disease such as tuberculosis may hide and shun treatment from medical professionals. It also prevents help-seeking behaviour from these communities by disengaging with the frontline workers and volunteers who are actively on the ground to provide support. This form of isolation fuels a vicious cycle that can spiral the epidemic out of control. For example, an individual living with HIV who is untreated is more likely to spread the disease to others as compared to an individual living with HIV with complete adherence to treatment. Similarly, an individual with a refugee status, who would typically live in cramped living spaces alongside other adults and children, may inadvertently spread tuberculosis to other community members sharing a common living space.

Working on the frontline with at risk communities can bring volunteers and frontline workers face to face with individuals and circumstances that challenge their values and beliefs. In order to prevent the disengagement of working with at risk marginalized communities, frontline workers and volunteers are required to check on their own value systems so that they prevent themselves from stigmatizing their clients in the first place. Although it is common for HIV/AIDS organizations to employ frontline workers and volunteers from the key affected populations, not all members of the key affected population are suited to work directly with people living with HIV or HIV/AIDS prevention work due to internalized or externalized prejudices towards the disease or towards the community itself. Despite the medical advancement on antiretroviral therapy (ART) which allows patients to live a relatively normal life and subsidizes in medication provided by certain countries, there is still a lingering fear of getting infected due to implications towards employability, education, and even migration. In the same way, in the refugee service provision arena, migration is a heavily discussed topic riddled with strong political undertones which can impact opinion held by citizens and foreign nationals providing service. There also exists other political, religious and ethnic prejudice within the refugee community which can cause other challenges in service provision and cooperation with community members. Therefore, all frontline workers and volunteers are usually required to attend a desensitization training to learn the jargons used within the community and methods in providing accessible service using simple language. At the same time, they are also made aware of the different levels of stigmatization and prejudice experienced by the community and how they can avoid doing so to their clients.

The identities of frontline workers and volunteers themselves do play a role in combating stigma and discrimination in their line of work. This can assist in service provision and in building bridges between communities. In the case of key populations affected by HIV and AIDS, most of them come from the same population as the clients and therefore tend to have a high capacity to understand and empathize the double discrimination that most of the clients face. This is common among men who have sex with men (MSM) and transgenders (TG) living with HIV where their sexuality as well as their HIV status is seen as an anomaly to the common population. Frontline workers and volunteers who are from the refugee community can increase the capacity of prevention of more serious health and mental health issues within the community through outreach programs. Additionally, having frontline workers and volunteers who are able to speak more than one ethnic dialect would greatly improve in building bridges between communities and in increasing access to services due to ease of readily available translation services.

However, it is possible that frontline workers and volunteers may over identify with clients. Examples of this include cases where the frontline workers or volunteers are HIV+ themselves or have had similar experiences of being separated from families, having serious health issues or mental health challenges. Frontline workers or volunteers who hold a refugee status themselves are at particular risk of becoming enmeshed and blurring the lines with clients as they may share similar experiences in migration, violence and loss. While this can be an issue in objective and efficient service provision, at the same time, their identities and experiences are positive assets since the workers can use them to attune to their clients' needs through peer outreach programs and support groups. Therefore, frontline workers and volunteers living who strongly identify with clients arc required to walk a fine line between helping the client and getting too involved with the client's journey in which failing to do so can result in burnout.

It is also interesting to note that most frontline workers and volunteers in the HIV/AIDS industry do report a change of dynamics between their friends within the community and themselves once they identify themselves as part of the workforce in an HIV/AIDS organization. Most of them have developed a sense of responsibility to advocate harm-reducing behaviours to their circle such as the usage of protection during sex, regular HIV testing, and introduction of needle exchange programs or methadone maintenance therapy (MMT). Usually, this can result in mixed reactions from their social circles. They are seen either as a carrier of bad news or a source of accurate information. For example, a common response towards a HIV/AIDS worker providing information on HIV/AIDS in an Internet forum can range from ignoring the information, denying the information, or asking more about the accuracy of information.

This experience also extends to other forms of interaction within the workers' social circle as well. Since the LGBTQ community is rather small and inclusive, it is highly likely that they will know each other or bump into each other in community-friendly areas. This includes healthcare centres such as hospitals or clinics. So, imagine the surprise and shock of frontline workers and volunteers should they bump into their friends unexpectedly in a hospital known for treating HIV/AIDS patients. The shock goes both ways since they weren't expecting the friends to be diagnosed HIV+. For some, a sense of guilt exists when the knowledge that a member of their social circle gets infected with this disease since they feel that they should have tried harder in providing information and guidance. For others, they are able to adapt to a new form of boundaries which acts as a protective barrier that can assist them in remaining objective in the light of such news. In fact, it is most likely that they use their resources and contacts to assist their friends in getting the best option for treatment. The same situation exists within working with refugees as an official may shop or dine at a place where refugees are the floor workers. A refugee who is working as a translator that has to deliver the news of a rejected refugee status application may also experience guilt and helplessness in delivering this news and may even experience aggression or discrimination within their community. These are circumstances that can further entrench the power gap that lies between a citizen or foreign national who is in a power of authority above refugees who are undocumented and are not legally recognized. It can also evoke feelings of bitterness, anger and even community hostility in the latter case as it can be seen that the translator did not do enough to assist the case.

From our experiences working with this population as counsellors and testers, a certain degree of openness and non-judgment is required in order to combat the ingroup versus outgroup mentality which can rapidly form and create further barriers to service provision. For those from the heteronormative society, since we identify ourselves as part of the heteronormative group with a HIV- status, there is always a possibility that clients may view us as part of the main 'society' – the society that shuns and persecutes them for being different. Most frontline workers and volunteers who work with refugees are typically made up of citizens of a country or foreign nationals which can already produce a power distance between service provider and service user. Therefore, in order to create a safe space for the clients, the basic principles of counselling are intermingled with the knowledge of the community lingo to ensure that the clients feel heard. Other than being aware of the differences between our own gender identities, citizenship, biological sex, cultural background, political background and HIV statuses as well as the impact of the differences towards our clients, we were also exposed to information regarding sexual health as part of our role in the frontlines. Indeed it is also important to be aware how our own worldview and values are impacted by what media popularizes and what laws and policies are in place in the respective countries. Also as counsellors, part of our duty is to provide accurate information and the importance of doing so in this industry cannot be undermined.

Perhaps, one of the common denominators among frontline workers and volunteers working with marginalized communities is their determination to end discrimination and stigmatization of the communities they work with. With key populations affected by HIV/AIDS there is a determination to end the stigmatization towards people living with HIV as well as getting members of the population to adhere to treatment. At the same time, they want to halt the spread of the HIV/ AIDS epidemic within their communities by passionately advocating for safer sex behaviour and harm reduction. For populations living as a refugee, frontline workers and volunteers work persistently and tirelessly at advocating for safety and protection of refugees as well as the provision of basic services to this population whilst they live in asylum. Advocacy for international cooperation amongst governments and to ensure the humane treatment of refugees as well as to decrease deportation are some of the efforts frontline and volunteers working with refugees persevere towards. In their line of work, they also do hear about stories of trauma, abuse, torture or separation and loss experienced by the clients on a frequent basis which can be hard on them. When both clients and organisations expect frontline workers and volunteers to take care of their needs, very rarely do we hear the question, 'Who is taking care of our frontline workers and volunteers's mental health?'. Stories of blatant prejudice and discrimination can sometimes incite intense emotions within the workforce due to the sheer amount of injustice faced by the community. Whether it is prejudice faced by legal and health systems or by one's own family and friends, working against systemic prejudice can be tiring as it may feel like one is constantly working against a brick wall.

Compassion fatigue among people in this type of workforce has yet to be researched in the Southeast Asia region, however it is a tangible concern due to the constant exposure of traumatized individuals or individuals in crisis daily. Being newly diagnosed with HIV or AIDS is a trauma – patients face the possibility of having health complications depending on the disease stage that they are diagnosed at. Major lifestyle changes are to be expected. Patients also have to consider their future post-diagnosis when it comes to employment, eligibility of insurance plans as well as the relationships. Similarly, working with individuals who hold a refugee status can be draining as frontline workers and volunteers constantly work on managing crisis on all fronts (safety, health, employment) of mass cases in countries that may not have adequate legal or financial systems to provide the intervention and support needed. When frontline workers and volunteers manage cases like these on a regular basis, the trauma can become normalized thus lowering their empathy levels with their clients (Schiff & Lane, 2016). It is also possible that their own trauma can be heightened in their interaction with clients (Howard, 2012, as cited in Schiff & Lane, 2016). This is particularly rampant amongst frontline workers and volunteers who work with communities that live in unstable living conditions yet assisting individuals with trauma, gender based violence experiences and drug usage towards recovery and stability. Once vicarious trauma is coupled with constant burnout, it sparks the development of compassion fatigue among the frontline workers and volunteers (Cocker & Joss, 2016). This can be detrimental to both the workers and community since the workers' wellbeing is jeopardized thus resulting in sub-par performance in their duties.

Thankfully, support systems are available among peers and members of the community. In times of crisis and emergencies, it is common to see people of this workforce band together for emotional and mental support. Examples of such events include the death of a client after succumbing to complications related to HIV/AIDS, police raids in refugee community areas, refugee workplaces or even homes, as well as the detainment or capture of community members, hate killings, extortion by local citizens or authorities and anti-HIV and refugee statements made by prominent figures in the local society. When organizations who work with key populations stand together in solidarity and condemn discriminatory acts through press statements, it sends the message to the public that behaviours that encourage stigmatization are unacceptable. Commemoration events such as World AIDS Day and World Rfugee Day commemorate the lives lost to AIDS and highlights the importance of communities standing together to fight against societal injustices .

Frontline workers and volunteers working with refugee communities and populations affected by HIV/AIDS have unique experiences in their line of work since the communities affected by these issues have varied needs despite being under the same umbrella. Yet, they share the themes of combating stigmatization, empowering clients through support, shifting dynamics in social circles from the community as well as experiencing secondary trauma through shared experiences with their clients. It is important to acknowledge these experiences since they make up the identities of which the frontline workers and volunteers working with this community take pride in.

Mental Health Professionals and Their Role as Frontline Workers in Key Populations

Counselling and therapy are important components in any community service, especially those dealing with 'at risk' populations. Although most frontline workers would have been exposed to a basic training in basic counselling skills in order to help build rapport with the community members, mental health professionals are more equipped to handle tougher cases that require specific interventions suited to the individual's needs. This can range from crisis counselling, implementing specific intervention techniques to assist clients healing and coping, to group counselling.

One of the more common forms of counselling used in HIV/AIDS is prevention counselling (Kanekar, 2011). This covers risk reduction, pre-test and post-test counselling. Mental health professionals deliver psychoeducation and risk assessments to clients prior to a HIV or STI test in order to help them prepare for the test mentally and emotionally (Kanekar, 2011). Depending on the results of the test, the post-test counselling varies between encouraging clients to maintain their HIV- negative status through behavioural change or maintenance or, in the case of HIV positive status clients, by guiding the clients to the next steps they can take as well as referring clients to medical providers (Kanekar, 2011). It also includes encouraging clients to commit to safer sex practice as well as the importance of duty to warn current and previous partners. Counseling HIV positive clients, specifically HIV positive MSM, can uncover many issues such as shame, grief over the loss of health, anger and confusion on how to manage safe sex negotiation (Barrett & Logan, 2002). The mental health practitioner would need to be aware of the complexities of these issues and assist their client to navigate through these challenges.

Client-centered counselling is also used within this population. Due to the fact that HIV/AIDS is still viewed with prejudice in this region, clients who are diagnosed with HIV tend to face discrimination which can lead to increased levels of anxiety and depression (Kanekar, 2011). Despite the fact that HIV is a manageable disease, it introduces a lot of uncertainty and instability to other aspects of clients' lives such as relationships, employability, and even end-of-life decisions. Therefore, client-centered counselling is used to cater to the different needs of the patients. Person-centered therapy is commonly used to provide a safe and empathic space for the clients so that they can slowly work on their acceptance towards the diagnosis. Having that space can be liberating for some clients as they could have internalized their own prejudices towards themselves, therefore this enables them to process their own experiences at their own pace. Cognitive behavioural therapy is used to help clients be aware with their irrational thoughts and adapt these thoughts to more positive ones in order to bring in beneficial behavioural changes. This works well with clients who engage in repetitive testing more than the advised frequency (three to six months for 'at risk' clients) as they may have anxiety, faulty thinking and obsessive behaviours such as constantly checking the accuracy of the tests as well as being hypervigilant on their surroundings.

Providing mental health services and support for clients who hold a refugee status can be complicated as these clients face instability across their various areas in their lives. Many times frontline workers, including mental health practitioners would need to play multiple roles of advocate, social worker and psychological support in order to stabilize the basic needs of refugee clients. Assisting clients to adjust to their new reality of holding a refugee status may require mental health practitioners to take on an eclectic framework of working with refugees which implement both cognitive and expressive techniques. It would also include assisting clients to cope with complicated grief of not knowing the fate of family and friends who have been left behind or separated in the process of migration. At the same time, practitioners would need be aware that research on evidence based practice for refugee mental health is still in its emerging stages and would need be tailored specifically for the challenges faced in the country they are seeking asylum due to differing legal protection and implementation in refugee protection. A more in depth understanding and discussion on the background of refugees, challenges faced and recommended techniques will be further elaborated in a later chapter.

The Experience of Managing Frontline Workers and Volunteers in Key Populations

In the previous section, we spoke through the eyes of frontline workers and volunteers themselves – their perspectives, their motivations as well as the qualities that made them stand out in the profession. However, they do not work alone in an organization setting as they have the support from the middle management. Program managers and supervisors serve as the sounding board for those who work at the frontlines as they provide the standard operating procedures as well as input from the organization's perspective. They also act as gatekeepers of information as they assist frontline workers and volunteers in handling complex cases that require intervention from middle management. In order to develop the competencies of frontline workers and volunteers in their on-the-ground work, program managers and supervisor provide trainings on a frequent basis that covers topics ranging from soft skills to more technical support such as rapid HIV testing or rapid health screening during mobile clinics. Mental health support is also focused in the role of middle management, especially supervisors for social workers, outreach workers or volunteers who deal with clients directly. Due to the nature of the work, burnout rates are high among frontline workers and volunteers. Therefore, supervisors are usually tasked to detect and support those who are already displaying signs of burnout or compassion fatigue.

For middle management, recruitment of frontline workers and volunteers for this line of work focus a lot on the communities themselves. Not only do they provide job opportunities for members of the community who are rejected or discriminated due to their HIV status, they create a safe environment for the members of the community to support each other in their journey against the disease. However, this does not imply that people outside of the community are discouraged to join this industry. In fact, allies are seen as important in the fight against HIV and AIDS as they support and empower the community through empathy and giving them the means to work on their difficulties (Mavros, 2015).

Unfortunately, the same cannot be applied to refugees who are living in asylum as this community may have challenges in being fully employed. Instead, many organisations enlist the support of other refugees with above average English communication skills in providing translation across both international and local organisations as well as clinics. These refugees whose help is enlisted are usually concurrently trained in providing outreach and psychoeducation within their various communities. This is one way organisations work with refugees in providing empowerment and preventive networks within the community. However, most refugees do not work in these areas. It would be important to highlight that refugees do take on roles as cleaners, cooks, waiters and other hard labour jobs in order to provide for their basic necessities.

The dynamics between frontline workers and volunteers are important to acknowledge as well. There is a power difference between these two groups of employees, therefore it is common to have a frontline worker as a facilitator or lead of a group of volunteers whenever they do on-the-ground work. Resentment may be formed when the frontline worker finds the added responsibility of looking after the volunteers coupled with their main responsibilities as an extra burden or the volunteers experience a lack of appreciation or acknowledgement of their efforts. Therefore, it is important that program managers and supervisors address the more subtle needs of frontline workers and volunteers instead of focusing mainly on financial compensation and performance. Unfortunately, this is a common scenario faced by many community organizations in which the focus leans heavily on the organizational aspect of management. Although it is understandable since community-based organizations are faced with the challenges of limited funding, ignoring the human side of management does more harm than good in the long run.

Although the key populations – men who have sex with men (MSM), transgenders (TG), sex workers (SW), people who inject drugs (PWID), women and children living with HIV/AIDS – are under the umbrella of HIV/AIDS prevention, a common theme highlighted by the workers is the lack of communication between these populations and the 'silo' mentality practiced by them. Since the clientele for this issue usually originate from two or more key population, having the sense of competition and territorial behaviour among the population can be debilitating. For example, quotas or key performance indexes (KPI) have to be fulfilled in order for organizations to continue receive funding from international funds such as Global Fund and Department of Immigration and Citizenship (DIAC). The sense of competition that is created from this expectation can result in the restriction of information flow between organizations that could have been beneficial to the community that they serve in.

These behaviours also can be seen in middle management, especially in organizations that provide more than one program for the community. On one hand, frontline workers usually focus their attention 'downward' to the benefit of the key affected population that they serve in. On the other hand, middle management focus their attention 'upward' to the relationship building aspect between upper management and foreign co-workers or supervisors (Schuller, 2016). Such differences can disrupt the communication between the two important roles in any community work, resulting in services rendered below par.

Managing frontline workers and volunteers who are working with HIV/AIDS is no different from other humanitarian settings as well. By providing boundaries and organizational support to the frontliners, those involved in middle management keep the gears turning in the organization. Not only do they balance between the needs of the community with the needs of the organization, they are there as protective factors for the frontline workers and volunteers in the face of compassion fatigue and burnout. Therefore, they are needed as much as the frontliners in ensuring marginalized communities are provided adequate assistance and support in meeting their needs.

CURRENT CHALLENGES FACED IN WORKING WITHIN MARGINALIZED AND VULNERABLE COMMUNITIES

Over the years, countless of volunteer programs are offered globally which provide opportunities to serve in the Southeast Asian region. One just needs to type in 'volunteer at Southeast Asia' in any search engine and hundreds of volunteer tour organizations will appear on the screen. Yet, there has been a raised concern on the trend of 'voluntourism' in which foreign volunteers temporarily attach themselves to a local project while enjoying their holiday in the region (Kushner, 2016). Unfortunately, local communities have more severe issues such as child abuse and poverty that require longer term skilled labour,- skillsets that 'voluntourism' do not usually provide. Although frontline workers are usually in charge of screening and mentoring volunteers, the lack of manpower makes it hard for them to monitor these volunteers carefully.

One of the most prominent challenges faced in the Southeast Asia region is the lack of training that can further equip volunteers as well as frontline workers in tackling sensitive issues in the community such as violence, abuse, and mental health. It is difficult for members of these communities to depend on the authorities. This is due to several factors including lack of adequate legal frameworks, politically biased implementation of laws and fear of prosecution based on their status in the country. Therefore, members of marginalized communities are exposed to risk factors on a daily basis with a lack of external support. Volunteers and frontline workers are essential in this case as they are able to reach out to these communities easily without causing much distrust. However, a common gripe shared amongst individuals in the community service sector is that they feel as if they are grappling in the dark without much support. Incomplete referrals to other organizations, lack of communications between NGOs, and inconsistent training are cited by many frontline workers as well as volunteers as common challenges faced. For example, a study on reporting behaviours of child abuse among NGO workers in Southeast Asia revealed that reporting behaviours were not necessarily related to their own attitudes towards reporting nor to how much they trust the institutions they serve (Chuah, 2017). It is possible that external factors such as the lack of confidence towards their own training and structure on reporting systems influence the decision to reporting among these workers. Although some NGOs provide guidelines on cultural sensitivity and communication, it is challenging for both volunteers and frontline workers to ensure the guidelines provided are adhered to due to work constraints to provide dedicated mentorship.

The lax screening on foreign volunteers is also a cause of concern for many NGOs in Southeast Asia. With the recent expose of the paedophile, Richard Huckle and his illegal activities, including the rape of at least 200 children while disguised as a volunteer, child protective services, law enforcement and mental health professionals are on high alert on uncovering paedophile groups who may use a similar modus operandi to target children from vulnerable communities. This is one example of lax screening of volunteers which highlights an important bias frontline workers and managers need to be aware of. Various issues compound the challenge of screening potential volunteers including "white bias", and differences in experiential exposure due to sociodemographic backgrounds. It seems to be a pattern among Asian locals to view Caucasians in a favourable light and as more knowledgeable. Frontline workers are bound by stricter rules as compared to volunteers. Coupled with the lax screening of volunteers, this perception can be damaging to both the organization and the community since it can be exploited by people who may have a hidden agenda.

The existence of the Internet and its technological advancements has proven to be a commodity in the field of work. It is easier to dissipate information, gather data and reach out to community members now in the region as compared to two decades ago. The relative anonymity that the Internet provides to clients encourages help-seeking behaviour since it is seen a safer route to seek help, especially in countries where they will be discriminated or punished by the law. However, there is a downside to it. Accuracy of information provided is questionable to say the least since the sources of the information provided by blogs or forums cannot be verified. One of the common examples include misinformation about HIV information and prevention which can either induce unnecessary panic or expose clients to avoidable risks. With the rise of internet outreach programs in humanitarian work, frontline workers and volunteers are required to manoeuvre and adapt to a new landscape. Mahanta, Choudhury, Borthakur, Bhagabati, and Gogoi (2015) reported that even though communication media such as the TV, radio and Internet have contributed to the increased performance of frontline workers, poor knowledge levels can sabotage the effectiveness of services provided. This means that the use of technology in frontline work can be redundant without the knowledge to accompany it.

Internal challenges are faced as well. Job insecurity and monetary compensation are a few of the personal challenges frontline workers and volunteers face in this line of work (Ahmad, 2002). Coupled with the constant exposure to highly-stressful situations and time constraints, it is no surprise that frontline workers and volunteers are highly susceptible to burnout which can have long-term consequences towards mental health. Effective self-care practices among the frontliners have not been thoroughly looked into as well as protective factors that encourage these group of people to continue their service to the community.

These are just a few of the many challenges that frontline workers and volunteers face working in marginalized communities across the region. Since the political environment of the region can directly affect their work towards the community, being on the same page as the government can be more beneficial in the long run. However, this is not the case if the implemented policies are at direct opposition with the values practiced by the community organizations. For example, the legal persecution of transgenders and asylum seekers in Malaysia as well as the drug war in the Phillipines have garnered criticisms from the international humanitarian organizations for the blatant violation of human rights. In order to salvage the situation, not only the efforts to assist the affected communities have doubled, conversations with the government were attempted with little success. Yet, passionate frontline workers and volunteers are well-known for their persistence. Despite the challenges ahead, we see no signs of the frontliners faltering in their work with marginalized and vulnerable communities in the region.

RECOMMENDATIONS AND CONCLUSION

As the awareness towards social issues that are plaguing the marginalized communities rises in this region, so does the pressure faced by volunteers and frontline workers to ensure quality ethical service is consistently provided. To deal with the challenges faced within the communities, communications among NGOs are important to avoid the silo effect. The silo effect happens when there is a lack of information flowing within the NGO and outside of the NGO. Dependent on the size of the targeted marginalized community, the demand for services can exceed the manpower available to provide these services. Therefore, strong referral points are needed to fulfil these demands, especially when there are so few NGOs serving specific communities such as refugees and people living with HIV (PLHIV).

Having more conversations with other NGOs and the government can do wonders to the morale of the frontliners. Since unclear channels of communications are among the challenges faced by frontline workers and volunteers, it is imperative that the collective looks into effective communication systems internally and externally. Dialogues and forums in collaboration with government officials can help solidify better working relationships as well as clearing misconceptions on the roles of both parties. In the end, the community benefits the best when two powerhouses work together for a cause.

Equipping volunteers and frontline workers with training skills is also an area that can be further improved. With the current focus on training and empowering members of the communities, it is expected that the demand for skill training programs will increase in the region. Additionally, teaching community members to help and empower each other goes a long way in keeping programs sustainable when the volunteers or the frontline workers leave the community.

Mental health of the frontline workers and volunteers should be emphasized in the future as there is little covered on the practice of self-care among these group of workers in the region. Being overworked and constantly exposing oneself to secondary trauma can do more harm than good. Therefore, having mental health professionals in a community organization is vital to ensure that the frontline workers and volunteers are supported psychologically in their line of work. At the same time, mental health professionals can act as facilitators in case debriefings or even general debriefings especially in events that has caused grievous harm to the community that they serve.

In the end, marginalized communities exist because certain individuals are excluded by the society due to their identity or behaviours that are deemed unacceptable (CARE, 2014). When the bridge between society and these communities collapse, the isolation itself would bring more harm than good to society as a whole. The role of volunteers and frontline workers can bridge the gap so that both parties can benefit in the long run.

REFERENCES

Ahmad, M. M. (2002). Who cares? The personal and professional problems of NGO fieldworkers in Bangladesh. *Development in Practice*, *12*(2), 177–191. doi:10.1080/09614520220127694

ASEAN. (2016). *HIV in the ASEAN region: Second regional report on HIV & AIDS 2011 -2015*. Retrieved from http://asean.org/storage/2016/11/08ASEAN-Regional-Report-on-HIV-AIDS-1dec.pdf

AVERT. (2017). *HIV and AIDS in Asia & The Pacific regional overview*. Retrieved from https://www.avert.org/professionals/hiv-around-world/asia-pacific/overview

Bansal, S. (2012, December 2). Volunteers on the frontline of services delivery. *The Guardian*. Retrieved from https://www.theguardian.com/global-development-professionals-network/2012/dec/05/volunteers-frontline-services-delivery

Barret, B., & Logan, C. (2002). Counselling Gay Men and Lesbians: A Practice Primer. Brooks/Cole, Cengage Learning.

BBC. (2015). *Asia Migrants: Malaysia Orders Search and Rescue for Boats*. Retrieved from http://www.bbc.com/news/world-asia-32822508

Brassard, C., Sherraden, M. S., & Lough, B. J. (2010). Emerging Perspectives on International Volunteerism in Asia. *The International FORUM on Development Service. IVCO.*

Buscher, D., & Heller, L. (2010). Desperate Lives: Urban Refugee Women in Malaysia And Egypt. *Forced Migration Review*, *34*, 20–21. Retrieved from http://ezproxy.help.edu.my:2052/eds/pdfviewer/pdfviewer?vid=22&sid=a0d7a383-ea6a-4ec6-bd99-0ad8ad602574%40sessionmgr4008&hid=4205

CARE. (2014). *Marginalised Urban Women in Southeast Asia*. Retrieved from https://www.care.org.au/wp-content/uploads/2014/12/MUW-in-SE-Asia-Report.pdf

Chuah, S. M. (2017). *Reporting Behaviours of Children-Centric NGO Workers on Child Abuse in Southeast Asia* (Unpublished dissertation). HELP University, Kuala Lumpur, Malaysia.

Cocker, F., & Joss, N. (2016). Compassion fatigue among healthcare, emergency and community service workers: A systematic review. *International Journal of Environmental Research and Public Health*, *13*(6), 618. doi:10.3390/ijerph13060618 PMID:27338436

Hashim, J., Chongsuvivatwong, V., Phua, K. H., Pocock, N., Teng, Y. M., Chhem, R. K., . . . Lopez, A. (2012). *Health and healthcare systems in Southeast Asia*. Retrieved from https://unu.edu/publications/articles/health-and-healthcare-systems-in-southeast-asia.html

Human Rights Watch. (2017). *HRW: Deteriorating outlook for human rights in Southeast Asia*. Retrieved from https://www.voanews.com/a/human-rights-watch-southeast-asia/3674978.html

IntraHealth. (2016). *The case for frontline health workers in addressing non-communicable diseases globally*. Retrieved from https://www.intrahealth.org/sites/ihweb/files/files/media/the-case-for-frontline-health-workers-in-addressing-non--communicable-diseases-globally/NCDBrief.pdf

Jones, E. (2017). *Life in Limbo: The Refugee Experience in Southeast Asia*. Retrieved from https://www.trtworld.com/opinion/life-in-limbo-the-refugee-

Jones, G. W. (2013). *The Population of Southeast Asia*. Retrieved from http://www.ari.nus.edu.sg/wps/wps13_196.pdf

Jung, Y. (2010). *Successful Models on achieving the Millennium Development Goals in South East Asia* (Unpublished dissertation). London School of Economics and Political Science, London, UK.

Kanekar, A. S. (2011). HIV/AIDS Counseling Skills and Strategies: Can Testing and Counseling Curb the Epidemic? *International Journal of Preventive Medicine*, *2*(1), 10–14. PMID:21448398

Kushner, J. (2016, March 22). The Voluntourist's Dilemma. *The New York Times*. Retrieved from https://www.nytimes.com/2016/03/22/magazine/the-voluntourists-dilemma.html

Liu, E. S. K., Ching, C. W. L., & Wu, J. (2017). Who is a volunteer? A cultural and temporal exploration of volunteerism. *Journal of Human Behavior in the Social Environment*, *27*(6), 530–545. doi:10.1080/10911359.2017.1295715

Mahanta, L. B., Choudhury, M., Borthakur, S., Bhagabati, R., & Gogoi, P. (2015). Can communication media improve the KAP status of frontline health workers? A cross-sectional study on MCH indicators from Assam, India. *South East Asia Journal of Public Health*, *5*(2), 57–64. doi:10.3329eajph.v5i2.28314

Mavros, K. (2015). *The importance of being an ally*. Retrieved from https://www.forbes.com/sites/strategyand/2015/06/16/the-importance-of-being-an-ally/#5caacc1d35c9

McCloskey, L. A., & Southwick, K. (1996). Psychosocial Problems in Refugee Children Exposed to War. *Pediatrics, 97*(3), 394-398. Retrieved from http://ezproxy.help.edu.my:2057/eds/pdfviewer/pdfviewer?sid=7f55c8c8-f3d9-4f9-3a7afb1f9e507e30b%40sessionmgr105&vid=21&hid=111

MDG Achievement Fund. (2017). *Millennium Development Goals*. Retrieved from http://www.mdgfund.org/node/922

Patel, C. (2017, February 25). Time for ASEAN to take human rights seriously. *The Diplomat*. Retrieved from https://thediplomat.com/2017/02/time-for-asean-to-take-human-rights-seriously/

Pitsuwan, S., & Parameswaran, P. (2015). *Why Southeast Asia Refugee Crisis Matters*. Retrieved from https://thediplomat.com/2015/07/southeast-asia-refugees-in-crisis/

Posselt, M., Procter, N., Galletly, C., & de Crespigny, C. (2014). Aetiology of Coexisting Mental Health and Alcohol and Other Drug Disorders: Perspectives of Refugee Youth and Service Providers. *Australian Psychologist*, *50*(2), 130–140. doi:10.1111/ap.12096

Randle, M., & Dolnicar, S. (2012). Attracting volunteers in highly multicultural societies: A marketing challenge. *Journal of Nonprofit & Public Sector Marketing*, *24*(4), 351–369. doi:10.1080/10495142.2012.733668

Ross, M., Svajlenka, N. P., & Williams, J. (2014). *Part of the solution: Pre-Baccalaureate healthcare workers in a time of health system change*. Retrieved from https://www.brookings.edu/wp-content/uploads/2014/07/Healthcare-Workers-Report.pdf

Sahri, M., Murad, K., Alias, A., & Sirajuddin, M. (2013). Empowering Youth Volunteerism: The Importance and Global Motivating Factors. *Journal Of Educational And Social Research*, *3*(7), 502. Retrieved from http://www.mcser.org/journal/index.php/jesr/article/view/995

Schiff, J. W., & Lane, A. (2016). *Burnout and PTSD in workers in the homeless sector in Calgary*. Retrieved from http://calgaryhomeless.com/content/uploads/Calgary-Psychosocial-Stressors-Report.pdf

Schuller, M. (2016). *Humanitarian Aftershocks in Haiti*. Rutgers University Press.

Sidebe, M., & Singh, P. K. (2016). *Thailand eliminates mother-to-child transmission of HIV and syphilis.* Retrieved from http://www.searo.who.int/about/administration_structure/cds/piis0140673616307875.pdf?ua=1

Taylor, S. (2017). *Refugee Protection in the Asia Pacific Region.* Retrieved from http://www.refugeelegalaidinformation.org/refugee-protection-asia-pacific-region

The Guardian. (2015). *Malaysia Migrant Mass Graves: Police Reveal 139 Sites, Some with Multiple Corpses.* Retrieved from https://www.theguardian.com/world/2015/may/25/malaysia-migrant-mass-graves-police-reveal-139-sites-some-with-multiple-corpses

UNHCR. (2017). *Joint statement on the Rohingya refugee crisis.* Retrieved from http://www.unhcr.org/en-my/news/press/2017/10/59e4c17e5/joint-statement-rohingya-refugee-crisis.html

UNICEF. (2012). *Understanding the focus on young people from Key Affected Populations in Concentrated and Low Prevalence HIV Epidemics.* Retrieved from https://www.unicef.org/rosa/20121012_ykap(1).pdf

United Nations High Commissioner for Refugees. (2016). *Refugees in Malaysia.* Retrieved from http://www.unhcr.org.my/refugeeMsia.htm

United Nations High Commissioner for Refugees. (2017). *Asia and the Pacific.* Retrieved from http://www.unhcr.org/en-my/asia-and-the-pacific.html

United Nations Volunteers. (2015). *State of the World's Volunteerism Report 2015.* Retrieved from https://www.unv.org/sites/default/files/2015%20State%20of%20the%20World%27s%20Volunteerism%20Report%20-%20Transforming%20Governance.pdf

Vijayakumar, L. (2016). Suicide Amongst Refugees – A Mockery of Humanity Crisis. *Journal of Crisis Intervention and Suicide Prevention, 37*(1), 1–4. doi:10.1027/0227-5910/a000385 PMID:27033678

Chapter 7
LGBTQ+ Population in Asia Pacific (Malaysia):
LGBTQ+ Populace

Gianina Ginnie Kon
HELP University, Malaysia

Anne Chong Yuk Ming
Lodge International School, Malaysia

ABSTRACT

The topic of LGBTQ in Malaysia was chosen as this issue is relatively new (as compared to Western society) and perhaps not as open due to the different religious, cultural, and familial taboo surrounding it. Individuals who face a crisis in their sexuality, hence, face insurmountable challenges and conflicts and may need to seek help from the counselling/helping professionals. This chapter that focuses on LGBTQ+ population in general, and particularly in Malaysia, it is hoped that it would facilitate the relationship between the counsellor with a member of this particular population.

INTRODUCTION

It seems that today's society, its members are segregated into groups using subjective labels e.g. gender (male/female) religion, race, age, socioeconomic level, marital status and now there seems to be another "recognized" group based on the group members' sexual identity and orientation namely, the LGBTQ group. The origin of why groups are labelled accordingly is unclear but perhaps it is to accord the members certain rights and privileges (certain discounts, membership, services) but it seems more often than not groups/ members of a certain labelled group have received negative treatment from others ranging from being ignored to even being killed. While many groups have experienced one kind of prejudice or another, groups that have faced extreme forms of discrimination are those that are based on religion, race and at present the group based on sexual orientation and sexual identify, namely the Lesbian, Gay, Bisexual, Transexual and Queer or commonly known as LGBTQ.

DOI: 10.4018/978-1-5225-6073-9.ch007

While other groups that had faced discrimination have achieved some sense of equality and a less obvious the LGBTG is the latest group to battle for equality and general acceptance by others. In recent times the group has gained much exposure and this topic has been addressed through media in more liberal societies (Hollywood, Australia etc) and have gained much traction in the battle to be treated equally as their heterosexual counterparts, the LGBTQ population still face daunting and insurmountable challenges in more conservative and religious societies, particularly in Islamic societies like Malaysia . They face hostility from families and even capital punishment from authorities.

As a group, LGBTQ population is still in the pioneering days of its struggles to achieve equality or at its basic core, the right to live a "normal life" and recognition as its heterosexual counterpart. As such counsellors/prospective counsellors, who wish to journey with the LGBTQ clients, would want to gain some insight on the different aspects of this group. A brief outline on the following topics, though in no means an exhaustive list, could be helpful in helping counsellors offer and maintain a healthy helping relationship in which an LGBTQ client can find a secure, empathetic relationship. The sections below address the following

1. The historical journey of the LGBTQ
2. Vocabulary involving LGBTQ
3. Challenges in Muslim countries
4. Methodology
5. Evaluation of Methodology
6. Counselling in a Malaysian context

HISTORICAL JOURNEY OF THE LGBTQ POPULATION

In order to understand another's present situation, it would be useful to know the other's some background. So it is with getting to know and understand the LGBTQ. When did it come to be? What has been its important challenges? What is the present situation? Only then can client and counsellor be able to map out its future either a group or as an individual. This section will summarize evidence of LGBTQ existence in early history, treatment and attitudes towards LGBTQ and some victories gained by them.

Existence of Homosexuality /Transgender

Earliest recording of homosexuality goes as far back as 9600 BCE in Mesolithic art in Sicily and Zimbabwe shown in drawn figures of phallic male figures in pairs. There were also religious depictions of male homosexual intercourse.

There are figurines believed to have been drawn during the Bronze age (7000 BCE) around the Mediterranean area that depicts the "third sex", which is of male figure having female breasts or no distinguishable identifying sexual characteristics

Historical Figures

The first recorded same sex couple were Khnumhotep and Niankhkhnum who were Royal Egyptian servants.

Sappho was a Greek lyric poet (630-570 BCE) famous for her lesbian themes, Coming from an island called Lesbos, thus the term Lesbian was attributed to her. However she was exiled in 600 BCE.

Treatment /Attitudes Towards Homosexuals Through the Ages

Like its modern counterparts, LGBTQ population were with abuse and maltreatments ranging from exile to execution. If a person suspected of being homosexual, any sexual harassment would be ignored or at worst executed. In medical world, especially psychiatry, being an LGBTQ was considered a mental illness and was listed in the DSM until 1973. Among the treatments recommended were conversion therapy, electroshock therapy and ice pick lobotomies. In the realm of religion, LGBTQ especially homosexuals have been renounced. In the realm of Islam, homosexuals/transgender have received treatments ranging from being demonized to being beheaded.

Victories of LGBTQ

The LGBTQ population has gained much attention recently especially in Australia where same sex marriage is now recognized. This is a significant victory for a well fought fight for recognition and fair treatment. However, while this is important, there are also some important battles won by this group. Some of them includes decriminalizing of homosexuality as early as the 1940s in Iceland and Switzerland among them, support groups for homosexuals and transgenders were formed and recognized and in the early 1990s homosexuality was no longer considered an illness.

While there are more roads to be travelled by LGBTQ group, it can look back with pride at the long history and more importantly its journeys and victories which in turn will encourage LGBTQ in other more conservative societies to be more proactive in advancing their rights for recognition and fair treatment.

VOCABULARY INVOLVING LGBTQ

Sexual orientation to many explained as a pattern of emotional, romantic and sexual attraction towards preference gender such as women to men, women to women or men to men or sometimes women to men and women as bisexual. To support that facts, researcher Susan & Vickie stated that sexual orientation does includes self-identification, life preferences, emotional, social, sexual fantasies, sexual behaviour and sexual attraction.

The term LGBTQ stands for Lesbians, Gay, Bisexual, Transgender and Queer. The "T" in LGBQ also stands for gender non-conforming and for those individuals that doesn't consider or conform to any particular identity associated with the gender by birth. Similarly, Queer stands for individuals that doesn't identify themselves as female or male which can also be called as "genderqueer". However, under the umbrella of LGBTQ+ there are so many various terminology that not many people understand and know about. Sometimes, this may create confusion of the LGBTQ+ members as they didn't know how to identify "self-sexuality". The phrase "gay" has been used so often to called same sex attraction and it is the generic term for all. Moreover, it is important to differentiate these terms to avoid confusions among the gay communities. The signature "(+)" as part of the acronym symbolize all other kinds of sexuality out there such as asexual, pansexual etc. as part of the PLUS. It was adding on to make everyone feel welcomed and put to stop closed focus mind on sexuality.

These terminologies were taken from a multicultural LGBTQ affairs to specifically understand the terms under these huge communities. And some was drawn by other LGBT Centers (Syracuse University, UC Berkeley, UCLA and Ohio University), The Brown Boi Project and trans-academics.org (University of Florida: Multicultural & Diversity Affairs, 2017).

- Biological sex/assigned sex

A medical label used to categorize people according to their chromosomes, hormones, genitalia and secondary sex characteristics (breasts, body hair, etc.). Usually assigned at birth as "male" or "female" by a doctor, though there are many variations outside of that socially-constructed binary (i.e. intersex).

- Gender

A socially constructed identity centering around notions of" masculinity," "femininity" and "androgyny," which includes aspects of identity and expression.

- Cisgender

Term used to describe an individual whose assigned biological sex aligns with their expected binary gender identity. Considered to be opposite of "transgender." *Example*: A person whose sex assigned at birth is "female" and identifies their gender as girl or woman.

- Cross Dresser

A person who enjoys dressing in clothing typically associated with the other of the 2 socially-sanctioned genders, but who generally have no intent to live full-time as the other gender. The older term "transvestite" is considered derogatory by many in the United States.

- Drag

The theatrical act of dressing in gendered clothing and/or adopting gendered behaviors as part of a performance (usually clothing and behaviors not typically associated with your own gender identity. Can be done for entertainment, as parody or to make a political statement. Does not indicate performer's sexual orientation or gender identity.

- Gender expression

The way an individual conveys (or is perceived as conveying) their gender, including their choices in clothing, hairstyles, mannerisms, communication patterns, social roles, etc.

- Gender identity

A person's own understanding of themselves in gendered categories such as woman, man, boy, girl, transgender, genderqueer, etc. How an individual feels inside and believes themselves to be.

- Gender dysphoria (formerly referred to as Gender identity disorder)

A diagnostic label included in the Diagnostic and Statistical Manual of Mental Disorders (DSM-5) to describe when a person identifies as a different gender than the one they were assigned based on their birth sex. This diagnosis is usually required so a trans person can receive hormone replacement therapy, sex affirmation surgery and/or revised gender and sex markers on their identification.

- Genderqueer

An identity label sometimes claimed by people whose gender identity does not fit into the culturally accepted man/woman binary. May be characterized by the desire to challenge norms of gender roles and expression, to "play" with gender and/or to express a fluid gender identity.

- Intersex

Term to describe a person whose sex assigned at birth does not neatly fit into the socially accepted binary of "male" or "female," because they have genitalia, hormone production levels and/or chromosomal makeups that are ambiguous or non-binary.

- MTF/M2F/MTF and FTM/F2M/FTM

Terms used to indicate the direction of a trans person's transition and/or identification change. Usually means male-to-female, male-toward-female, female-to-male or female-toward-male.

- Passing

Being perceived by others as the gender you are aiming to present as. Usually used to describe if a trans person is able to live convincingly and publicly as the gender they identify as.

- Pre, Post and Non-operative (OR-OP)

Terms used to describe a transgender or transsexual person's intentions or status regarding sex affirmation surgeries.

- Queer

An umbrella identity term used by people who do not conform to norms of heterosexuality and/or the gender binary. A reclaimed slur, often used with a political connotation.

- Sex affirmation surgery or Sex reassignment surgery or Gender confirmation surgery

Surgeries to change the sex characteristics of one's body, including genitals and/or secondary sex characteristics. Often misunderstood as being a single surgery that makes all body modifications, but the reality is that there is no "*one*" surgery or procedure.

- Transgender or Trans

An identity label used to describe a person whose gender identity does not align with the socially expected one according to their sex assigned at birth. Often used as an umbrella term to include people who transgress gender norms, including cross dressers, genderqueer people, trans women, trans men, bigender or polygender people, etc.

- Trans Man or Transgender man or Transexual man

A person who has transitioned their identity from woman to man, and sometimes their body from female to male.

- Trans Women or Transgender woman or Transexual Women

A person who has transitioned their identity from man to woman, and sometimes their body from male to female.

- Transition

The process of changing one's sex or gender, socially (e.g. changing one's name, clothing, makeup, hair, pronouns) and/or medically (e.g. hormones and/or surgery).

- Transexual

A person who usually experiences a strong and persistent feeling that their body and assigned sex are at odds with their gender identity. These individuals often (but not always) desire to change their bodies to reduce this dysphoria. Since this term comes from the medical establishment, many people choose not to identify with it.

- Two-spirit

Identity label used within many American Indian and Canadian First Nations indigenous groups to describe an individual that possesses both "masculine" *and* "feminine" spirits. Coined by contemporary LGBT Native Americans to describe themselves and the traditional roles they are reclaiming.

- Ze/Hir

Gender-neutral pronouns. Can be used similarly to she/her, he/him or they/them.

- Asexual

An identity label sometimes claimed by people who do not experience sexual attraction. This differs from celibacy or abstinence, which are behaviors. Often used as an umbrella term to encompass identities such as aromantic, demisexual, grey-A, heteroromantic, homoromantic, etc.

- Pansexual

An identity label sometimes claimed by people who experience sexual attraction across the spectrums of gender identity, biological sex and sexual orientation.

- Lesbian

An identity label sometimes claimed by woman-identified people who form their primary romantic and sexual relationships with other woman-identified people.

- Bisexual

An identity label sometimes claimed by people who are sexually attracted to two (or more) sexes or genders, not necessarily equally or simultaneously.

- Gay

An identity label sometimes claimed by man-identified people who form their primary romantic and sexual relationships with other man-identified people.

- FAAB OR AFAB

Abbreviation for “female assigned at birth” or “assigned female at birth.”

- MAAB OR AMAB

Abbreviation for “male assigned at birth” or “assigned male at birth.”

- Polyamorous

An identity label sometimes claimed by individuals that recognize their ability to be in multiple loving and honest sexual and/or romantic relationships at the same time.

- Aggressive (AG)

An identity label claimed by some African-American and Latin@ masculine of center lesbians. Some use “stud” as a synonym.

- Same gender loving (SGL)

A term sometimes used by Black women who love women and Black men who love men. Emerged in the 1990s to provide people in the African-American and Black communities an alternative way to discuss their identity, outside of white-centric terminology.

- QPOC/QTPOC

Abbreviation for "queer people of color" or "queer and trans people of color."

- Undocuquer

Identity label claimed by some individuals in the United States who are both queer and undocumented to show that those two aspects of their identity are not only intersectional, but also inseparable.

- Down Low (DL)

A term originating from the African-American community to describe a man who usually identifies as heterosexual but also has sex with men, often secretly.

- Butch

A person, often—but not always—a lesbian or queer-identified woman, that identifies strongly with "masculinity." Has been used historically in a derogatory manner.

- Femme

A person, often—but not always—a lesbian or queer-identified woman, that identifies strongly with "femininity."

- Transmasculine

A trans person whose gender expression is primarily "masculine." Often includes trans, transgender and/or transexual men.

- Transfemine

A trans person whose gender expression is primarily "feminine." Often includes trans, transgender and/or transexual women.

CHALLENGES IN THE MUSLIM WORLD FOR LGBTQ AND COUNSELLORS

As stated earlier, LGBTQ population and potential clients face daunting and insurmountable challenges in the Muslim world. Being aware of these real and potentially deadly challenges would serve counsellors well in order to help clients make safe choices and live fuller lives in spite of their situation. Challenges can be classified into 2 groups:

1. Muslims who are LGBTQ Members

Islam in its teachings and in its holy books condemns homosexuality as unnatural and sinful. Those involved in unnatural sexual acts are vehemently condemned and in some countries they live in fear of capital punishments which can include caning in public and execution (stoning). Practising and devout Muslims face internal conflict between their sexual tendency and the demands of their religion. They not only live in fear of rejection by society and families but also fear of possible legal and religious condemnation and punishment. Muslims who belong to this group could face issue of negative self-concept and self-identity.

2. Muslim Counsellors for LGBTQ Clients

While counselling of this population enters the realm of multicultural counselling with its inherent challenges, Muslim counsellors face additional dilemmas. Questions they constantly face include: Will they be able to balance between ethical and legal standard codes? Will they be able to conduct a value – neutral stance relationship with the clients or is this the time to initiate a proper referral process.

RESEARCH METHODOLOGY OF LGBTQ POPULATION IN MALAYSIA

Introduction

To gain a deeper understanding and wider knowledge of the experiences faced by LGBTQ+ population in Malaysia with the purpose of gaining more insight into their experience and world view; we have decided to conduct a research by giving out electronic survey to individual whom struggles about their sexuality under the umbrella of LGBTQ+. The population were mainly gathered from Malaysian LGBTQ+ populace.

Research Designs

Research Purpose

The purpose of this study is to explore the LGBTQ+ populations in Malaysia on their personal journey about their sexuality and expectations from counselor in Malaysia. Counselor in Malaysia aren't trained to participate in the lives of LGBTQ+ population because of the stigmatization. Which may lead to the lack of understandings in the LGBTQ+ aspects. Mostly, from the LGBTQ+ member's perspectives some may not be comfortable in opening their sexuality in the counselling session because of the potential social judgement from counsellors. These findings would help counsellor in Malaysia to gained better understandings about the LGBTQ+ expectations in a counsellor.

Research Approach

The nature of our findings is predominantly sensitive therefore, for us to collect specific information, the main study instrument was an anonymous online survey by google forms. The questionnaire consisted of two sections: (1) Background information and (2) open-ended questions that allowed subjects to respond with their personal perceptions and rich experiences.

Online anonymous surveys that included both closed and open-ended questions were proposed to individuals who self-identified their sexual orientation under the LGBTQ+ umbrella. According to (Cowan, 2007) the practice of purposive sampling helped in gathering the LGBTQ+ perceptions of their sexual minority status and what expectations they wanted from a counsellor.

Research Strategy

The aim of the sampling strategy was to find a distinct sample in terms of sexual identity and their involvement in the LGBTQ+ groups. There were several challenges when associated with sampling the LGBTQ+ population in Malaysia because of the illegality in the country. One of the biggest challenge was the insufficient response rate due to fear of voice out. The current attitudes towards the LGTBT+ individuals in Malaysia may face social isolation and discrimination, thus this population was very hard to find, difficult to reach and very unwelcome towards giving opinions (Sullivan & Losberg, 2003). Because of these encounters non-probability sampling was used (Sullivan & Losberg, 2003). Precisely, a snowball strategy and purposeful was used. The hard to reach population allowed us to purposeful send out electronic surveys to specific LGBTQ+ groups in social media were reached. At the same time, by incorporated snowball approach, individuals could contact other LGBTQ+ members who aren't involved in any organization or groups in the social media. In this study, internal validity is more realistic to achieve than external validity. Because using non-probability sampling restrict generalization of the findings. To get a huge sample with this population it was not achievable thus, overall generalizability was considered more important in this segment.

Population and Sampling Design

Populations

For this chapter, we have come to gather population from Lesbians, Gay, Bisexual, Transgender and others in social medias such as groups in Facebook. However, we are not able to have a solid number of participants because of the social nature of this study which we endeavored to minimize potential harm and danger to those in response to self-identification. The sample chosen for this study are anonymous and volunteered from all LGBTQ+ members in Malaysia. There are no specific sample targeted in this area as we aimed to get information only with those who are willing to do so. At the same time, online survey was distributed to social medias organizations and we snowball from there.

Sampling Method

In this study, we used snowball sampling because the population we were exploring were hard to reach groups. This kind of populations that can be hard to reach display some sort of social stigma, illegal behaviors and social marginalized. For that reason, this sampling technique helped us to gain access to such population in Malaysia.

Sources of Data Collection

This research was conducted using anonymous (Schuh et al., 2001) stated that online surveys that incorporated open ended and close questions permissible more in-depth exploratory which leads individuals to deliver their personal thoughts, attitudes and experiences. Self-identified individuals as Lesbians, Gay, Bisexual, Transgender or others are subjective to privacy and are permit for more personal disclosure. The purpose of the data collection in this case was to understands their journey on their challenges and how a counsellor can understand what they are request for.

Limitations of Methodology and Ethical Considerations

Ethical concerns were exceptionally important in sampling and data collection phase as it only self-volunteering based. All correspondence from participants who expressed an interest in participating in the research must do it at their own will. Thus, it causes small data collection from the study. Another limitation was that we only used one social media to reach out to participants which have causes limited resources and detailed on the study. It would have been a better study if we reach out to specific LGBTQ+ activist in Malaysia to participate along with the study which may have allowing us to have more data and sample.

DATA ANALYSIS AND FINDINGS

Quantitative Data Analysis and Interpretation

In this study, the researcher was hoping to find answers towards three research questions. First, were there challenges for LGBTQ+ respondents to come out? Secondly, how can a therapist come in to help with the presenting issue? Thirdly, what are the expectations from the LGBTQ+ communities when reaching out for help from a therapist in Asia? Ought to understand their challenges in seeking for help especially in Asia Pacific. There were also multiple questioned given to demonstrate out their level of comfort in seeking for help and learn to understand what can therapist do to be more understanding towards this group of minorities.

The first thing participant were asked in the questionnaires was to self-define their sexual identities. Figure 1 showed the classification of partakers sexual orientation. This questionnaire was only allowed LGBTQ+ self-classify individuals for taking part of the survey which means Heterosexual individual couldn't partake in this study. In this table, it showed that the highest majority sexual orientation is Gay and lesser is Queer. As it also displayed there were none Transgender participating in this study. This had showed us that the Transgender communities may have become closed due to complications they had to face with Malaysia legal bias. "How life is" (2017) contend such tragedy or murder had happened in Malaysia on the Transgender communities therefore, it had shocked them. It is understood that it is only fair for them to participate in this study

In the next section, participant was requested to answer at what age they learned about their sexuality. As it displayed in Figure 2, most LGBTQ+ members found out their sexuality at Adolescence from age 12-18 years, next highest was during school age from 5-12 years and some found out about their sexuality

Figure 1. Demographics of participants' sexual identities

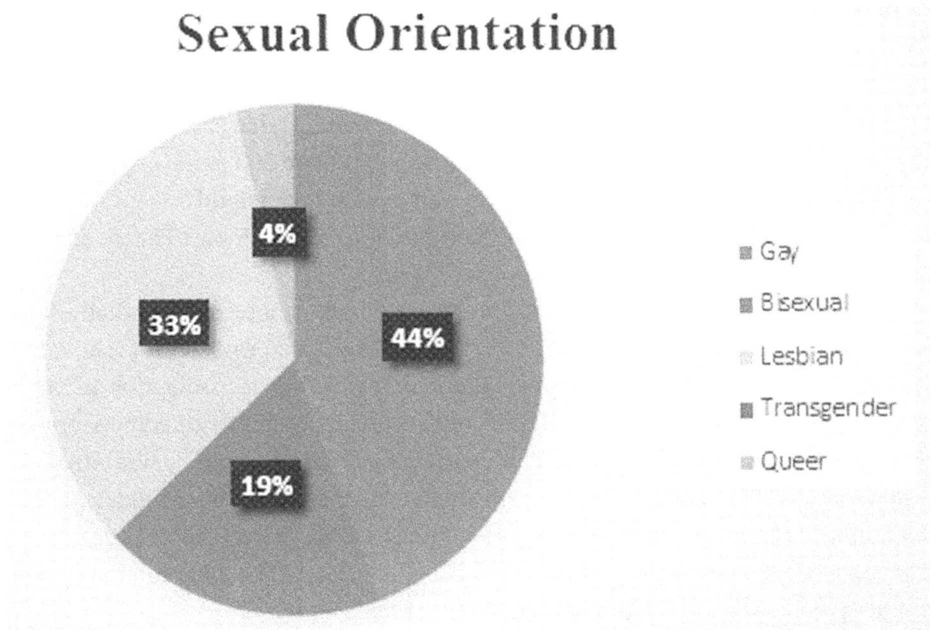

**For a more accurate representation see the electronic version.*

Figure 2. Participants discoveries on their sexual identity initial age

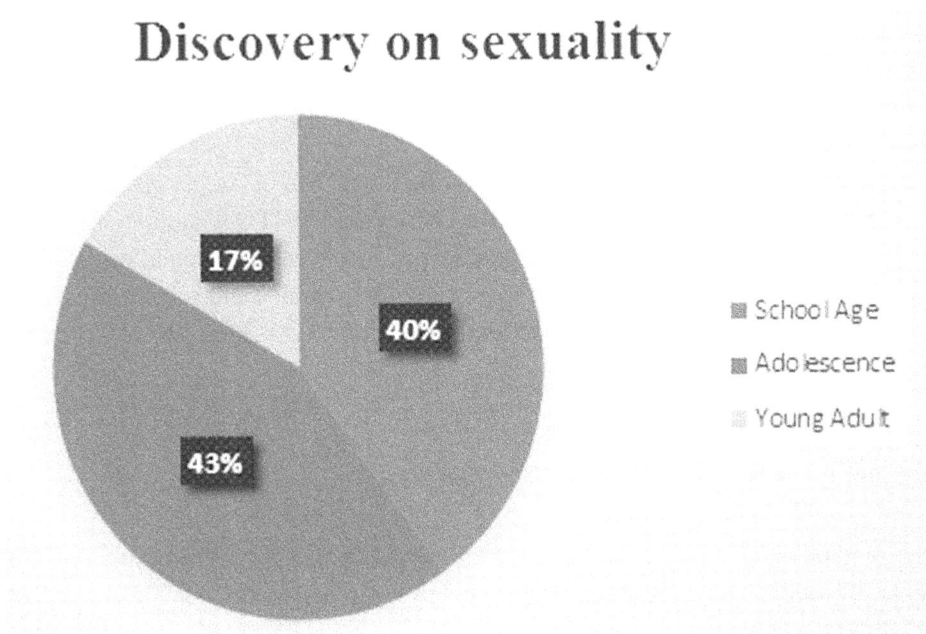

**For a more accurate representation see the electronic version.*

during young adulthood range from 18-40 years old. Majority are opened about their sexuality, especially to those whom participated in this study but some aren't because of social judgement from the society.

The second part of the questionnaire, participants was asked to briefly explain if they are opened about their sexuality what are their experiences in coming out to their loved ones. Most of them would come out to their peers first before family members and some still comfortable staying in the closet. However, some has shared that they came out naturally by being who they are and some expressed that they were out by physical appearance. Next, when researcher attempted to understand how participants view their own sexuality most LGBTQ+ individuals mentioned that it is part of their identity and comfortability being the person they are born to be.

The third part of the questionnaire, was to asked participants about their challenges as being LGBTQ+ in Malaysia and how can mental health therapist in Malaysia provide professional help to them. The common challenges the LGBTQ+ members are facing was the discrimination in Malaysia, act on love such as expression to loved ones, acceptance, religion, marriage, self-esteem, depression, anxiety, panic attacks, career, social pressure, sexual health (HIV&STI) and mental health issues. Next, the expectation from the LGBTQ+ member to seek help are to have therapist who can relate to their sexuality, understanding, non-judgmental, comforting and genuine guidance. Lastly, the major expectations from this minority was to raise more awareness on LGBTQ+, provide support for the minority and educate society about people like them to help in understanding their nature.

Summary and Recommendations

To conclude this study, the researcher has found that there would be a significant amount of challenges in the therapy setting for therapist to understands LGBTQ+ struggles and expectations. The data collection was used to draw inferences about LGBTQ+ perspectives on reaching out to a therapist when needed help. Not many would seek help because of the fear of being judge and discriminate. There are many conclusion that can be drawn from this findings, the anonymous participants are seeking for a professional help to meet their quality of life.

The fight for equal rights in Malaysia are clearly hard because of the nature of the country. However, with a higher education many citizen may learn about the LGBTQ+ nature. One recommendation that was suggested by the participants was to practiced subjects such as sexual orientation and sexual identity in schools to carry awareness to the students, families, friends and society. Apart from that, one suggested a course about LGBTQ+ for counsellors/therapist to partake to achieve richer understanding about the LGBTQ+ individuals.

EVALUATION OF THE RESEARCH METHODS

The research method used on the LGBTQ population was self-report. While it is a viable method of gathering data, it would serve counsellors well to note the strengths and weaknesses of this method of research.

- **Strength:**
  - Respondents give descriptions of their feelings and opinions. It's not scientific so it is easily understood by individuals not in the psychology field.

    - Self-reports are replicable: can be given to populations in other areas.
    - Results can be shown in tables and graphs: Quantifiable.
- **Weaknesses**
    - There are also inherent weaknesses in this type of research. Among them are
    - As it is not scientific, it may not be reliable and valid.
    - Respondents may not answer as accurately due to certain factors: embarrassment, uncertainty and mood at the time of answering the questionnaire embarrassment, or uncertainty

While this research has proven useful and information, it would serve counsellors well to practice a little caution while considering the results.

Future of LGBTQ

The future for LGBTQ+ in Asian pacific may not seem to be brighter than the westernize country such as the U.S.A or European country. However, there will always be a constant movement and hopes in Asia pacific for the LGBTQ+ communities. The first Asia pacific country that was acknowledging same-sex relationship was Taiwan although the polls was not strong enough to win the legislation but the acceptance has grown rapidly since year 2001. However, Thailand once beat Taiwan as the first place in Asia to engaged in same-sex marriage law but wasn't able to pull through accordance with the law. The second country that may have a brighter future for the LGBTQ+ communities are Singapore. The annual event "Pink Dot" for 9 years has increased in numbers and the communities were seen to bring relatives along to support the pride celebrations.

Counties with a strong religious background such as Indonesia and Malaysia would find it hard to approve same-sex marriage laws because it lives by the Islamic rules. It was said that countries such as China, Laos, North Korea and maybe Singapore are unlikely to legalize same-sex marriage in full because of the authoritarian styles that would restrict a civic activism. In 2015, Vietnam legalized same-sex marriage but it was never followed up with the enforcement.

REFERENCES

Cochran, S. D. (n.d.). Lifetime Prevalence of Suicide Symptoms and Affective Disorders Among Men Reporting Same-Sex Sexual Partners: Results From NHANES III. *American Journal of Public Health*, *90*(4), 573–578. PMID:10754972

Cowan, G. (2007). *Understanding and conducting research in education: A user-friendly approach* (2nd ed.). Dubuque, IA: Kendall/Hunt Publishing Company.

How life is tough for transgender in conservative Malaysia, who face violence, religious and official bias, and abusive media. (2017, November 15). *South China Morning Post*. Retrieved from http://www.scmp.com/lifestyle/article/2119847/how-life-tough-transgenders-conservative-malaysia-who-face-violence

Schuh, J. H., & Upcraft, M. L. (2001). *Assessment practice in student affairs: An applications manual*. San Francisco, CA: Jossey-Bass.

Sullivan, G., & Losberg, W. (2003). A study of sampling in research in the field of lesbian and gay studies. In W. Meezan & J. I. Martin (Eds.), *Research methods with gay, lesbian, bisexual, and transgender populations* (pp. 147–162). Binghamton, NY: Harrington Park Press. doi:10.1300/J041v15n01_10

University of Florida, Multicultural & Diversity Affairs. (2017). *LGBTQ Terms and Definitions*. Retrieved from https://lgbtq.multicultural.ufl.edu/programs/speakersbureau/lgbtq-terms-definitions/

APPENDIX

Survey Questions

Background Information

1. Gender: F/M/
2. Age:
3. Race:
4. Sexual Orientation: L/G/B/T/Q/+ (others)
5. When did you find out about your sexuality?
   School Age: Adolescences: Young Adulthood
6. Are you open about your sexuality? If yes,
   No; Yes
7. How did you come out and explain briefly about the process?
8. How do you perceive your sexuality?
9. How did you came out and explain briefly about the process?
10. What are the common challenges you face being one of the LGBTQ+ members in Asia, specifically in Malaysia?
11. What concern you most about your sexuality?
12. How would you get help/seek help in expressing your sexuality?
13. Do you have concerns/issues you would like to voice out regarding your sexuality?
14. What can we do as counsellors/therapist to help you as a client when it comes to your sexuality?
15. What do you want you want counsellors/therapist/society to understand about your sexuality?
16. What can we do differently to help the LGBTQ+ community?

Chapter 8
Counseling Refugees

Ann Nunis
HELP University, Malaysia

ABSTRACT

This chapter discusses the plight of refugees, the challenges faced, and the psychosocial impact of said challenges. It further provides practitioners with a review of coping methods utilized by refugees throughout the refugee journey in order to highlight possible protective factors practitioners may build on in the provision of mental health services. Lastly, the chapter provides an overview of current therapeutic frameworks that are culturally sensitive for counselling refugees, the challenges in the provision of mental health services, and techniques utilized by practitioners in the delivery of mental health services through evidence of research and case-based examples.

INTRODUCTION

Being a refugee is usually considered a temporary situation (El-Sharaawi, 2015). Yet, due to political and environmental situations that impact the flow of migration around the world, being or living as a refugee is met with persistent instability and the consistent need to re-conceptualize a situation of exile and transit in an environment that places little within the direct control of refugees themselves. This also includes a suspension of future plans for education, financial security and building a family with no way of knowing when a durable solution will be reached. Currently, the United Nations High Commissioner of Refugees (UNHCR) has recorded the highest amount of displaced persons across the world since World War II (UNHCR, 2016). The rise of displaced persons and persons seeking asylum across the world has led to increased efforts to alleviate this growing crisis. However, although the crisis of refugees is not new, knowledge is still emerging on evidence based therapeutic frameworks and techniques in providing mental health and even social work services to this group of persons.

This chapter aims to provide a background understanding for mental health practitioners on the plight of refugees, the challenges faced and the psychosocial impact of said challenges. It further aims to provide practitioners with a review of coping methods utilized by refugees throughout the refugee journey in order to highlight possible protective factors practitioners may build on in the provision of

DOI: 10.4018/978-1-5225-6073-9.ch008

mental health services. Lastly, the chapter provides an overview of current therapeutic frameworks that are culturally sensitive for counselling refugees, the challenges in provision of mental health services and implications for practice.

BACKGROUND

To date, there are 67.75 million displaced persons in the world, the largest number since the end of World War II (UNHCR, 2018a). A majority of this number is made up of refugees. Refugees are one of the biggest crises amongst modern day issues. Each day, masses of individuals and families seeking asylum are forced to leave their homes in search for safety. Some make a long journey on foot or are smuggled into vehicles across country borders. Others even brave the journey by sea in the hopes of landing on more welcoming shores. Many risk their lives and are separated from family and friends in the process.

The term "asylum seeker" and "refugee", although used interchangeably, have different operational definitions. An asylum seeker is an individual who is seeking international protection but whose claim has not been confirmed by the UNHCR (Phillips, 2011). For example, an individual escaping armed conflict in Myanmar may cross the border into Thailand or Malaysia seeking asylum and protection, however is not referred to as a refugee until he or she has completed a refugee status determination process by the UNHCR. On the other hand a refugee as defined by the United Nations 1951 Convention Relating to the Status of Refugees and the 1967 Protocol, is a person who

owing to a well-founded fear of being persecuted for reasons of race, religion, nationality, membership of a particular social group or political opinion, is outside the country of his nationality and is unable to, or owing to such fear is unwilling to avail himself to the protection of that country...or is unwilling to return to it. (UNHCR, 2010, p14).

Examples of these reasons include evidence of discrimination and violence towards ethnic minorities, LGBT community or even arrest and detention of individuals who voice opinions opposing that of the government in their home country. The convention also states that refugees should at the minimum be accorded the same rights given to foreign nationals living legally in a country (Arshad, 2005). However, in implementation, the likelihood that refugees have access to the same rights as foreign nationals is not only dependent on the migrant laws of a country but also each country's adherence to international humanitarian treaties and declarations.

The experiences that comprise the asylum seeker and refugee journey can be complex to understand. This journey involves the forceful uprooting of an individual or group of persons from their home country to begin an uncertain journey in the search for safety (Vogel, 2016). The journey of a refugee often involves a lack of certainty of a foreseeable future for a protracted period of time. Refugees can live for several years without recognized documentation, stable financial income and the ability to plan a secure future.

The refugee journey has been conceptualized by researchers in three stages; preflight, flight or asylum and resettlement (Gonslaves, 1992). Preflight is defined as the stage where refugees or asylum seekers are still living in their home country (Wessels, 2014). The flight period, on the other hand, is characterized by a physical relocation to a country of asylum where refugees await a long term solution (Bhugra & Jones, 2001; Wessels, 2014). Lastly, resettlement is the stage where refugees are relocated to a host country where they will be able to live in the long term (Wessels, 2014). However, resettlement is not the only option. There are three potential durable solutions for refugees; voluntary repatriation back to their home country, local integration into the country of asylum, or resettlement (Horyniak, Melo, Farrell, Ojeda, Strathdee, 2015). At the same time, only 1% of the world's refugees are resettled to third countries (Phillips, 2011). The question then remains, what is the fate of the remaining 99% who do not attain resettlement is an area of concern for both humanitarian and mental health groups? These individuals usually are faced with continued ambiguity and instability on the result of their status with no possibility of knowing when they will have a conclusion to their living their life in asylum.

Refugees are also at risk of developing mental health issues due to trauma and stress experienced throughout the journey. Research has suggested that 9% of adult refugees and 11% of child refugees have symptoms consistent with post-traumatic stress disorder, otherwise known as PTSD (Schweitzer, Brough, Vromans & Asic-Kobe, 2011). A meta-analysis of psychiatric surveys has shown that adult refugees living in Western countries are ten times more likely to develop PTSD, placing them at a higher vulnerability to substance abuse and suicide (Fazel, Wheeler, & Danesh, 2005). At the same time, the provision of mental health treatment for refugees across the world is met with various challenges due to the lack of interpreters and psychometric assessments that are available in relevant languages (Ullmann, Barthel, Tache, Bornstein, Licino, & Bornstein, 2015). The shortage in availability of a comprehensive and multicultural approach to providing mental health for refugees is also part of the issue that magnifies the challenges in ensuring refugees are able to access mental health services.

Psychosocial Impact

Throughout the journey of a refugee, refugees face various complexities. The constant state of limbo and lack of stability causes the experience of time to become an altered state where the future is uncertain and day to day living becomes unstable due to this experienced sense of limbo (El-Shaarawi, 2015). Refugees and asylum seekers alike face various issues of harassment, threat of arrest and detention, exploitation, discrimination and vulnerabilities to gender based violence and development of illnesses. Communicable illnesses, such as tuberculosis, have an increased likelihood of spreading due to overcrowded living spaces. Furthermore, refugees and asylum seekers typically have preexisting mental health conditions due to pre-flight trauma and experiences such as extortion by traffickers, abuse and harsh physical conditions during the long journey to safety (Mann & Fazil, 2006).

Protection Issues

What can further compound the stressors refugees face is that not all countries recognize refugees and asylum seekers. Although many countries are signatories of the 1951 Convention and the 1967 Protocol, there are still other countries who are not members to these conventions. In Southeast Asia, UNHCR works alongside various governments to address the issues of migration flows across sea and land. Unfortunately, most countries in Southeast Asia have are not signatories to the 1951 Refugee Convention and its 1967 Protocol. Countries who are not signatories include Thailand, Malaysia and Indonesia. This means that thousands of refugees in these countries live without the right to work and without the guarantee of protection and safety. Therefore, it leaves hundreds and even thousands of refugees and asylum seekers with a legal system that lacks the protection structure to ensure basic rights and safety for them. As part of providing a framework that all governments can use as a baseline governments have adopted and signed various international treaties The Bali Process on People Smuggling, Trafficking in Persons and Related Transnational Crimes as well as adaptation of the Child Rights Convention, Convention on the Elimination of all Forms of Discrimination Against Women (CEDAW) and the Universal Declaration of Human Rights are some of the international treaties adopted by some Southeast Asian governments. However, countries as these are international treaties that do not carry legal consequences if not met, the majority of these countries often ignore the application of these treaties on migrants, particularly migrants who are undocumented or are considered illegal; a category that many refugees unfortunately fall into.

Although refugees living in asylum are removed from the immediate danger and violence of war in their home country, persistent challenges are faced as refugees experience restricted movement in camps and an uncertain future without work or the provision of education for their children (Farzana, 2016). At the same time, the experience of refugees in different asylum seeking environments may present refugees with varied concerns for safety and mental health. For example, refugee camps offer the possibility of greater safety and higher access to basic needs of food and shelter (Shakespeare-Finch, Schweitzer, King & Brough, 2014). Also, there may be other challenges refugees face in these environments. Asylum centres, for example, may increase the risk of ethnic conflict and the development of mental health issues due to the isolation and segregation within the centre (Lauritzen & Sivertsen, 2012) Additionally, the increased time spent waiting for a result at asylum centres made it challenging for asylum seeking children to develop positively in a space where safety and health are compromised. Furthermore, refugees in Southeast Asia typically live as urban refugees in cities and towns allowing them to blend into daily life amongst locals but without the same rights, access to services and protection as locals. Typically urban refugees were made up of single, young, male refugees (Crisp, 2017). However, urban refugees are increasingly made up of refugee community demographics including elderly, unaccompanied minors, single females and young families. This implies that there is an added risk posed not only in safety, but also in susceptibility to raids, arrest, extortion, gender based violence, and family cohesion.

Other protection issues can impact the mental health of refugees and asylum seekers. Isolation, fear of deportation and the possibility of being separated from family members caused the highest distress for refugees asylum centres (Sourander, 2002). Other mental health stress reactions such as depression, despair, anxiety, shame at surviving, anger were reported to be experienced during the asylum seeking period due to living with the constant threat of death and violence (Knezevic, Olson, 2014). The culmination of detention, ongoing discrimination and economic hardships can generate stress and a sense of hopelessness in refugees, which can lead to suicide (Vijayakumar, 2016).

Generating a Stable Livelihood

Creating a stable livelihood is another challenge faced by refugees in asylum that can contribute to mental health issues. Refugees tend to face difficulties in gaining employment whilst seeking asylum which may induce further psychological issues such as disturbed sleep patterns, low self-esteem, anxiety, depression and family violence (Mann & Fazil, 2006). Refugees living in a camp tend to find it difficult to gain sustainable methods in providing food and amenities due to an unemployment crisis experienced by refugees (Sarfo-Mensah, 2009). Refugees in camps usually have limited equal access to resources as compared to citizens of a country. Local organisations, including international and regional organisations, may be unable to provide sufficient support through provision of food and other basic necessities. Thus, providing a livelihood is not only an issue due to an individual holding a refugee status but also due to resource restraints of intervening organisations and the political climate of the relevant host country.

Language Barriers

Language is one of the most common challenges refugees face once they have left their home country. Refugees who experienced more language difficulties report higher anxiety symptoms, indicating that issues with acculturation is one of the most salient factors in post-migration well-being (Kartal & Kiropoulos, 2015). This can happen at any point of the refugee journey once an individual has left his or her home country. With the lack of English communication skills to assist them in integration to a host country, many refugee parents instead rely on their children to provide translation for them when accessing services (Francis & Yan, 2016). Consequently, youths who had resettled with their families experienced a reversal of roles when it came to language and skills as the youths now had to provide communication support to their parents who had lower proficiency of the English language. This reversal of roles also meant that adult refugees lose the important social roles once resettled to a new country. This may include loss of roles such as a spouse, parent or child through separation or death or even occupational roles and cultural peacemakers or teachers (Goodkind, Hess, Isakson, LaNoue, Githinji, Roche, Vadnais, & Parker, 2014). As you can see, being a refugee can not only impact an individual's livelihood and protection but also the cohesion and wellness of the family unit, an area of life that could act as a protective factor but could serve as a perpetuating factor to stress or mental health issues.

Survivor Guilt

News of increasing conflict in their home country may also lead refugees to experience survivor's guilt as refugees may compare the dangerous circumstances loved ones in their home country may face to their own relative safety (Bemak & Chung, 2017). Many refugees naturally continue to be anxious about the safety of their loved ones who have remained in their home country. They may even feel guilty for not doing more to take their loved ones with them. Others may remember the experiences of violence they witnessed or have known to happen to their own loved ones. Still others may have the shock of finding out that a loved one has been arrested or killed by news on social media. These are issues that can complicate the process of grief, trauma and ultimately the mental health of refugees who have left their home country.

Coping Methods

However, despite the unstable circumstances surrounding refugees that continue for an unpredictable period of time, some refugees have found ways to cope with these difficulties. Being future oriented (Borwick, Schweitzer, Brough, Vromans, & Shakespeare-Finch, 2013; Mann, 2010), being able to utilize cultural traditions and community networks (Knezevic & Olson, 2014; Akinsulure-Smith, Dachos & Jones, 2013), and religious practice (Earnest, Mansi, Bayati, Earnest, & Thompson, 2015; Shakespeare-Finch, Schweitzer, King & Brough, 2014) are some of the factors that have helped refugees to cope with new environments. Although most of these coping methods are common amongst resettled refugees, similar findings were also found by the author amongst refugees in asylum, who also relied on community support, religion, self-directed coping and focusing on their future in order to cope with the long and dangerous type living in asylum (Nunis, 2017).

Although the utilization of positive coping methods is widely reported, there also exist reports of negative coping methods amongst refugees. For example, Rohingya refugee youth living in a refugee camp in Bangladesh frequently became involved in drug usage, alcohol consumption and gambling (Farzana, 2016). Higher alcohol prevalence amongst male Middle-Eastern government assisted refugees than female government assisted refugees in British Columbia (Miremadi, Ganesan & McKenna, 2011). The impact of an unstable livelihood on mental health was also seen amongst female Iraqi refugees who were vulnerable to experiencing domestic violence if they had no finances upon arrival in a country of asylum and had borrowed money in Syria (Tappis, Biermann, Glass, Tileva & Doocy, 2012). Similarly, urban refugees working in a factory in Mizoram resorted to alcohol usage and family violence when male family members were unable to protect their families or provide basic necessities whilst seeking asylum (James, 2010).

The Situation in Malaysia

As of February 2018, the number of registered refugees and asylum seekers under the UNHCR mandate in Malaysia was at a total of 154, 400 (UNHCR, 2018b). However, it would be important for readers to bear in mind that this number is not inclusive of asylum seekers who are yet to receive recognition by the UNHCR as a person of concern to their mandate. A majority of registered refugees and asylum seekers are of Myanmar nationality, however, refugees and asylum seekers from Yemen, Somalia, Sri Lanka, Iraq, Afghanistan, Palestine and other countries also make up the total number. Additionally 40, 540 children of the total number are below 18 years old (UNHCR, 2018).

The phenomenon of refugees in Malaysia paints a different set of challenges for asylum seekers and refugees as Malaysia is not a signatory to the 1951 Convention Relating to the Status of Refugees or the 1967 Protocol Relating to the Status of Refugees (UNHCR, 2017a). Malaysia further lacks domestic law that details the rights and protection for an individual of an asylum seeker or refugee status. Instead this group of individuals is classified as illegal immigrants under the Immigration Act thus making them vulnerable to arrest, detention and possible deportation (SUARAM, 2014). Although holding a UNHCR card provides a measure of protection and the hopes of being resettled to a third country, it does not guarantee absolute protection or access to benefits in Malaysia (Alexander, 2008). Due to this, refugees in Malaysia determine the likelihood for safety and protection by negotiating their place of living, typically in either remote jungle areas such as plantations or pockets of the úrban sites' made up of low cost apartments (Nah, 2010). A country that faces a similar situation is Indonesia. Some of the major challenges faced by asylum seekers and refugees include financial difficulty, health issues, lack of security, gaps in continuing education for their children as well as mental health problems (Ali, Briskman, & Fiske, 2016). This then produces a domino effect of being exploited in and out of the workplace including exploitation by authorities and lack of access to education, medical attention and equal and fair work environment.

As Malaysia is not a signatory to the Refugee Convention or the 1967 Protocol, refugees in Malaysia are subject to being arrested and detained by authorities. Refugees are frequently subjected to raids at their workplace or residence, even in public areas, on a daily basis (Alexander, 2008). Rohingya asylum seekers and refugees in Kuala Lumpur have reported being stopped by authorities and having to pay bribes to avoid being arrested, with men being stopped to a higher frequency than those deemed vulnerable such as women, children and the elderly (Wake & Cheung, 2016). The lack of legal status also compounds the ability of refugees to earn a living whilst awaiting a long term durable outcome. Refugees frequently work in informal work areas in what the United Nations High Commissioner of Refugees has classified as 3D jobs – dirty, dangerous, difficult (UNHCR, 2011). Working in these fields further compromises the safety of refugees, in particular female refugees who are frequently sexually harassed and exploited by their employers (Buscher & Heller, 2010).

Furthermore, as refugees legally fall under the broad category of migrants, they are not privy to the right to health access (Health Equity Initiatives, 2010). Issues with communication due to language barriers at health facilities impede access to medical care. It was further reported that a number of refugees displayed PTSD symptoms such as flashbacks, difficulty sleeping and anger outbursts. Additionally, refugee children are not entitled to education in government schools in Malaysia due to their status as an undocumented child and as a refugee (SUARAM, 2015). Refugee children are however able to receive alternative education through community schools run by local NGOs or the refugee community that usually operate out of flats or shop houses (UNHCR, 2017b). However, these alternate routes of education frequently face resource constraints such as qualified teachers, salaries to pay teachers and materials to teach (Health Equity Initiatives, 2010).

Issues such as this can impede the emotional well-being of refugees as this places barriers in other social domains. A research by the author on refugees in Malaysia revealed that refugees face protection and psychosocial issues which impact their mental health well-being (Nunis, 2017). These issues include difficulties in ensuring safety for themselves, ensuring a sustainable livelihood and coping with the psychological impact of pre-migration factors and current living factors. The status as an undocumented person left urban refugees in Malaysia vulnerable to extortion, arrest, and to be taken advantage of by locals. The loss of education opportunities, high medical fees and low salaries were factors that made it difficult for refugees to provide a sustainable livelihood for themselves and their families. This led refugees within the sample to have a decreased sense of self and symptoms similar to post traumatic stress disorder and depression. While some refugees were able to depend on religion, family and community support as well as future oriented thinking to cope with the persistent instability and challenges, some instead turned to alcohol to numb their difficulties. Other families who are unable to gain a sufficient income to look after their families may give their children, particularly female children, to others either in marriage or for labor in order to better provide for the child who leaves and for those who remain.

Working With Refugees

While there have been increased efforts to study and produce evidence based practice for working with refugee clients, research is still in its emerging stages. Most research on the refugee journey and interventions highlight the experiential journey of refugees, particularly during the resettlement stage of the journey. Research has further focused on refugees based in Western countries. Few research efforts have focused on highlighting the delivery of mental health services and interventions through a multicultural lens. Thus, there is less emphasis on a coherent framework to interpret and apply multicultural sensitivity to the provision of mental health services for refugees.

There is no specific model applicable to all refugee cases. This is a group that is diverse, not only in sociodemographics but also in the type of migration experiences and reaction to these experiences, therefore being able to understand the nuances of each individual's journey is imperative in working with refugees. It would be first beneficial to conceptualize the social, legal, and psychological issues surrounding refugees. An example of an approach that would assist is the humanistic approach. Maslow offers a theory to understand this through the motivational theory of the hierarchy of needs (Corey, 2013). Humans would need to first adequately satisfy the basic needs of food, water and security in order to attempt to meet other psychological and self-fulfillment needs. the case of refugees, basic needs are consistently not adequately met, causing these individuals to cycle back and forth in an attempt to meet basic needs for their families and selves whilst also trying to maintain psychological needs. In the case of refugees, it is a daily struggle to meet their basic needs which are rarely consistently adequately met. Due to this, it may make it challenging for practitioners to work on addressing the emotional and cognitive impact of migration experiences as they may need to first address the stress and anxiety of dealing with current environment challenges within the host country. In fact, this may even deter refugees from seeking out mental health services as it is not deemed high on the list of priorities or needs.

Practitioner Self-Reflection

One of the first questions practitioners should ask themselves before working with a client from a refugee background is "How do I feel about migrants and refugees in my country?" and subsequently "What do I believe the government should do about unauthorized immigrants in my country?" (Villalbla, 2009). Without reflecting on their personal opinions and beliefs of these issues, practitioners may be in danger of being bias, hostile or insensitive to a refugee client which will impact the therapeutic alliance and wellbeing of the client. Practitioners would also need to prepare themselves by reading news articles on the developments specific to the country of origin before beginning an intervention. It would be useful to watch videos or read other resources on the cultural practice of a country, ethnic or religious group.

In today's fast paced virtual world, global news is readily available to the public through both print and social media platforms. These platforms make available both overt and covert political messages around the clock. (Bemak & Chung, 2017). Therefore, it may be possible for mental health practitioners to experience political countertransference which is a negative reaction towards migrants or refugee populations (Chung, Bemak, & Grabosky, 2011). Furthermore, heated debate usually surrounds the issues concerning migration and refugees which can give rise to a culture of fear of foreigners and the possibility that they may be terrorists (Bemak & Chung, 2017). This may affect mental health practitioners on a conscious or subliminal level thus inhibiting their work with refugee clients. Practitioners working with refugees must be keenly aware of their own political knowledge and value system in order to prevent buying into xenophobia and intolerance (Chung, Bemak, & Grabosky, 2011).

Adopting a Culturally Sensitive Lens

Therapy frameworks have long been criticized for being coined from a primarily Western and Caucasian perspective. While the core principles of these frameworks are important to understand in the application of techniques, it is also important to adapt strategies to fit multiple cultural backgrounds and issues. Over recent years, research has increasingly focused on identification of cultural variation in trauma and recovery models in order to make informed treatment approaches.

Cultural Formulation Interview

One of the results of this is the Cultural Formulation Interview (CFI) which has been included in the DSM 5. The CFI offers an assessment tool to assist practitioners during initial assessments in exploring cultural and social issues relevant to the client's cultural background (Crock, 2015). Although not all practitioners would utilize this but an understanding of the categories covered in understanding a person's cultural background would assist providing an example of factors to consider not only during the initial assessment but also throughout the therapeutic process.

Multiphase Model of Psychotherapy, Counseling, Social Justice, and Human Rights

The Multiphase Model of Psychotherapy, Counseling, Social Justice and Human Rights coined by Bemak and Chung (2017) is a framework that allows mental health practitioners to take into account various factors when working with refugee clients. This framework is made up of five phases; 1) the mental health education, 2) individual, group and/ or family psychotherapy, 3) cultural empowerment, 4) indigenous healing as well as 5) social justice and human rights. These phases may be used concurrently or sequentially. The MPM emphasizes the importance of core therapeutic principles including the introduction and education on basic therapeutic practice such as confidentiality, intake assessments, interpreter role and the counseling process. Although explained in the initial phase, these concepts may be reintroduced continually throughout the therapeutic process. The MPM further highlights the importance of practitioners being familiar with the difficulties in acculturation and to adopt a more case management approach in ensuring refugee clients are able to manage their practical problems such as transportation, medical care and housing. At the same time, practitioners need to be cautious of being totally absorbed in becoming a case manager but rather an information guide to support adjustment.

Mental Health Psychosocial Support Model

Humanitarian agencies have also recognized the importance of mental health interventions and psychosocial support, especially in emergency setting. The Inter-Agency Standing Committee (IASC) has created the Mental Health Psychosocial Support model which captures the importance of inter-agency collaboration in humanitarian emergencies. In this context, emergencies are not constricted to pre-flight but also the disruption of livelihood, family and community structures which plague the life of a refugee. An important point highlighted is the need to focus on local supportive resources and access to said resources instead of focusing solely on the pathology of an impacted group. Bridging a partnership alliance with community organisations and refugee communities can help to reduce isolation and increase social integration (Rousseau, Pottie, Thombs, Munoz, & Jurcik, 2011). Although geared towards humanitarian health workers, it is applicable for other agencies and persons working with refugees to have an understanding of the importance of engaging various organisations and most importantly communities in supporting mental health and psychosocial well-being during emergencies. Figure 1 shows the mental health and psychosocial support (MHPSS) intervention model recommended by the IASC.

The IASC guideline has been found to be particularly useful in practice especially in areas where refugees live as urban refugees.

The Translator as Part of the Therapeutic Process

Working with a translator in delivery of mental health services will require more time allocation. Practitioners cannot ignore the importance the translator plays in building a therapeutic alliance with the client. In fact, research has shown that a good working alliance where all parties establish trust and team support built the foundation for successful therapeutic outcomes (Mirdal, Ryding, & Sondej, 2012). Practitioners will need to take into consideration time constraints when planning each therapy session. It

Figure 1. Mental Health Psychosocial Support (MHPSS) Model

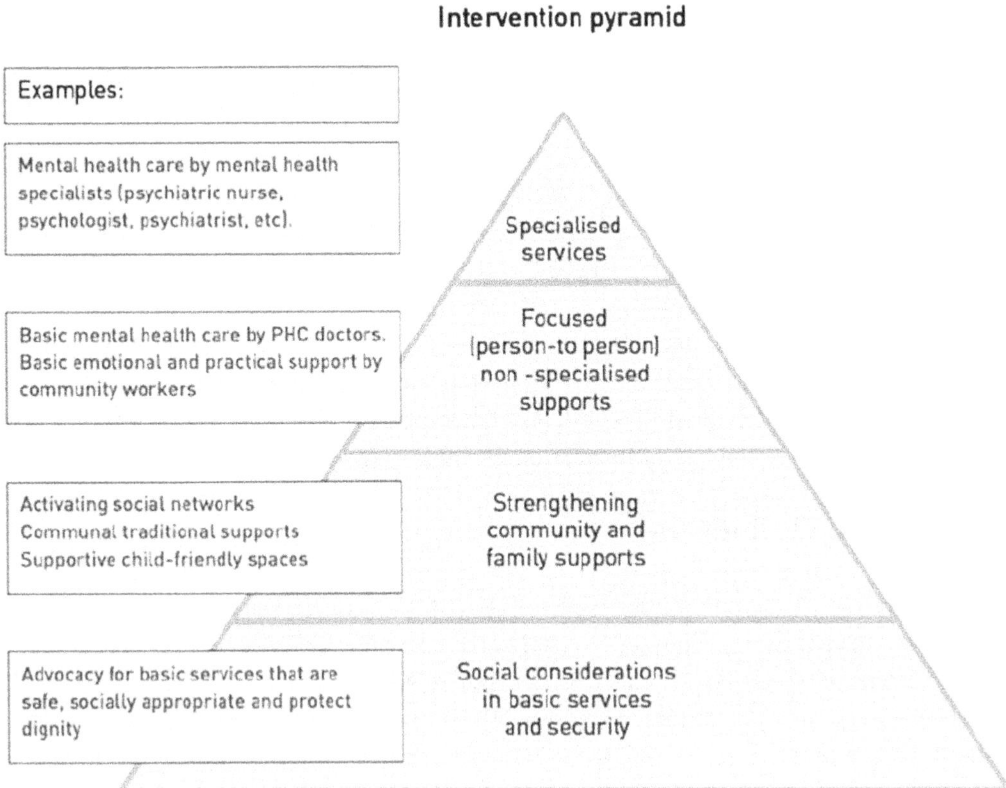

would be useful for practitioners to utilize an extra ten minutes at the beginning and end of each session to develop a working alliance with the translator. The pre-therapy session should be used to review the aim of the session, as well as to clarify technical terminology and cultural factors (Tribe, 2002). Furthermore, practitioners should remember that some translators may hold a refugee status themselves and can thus be vulnerable to vicarious trauma from listening to the client's story in therapy. Thus, it would be recommended to treat the post-therapy session as a debrief session for the translator and practitioner.

If practitioners are working with translators who also hold a refugee status, there is a possibility that practitioners may be able to enhance their knowledge on the current contextual issues and cultural beliefs that may be pertinent to a client. Maintaining openness to feedback from the translator and being curious about the client worldview can help to build a working relationship with the translator while also deepening knowledge of the refugee world. This can be done by utilizing extra time before and after a session for discussion. At the same time, some clients may not be comfortable working with translators who are from the same community as they may share the same living or community spaces which can cause clients to be unsure if information from the session will be divulged to other community members. Practitioners would need to be alert to any discomfort or less forthcoming clients for issues such as this.

It is important to bear in mind that the constructions of psychological health may be culturally different to those entrenched in psychological theories and modalities that are rooted in Western ideologies. For example, words such as "depression" or "self-awareness" may not have an equivalent in some Myanmar dialects. Often times, words such as this will need to be explained by the emotive content of the word or by using an analogy in order to be understood by the client. Therefore, attempt to use simple words in session. Instead of saying "That must be very depressing." You could choose instead to say "That must have made you very sad/ hurt you a lot." This will greatly assist the interpreter in explaining psychological constructs and the different levels of emotion to the client. Complicated words may confuse the client and could increase the power distance felt between a client and a practitioner who have varying levels of English fluency. Hence, it will also assist the client in understanding and explaining their concerns, thoughts and feelings and can contribute to a stronger therapeutic alliance.

As practitioners we are used to speaking seamlessly with our clients in a language exchange both practitioner and client are fluent in. Translators, however, are not necessarily as fluent in English or other mainstream languages a practitioner would be familiar with. Therefore, translators may not be able to remember all of what the practitioner says, especially if it has been said in long sentences with complicated jargon. Attempt to pause after two to three sentences. Translators need time to translate your thoughts and words to the client. It would also be helpful to keep sentences as short as possible in order to increase ease and efficiency of translation during the session.

Interventions and Techniques

In working with refugees, it would be difficult to ignore the external events and living conditions that take place in the everyday lives of refugee clients (Mirdal, Ryding & Sondej, 2012). The issues in gaining an income, acknowledged refugee status, and accessing health and education, as well as the possible experience of exploitation, discrimination and violence perpetrated by local citizens or within the community all contribute to the progress refugee clients can make within the limited therapeutic sessions we have with them. Hence, it is important to consider taking an integrated approach in order to meet the layered experiences and challenges faced by refugee clients. Commonly used approaches include cognitive behavioral, humanistic and psychodynamic approach (Schweitzer, van Wyk,& Murray, 2015). Additionally, cognitive behavioral therapy (CBT), narrative exposure therapy (NET), eye movement desensitization and reprocessing (EMDR) and testimonial psychotherapy have been recommended therapies for working with refugees (Ehnholt & Yule, 2006). However, though refugees come from a homogenous experience of fleeing persecution, each individual may have a very different experience and response to the experiences they have had. These techniques could also include expressive work such as imagery, metaphors, storytelling and psychodrama. An overview will be given for several of these approaches, however, practitioners should bear in mind that research is still emerging in this arena and that the following approaches are not the only ones that may be applicable for working with all refugee clients.

Humanistic Approach

As mentioned before, the therapist ability to connect with the client plays a major role in successful therapeutic outcome. Reflecting the core Rogerian conditions of congruence, unconditional positive regard and empathic understanding would be a basic foundation in working with refugees which need to be done in alliance with the interpreter. Being genuine and authentic have been shown to be the main underlying component in working with refugees which can be the foundations in providing a sense of safety to refugee clients who have had complicated experiences of loss, violence and trauma (Schweitzer, van Wyk, & Murray, 2015). Further, implementing equality between client and practitioner is imperative, particularly in working with refugees. A power distance would keenly be felt in this context where the practitioner is not only deemed more knowledgeable but is also an individual with more rights in the host country. Refugees may be more inclined to feel indebted or the need to comply or withhold information for fear of either not receiving further assistance or incurring other protection issues. Whilst implementing these core principles can assist in building a therapeutic environment favourable to a successful outcome, it would be important to note that practitioners may at times need to take on a more directional approach with refugees, particularly in crisis situations or in advocating on a larger sphere for refugee rights or access to basic needs.

Person Centered Therapy has also been expanded to include person centered expressive art therapy (Corey, 2013). This technique builds on the creative process as a way to transform and heal and ultimately personal growth by integrating the cognition, emotion, bodily and spiritual factors of an individual. Integrating expressive techniques with other therapeutic frameworks may be necessary especially if working with clients who find it difficult to verbalize thoughts and emotions. An overview of expressive techniques will be provided later in the chapter.

Behaviorism Approach

There are concerns that exposure techniques may not be best suited to treatment of trauma in refugees. Exposure techniques often focus on one traumatic event which is not applicable to refugees who have intersecting and complex trauma histories. Additionally, refugees typically receive treatment whilst still in unstable situations in new host countries which further complicate the ability to treat one issue whilst the client is facing a myriad of other threats. However, EMDR has shown improvements in PTSD rates amongst Syrian refugees who showed improvements on the Impact of Events Scale -Revised (IES-R) and Beck's Depression Inventory (BDI) (Lehnung, Shapiro, Schreiber, & Hofmann, 2017). At the same time, bear in mind that refugee clients come from different cultural background and may have difficulty in verbalizing their experience and emotions surrounding a traumatic event. Adopting a trauma-focused psychotherapy approach combined with art therapy has been shown to be more effective in reducing trauma symptoms than only relying on trauma-focused psychotherapy (Schouten, de Niet, Knipscheer, Kleber, & Hutschemaekers, 2014). Furthermore, it would be important to implement a phased method of treating PTSD. Phase one would first require a removal or minimising of risk of trauma, providing coping methods to reduce symptoms and skills training. Only then can the second phase of processing traumatic memories and third phase that focuses on social and psychological reintegration take place (Heide, Mooren, & Kleber, 2015). Whilst it may be challenging to totally remove the risk of trauma, practitioners can work on assisting clients to source for other networks that can provide some support for their basic needs. Examples include safer living spaces, supportive community organisations or members or medical assistance.

Cognitive Behavior Therapy

Culturally adaptive CBT model, or CA-CBT, may be more effective in working with refugee clients (Hinton, Rivera, Hofmann, Barlow, & Otto, 2012). This model highlights the role of arousal and somatic symptoms using an arousal triad to explain how physical symptoms are produced as well as a multisystem model to show how therapeutic techniques can improve physical symptoms. It may also be particularly useful in addressing PTSD amongst Southeast Asian refugees by explaining catastrophic thinking of physical sensations and the spiral of panic (Hinton, Chhean, Pich, Safren, Hofmann, & Pollack, 2005). Many refugee clients may not understand the physical distress and its link to other internal emotional and cognitive distress. This could be due to lack of mental health knowledge, literacy rate, access to education or cultural beliefs. An example of this is a young woman living as a refugee who was diagnosed with depression and generalized anxiety but who also experienced seizure like symptoms and tremors for many years. It was only after several sessions did she reveal that she had deep fear of being abandoned by her partner due to previous issues of infidelity. This also led to issues of not feeling worthy enough for her partner. Coupled with the unstable and harsh realities of living as an urban refugee and coping with separation from family, it had led to other relationship discord. This had a profound effect by manifesting as conversion disorder in order to gain affirmation in the form of care and attention from her partner. By working through the emotional and thought pattern she had and providing relaxation techniques, symptoms of seizure and tremors gradually decreased.

Mindfulness Therapy

The practice of mindfulness training has been shown to be effective in reducing PTSD rates (Marzabadi & Hashemi, 2014). By addressing health from a biopsychosocial approach by assisting an individual to understand their emotions, to accept experiences as it is and to focus their attention it assists refugee clients in building a holistic understanding of the experiences they have had. It also assists in better understanding physical symptoms and therefore a more coherent mindset towards leading a more efficient life outside of therapy. This may be a more appropriate technique in working with refugee communities who experience panic attacks, anxiety and to combat some PTSD symptoms as it introduces the concept of mental health and its effect on the body thereby affirming the manifestation of psychosomatic symptoms.

Narrative Therapy

As previously mentioned, exposure techniques may not necessarily be applicable to refugee clients as these techniques usually address one traumatic experience at a time. However, the creation of an exposure technique that combines individual narratives coined as Narrative Exposure Therapy (NET) has shown to be effective with refugees and asylum seekers. NET was originally designed to provide intervention for survivors of organized violence when faced with limited professional resources to address their needs (Hijazi, Lumley, Ziadni, Haddad, Rapport & Arnetz, 2014; Schaur, Neuner & Elbert, 2005). It is a short term therapy meant for individuals suffering from PTSD through emotional exposure to traumatic memories, and reorganizing said memories into a coherent and chronological narrative (Robjant & Fazel, 2010). Techniques include fusing emotional processing with expressive writing which may imply that clients whose cultural background value history telling may find this approach more socially acceptable (Hijazi et al., 2014). It has been found to be effective when used with both adults and children. At the same time, practitioners who are interested in employing this methodology may need to practice caution when working with refugee clients who live in a country that may not be socially or economically supportive of refugees as this may lead refugee clients to experience increased and consistent victimization and thus aggravate the original trauma experienced. The lack of medical attention, poverty, and malnutrition may restrict impact of any psychosocial intervention (Neuner, Schauer, Klaschik, Karunakara, & Elbert, 2004).

Expressive Techniques

Techniques utilizing art may be especially useful for clients who are less verbal and particularly for survivors of gender based violence and children. Providing clients with the space to express their emotions and thoughts in a non-verbal way will be useful. It can also provide clients a space to assert control of how they express themselves and a way to assert themselves. Art techniques utilized in therapy can also be a way for bridging the gap between refugee parents and their children communication especially when a family has newly arrived in a host country. Combining hope based theoretical framework together with art based techniques (producing a hope quilt, allowing children to take photographs of their lives) and then discussing these elements with the child and later their parents have helped refugee children and parents to be more aligned in hope and strength in order to assimilate better into a host country (Yohani, 2008). At the same time, art based techniques may need to be paired with other frameworks in order to facilitate the journey towards healing. There are several frameworks that have been found to be useful in combination with art techniques. One of them is solution focused art therapy (Moosa, & Koonrankot, 2017). Another is the usage of mandala art therapy in assisting refugees to find safety in a new host country by finding safety and reclaiming their identity and empowerment despite having traumatic migration experiences (Ely, Koury, Bennett, Hartinger, Green, & Nochajski, 2017).

Finding safety is a core issue for refugees living in asylum, particularly urban refugees who do not have the relative safety of a refugee camp to depend on. Previous group work utilizing art based techniques conducted by the author and a group of community health workers with a group of refugee women is an example of this. This group women lived in a high risk urban area that was known for high crime rate and densely populated with drug users. They spent most of the day alone at home with their children whilst their husbands were at work. Many had experienced assault and robbery. It was difficult for many of the group members to acknowledge difficult emotions including fear and even anger. One of the sessions included using plasticine to model their experience of being robbed or assaulted. Some art products included abstract forms and even prison bars. The emotions evoked during and after the activity were discussed and group members were then invited to do whatever they liked with it before collecting it into a basket. Some gently set it aside, others split it into two pieces thus showing the varying reactions each member had to their current situation. This was also processed. The activity allowed group members to acknowledge the emotions and stress they were experiencing towards their current context in a non-threatening and overly verbal way which is the beginning of finding emotional release and coping methods in the situation they were placed.

Implications for Practice

One of the first ideas you may have as a therapist working with refugees is to contact the respective embassy of your client. This is the least helpful approach to take. Many refugees have fled their home country for fear of their lives due to persecution at the hands of their government or fellow citizens. Thus, refugees are usually in fear that their embassy may locate them and taking action against them and their families (Tribe, 2002). Proceeding with this approach, especially without a client's consent, may impact the formation of therapeutic alliance and further deter the client from continuing to further sessions. Instead, consider contacting organisations such as United Nations High Commissioner for Refugees, and a range of local non-governmental organisations that cater to assisting migrants and refugees.

A main point highlighted by many researchers and practitioners in the medical and psychology field is the importance of psychoeducation for refugee clients and community members (Giacco, Laxhman, & Priebe, 2017; Dotevall, Winberg, & Rosengren, 2017). Providing psychoeducation may increase the likelihood that refugees will access mental health services during asylum or resettlement. This is inclusive of providing brief information on psychological issues refugees may experience and how to seek help. It is particularly important to provide psychoeducation when it comes to treatment adherence of psychotropic medication. This may include the need to include family or community members who can assist the client in adhering to treatment. For instance, a client who is experiencing psychosis will not be oriented to time, date or place and will need assistance from family, friends or community member in adhering to psychotropic treatment in order to reduce psychotic symptoms. Similarly, a client who is elderly and experiencing depression may not only need assistance in taking the right dosage at the right time but also physical assistance and increased emotional support.

Practitioners may be inclined to place clients from the same country in the same therapy group when conducting group therapy. This may be a risky strategy as refugees may have been forced to flee due to reports on their religious, political and ethnic views thus leading refugees to have mistrust towards members of the same national background. Refugees may also be anxious that their personal information may fall into the wrong hands and thus endanger them or the lives of their family in their home country (Tribe, 2002). However, it is not impossible for group therapy or support groups to succeed. For example, due to the nature of political unrest in Sri Lanka, Sri Lankan refugees may have more challenges building a supportive environment even within a support group. One of the key elements that assisted members of this group to move beyond initial prejudices and fears was the sensitive practitioner who understood the nuances of the political situation in Sri Lanka and chose instead to build on commonalities within the group. Building on common experiences of loss, violence and challenges experienced living as a refugee helped the members of this group to extend emotional support to one another.

Additionally, practitioners need to be alert to the impact of cultural patterns, both positive and negative, on a client (Bala & Kramer, 2010). Whilst practitioners should be aware of cultural practices and differences of a client's background, it should not necessarily stop practitioners from addressing and even challenging the negative impact of cultural practices and beliefs. In order to do so, practitioners may need to consult with members of the same ethnic community, including trusted family members or friends of a client in understanding and possibly challenging certain beliefs and behaviors. For example, while some cultures may be more open to a husband physically reprimanding his wife, in many countries this is defined as domestic violence. Most Southeast Asian countries view this as a crime and have legal ramifications. Practitioners may need to confront the seriousness of these actions and its legal and practical implications in the host country. Likewise, some countries may be more open to indulging recreational use of drugs. Again, these are behaviors which can not only negatively implicate a client in the eyes of the law but can also induce negative coping methods which can lead to other mental health challenges such as addiction and drug induced psychosis. As a consequence of this, it can add issues in maintaining a job, income and also decrease the cognitive functioning of an individual. Additionally, it may affect the likelihood of resettlement as a durable solution for the client as countries of resettlement have strict criteria on the sociodemographic and health background of refugees accepted.

Furthermore, services and interventions for refugees are usually clustered within certain geographical areas. Most organizations offering medical, legal and protection services for refugees are clustered around major city centres. This is inclusive of UNHCR that may only have one branch office in some countries. This can leave many refugees with limited knowledge and access to much needed services.

As an illustration, refugees who work in plantations or on fishing boats may have the tendency to have drug misuse issues as a result of working in lonely spaces for long hours. However, due to their far out location, they would have low knowledge on the signs on addiction and withdrawal and how to intervene in such cases. Besides this, refugees needing assistance would need to travel to these areas in order to access much needed service. This can cause many issues for refugees as their safety may not always be guaranteed when travelling, particularly if they are undocumented or living in a country that does not recognize refugees. It would also impact their finances as they would need to utilize their meagre salary in order to take leave from work for several days to conclude their appointment. Complications such as this can result in many refugees choosing to ignore health or mental health ailments until it has become too serious to ignore often times to the detriment of the individual.

In spite of the various experiences and challenges refugees face throughout their journey it is imperative to highlight that not all refugees, though having experienced major loss and even violence, will need therapeutic intervention. Although most refugees share similar experiences, not all experience significant mental distress as a consequence. It would be practical to first consider the individual's journey, current contextual factors and personality traits before concluding the existence of mental health issues. Drawing from the IASC's MHPSS system, it would be then important to draw on protective factors and preventive measures within the community and individual's life that can assist the client in coping with current challenges.

As mentioned earlier in this chapter, refugees themselves do endeavor to find ways to cope. Some of the factors practitioners may consider are community networks and religion (Nunis, 2017). Refugees typically have a network of contacts and even ethnic and religious organisations specific to their background. It would be beneficial to understand the network of refugee communities and build liaisons with them in order to work together on outreach and support in challenging cases. Local religious organisations are another resource a practitioner can tap into for both community and development support. Further, some refugees may have strong religious or spiritual beliefs. Having a firm belief and faith in God's plan has helped refugees, particularly refugees living in asylum, feel comforted and maintain a sense of hope (Nunis, 2017). These are examples of support systems and coping methods that may exist that can further assist refugee clients. At the same time, not all refugee clients may find these options helpful. Exploring a client's networks and coping mechanisms whilst being aware of cultural differences would be most important in order to help build preventive and supportive measures.

Practitioners would also need to take on a more assertive role in advocating for multi-lingual instrument measures, mitigating social and institutional discrimination, conducting culturally appropriate outreach and placing the client as the cultural expert (Villalbla, 2009). It would be difficult for practitioners to ignore the contextual issues that exacerbate the mental health of refugee clients whilst also attempting to provide services without first understanding the complexity of the social, health and community issues of the refugee client. Practitioners should be prepared to take on a more assertive in advocating for change whilst maintaining the confidentiality of the refugee clients they work with. This includes building networks with both local and international organisations, local refugee communities as well as promoting for the availability and access of services and safe spaces.

FUTURE TRENDS AND CONCLUSION

Moving forward, practitioners would need to take on more assertive roles in ensuring that culturally appropriate interventions for working with refugees and migrants continue to reflect the diversity of the population they work with. More services and information on services should be disseminated to refugee communities and agencies. However, practitioners should keep in mind that not all refugees are fully literate therefore practitioners would have to find different ways of communicating this information, such as pictorial pamphlets or videos (Giacco, Laxhman, & Priebe, 2017). More importantly, practitioners should also be aware of culturally appropriate ways emotions are exhibited before being too quick to diagnose a refugee client.

In the current climate of heated political debate around the refugee crisis and migration policies, practitioners must endeavor to focus instead on the human behind the label of a refugee. Understanding the human aspect of various pre and post migration experiences and current contextual issues should be one of the main aims of practitioners. Practitioners would need to make consistent effort towards understanding patterns of migration, political background of refugee home countries and being adaptable when working with refugee clients. Further, increased efforts should be made in publishing culturally appropriate evidence based strategies in working with refugee clients in order for practitioners to be able to assist clients to cope and heal better throughout the migration journey.

REFERENCES

Akinsulure-Smith, A. M., Dachos, N., & Jones, W. L. (2013). Nah We Yone's De Fambul Camp: Facilitating Resilience in Displaced African Children. *Journal of Immigrant & Refugee Studies*, *11*(3), 221–240. doi:10.1080/15562948.2013.801721

Ali, M., Briskman, L., & Fiske, L. (2016). Asylum Seekers and Refugees in Indonesia: Problems and Potentials. *Cosmopolitan Civil Societies Journal*, *8*(2). doi:10.5130/ccs.v8i2.4883

Arshad, A. H. (2005). *The Protection of Refugee Children in Malaysia: Wishful Thinking or Reality.* Retrieved from http://www.malaysianbar.org.my/human_rights/the_ protection_of_refugee_children_in_malaysia_wishful_thinking_or_reality_.html

Bala, J., & Kramer, S. (2010). Intercultural Dimensions in the Treatment of Traumatized Refugee Families. *Traumatology*, *16*(4), 153–159. doi:10.1177/1534765610369262

Bemak, F., & Chung, R. C. Y. (2017). Refugee Trauma: Culturally Responsive Counseling Interventions. *Journal of Counseling and Development*, *95*(3), 299–308. doi:10.1002/jcad.12144

Borwick, S., Schweitzer, R. D., Brough, M., Vromans, L., & Shakespeare-Finch, J. (2013). Well-Being of Refugees from Burma: A Salutogenic Perspective. *International Migration (Geneva, Switzerland)*, *51*(5), 91–105. doi:10.1111/imig.12051

Chung, R. C. Y., Bemak, F., & Grabosky, T. K. (2011). Multicultural-Social Justice Leadership Strategies: Counseling and Advocacy with Immigrants. *Journal for Social Action in Counseling and Psychology, 3*(1). Retrieved from http://www.psysr.org/jsacp/chung-v3n1-11_86-102.pdf

Corey, G. (2013). *Theory and Practice of Counseling and Psychotherapy*. Brooks/Cole.

Crisp, J. (2017). *An Inside Account of UNHCR's Urban Refugee Policy*. Retrieved from https://www.newsdeeply.com/refugees/community/2017/04/14/an-inside-account-of-unhcrs-urban-refugee-policy

Dotevall, C., Winberg, E., & Rosengren, K. (2017). Nursing Students' Experience with Refugees with Mental Health Problems in Jordan: A Qualitative Control Analysis. *Nurse Education Today, 61*, 155–161. doi:10.1016/j.nedt.2017.11.025 PMID:29207287

Earnest, J., Mansi, R., Bayati, S., Earnest, J. A., & Thompson, S. C. (2015). Resettlement Experiences and Resilience in Refugee Youth in Perth, Western Australia. *BMC Research Notes, 8*(1), 1–10. doi:10.118613104-015-1208-7 PMID:26054946

Ehntholt, K. K., & Yule, W. (2006). Practitioner Review: Assessment and Treatment of Refugee Children and Adolescents Who Have Experienced War-Related Trauma. *Journal of Child Psychology and Psychiatry, and Allied Disciplines, 47*(12), 1197–1210. doi:10.1111/j.1469-7610.2006.01638.x PMID:17176375

El-Shaarawi, N. (2015). Living An Uncertain Future. Temporality, Uncertainty, and Well Being Among Iraqi Refugees in Egypt. *Social Analysis, 59*(1), 38–56. doi:10.3167a.2015.590103

Ely, G. E., Koury, S., Bennett, K., Hartinger, C., Green, S., & Nochajski, T. (2017). "I Feel Like I am Finding Peace": Exploring the Use of a Combined Art Therapy and Seeking Safety Progam with Refugee Support Groups. *Advances in Social Work, 18*(1), 103. doi:10.18060/21130

Farzana, K. F. (2016). Voices of Burmese Rohingya Refugees: Everyday Politics of Survival in Refugee Camps in Bangladesh. *Pertanika Journal of Social Science & Humanities, 24*(1), 131–150. Retrieved from http://ezproxy.help.edu.my:2057/eds/pdfviewer/pdfviewer?vid=2&sid=690dc86c-c8bd-4fae-8c90-9e0e677b12ec%40sessionmgr102

Fazel, M., Wheeler, J., & Danesh, J. (2005). Prevalence of Serious Mental Disorderin 7000 Refugees Resettled in Western Countries: A Systemic Review. *Lancet, 365*(9467), 1309–1314. doi:10.1016/S0140-6736(05)61027-6 PMID:15823380

Francis, J., & Yan, M. C. (2016). Bridging the Gaps: Access to Formal Support Services Among Young African Immigrants and Refugees in Metro Vancouver. *Canadian Ethnic Studies, 48*(1), 77 – 100. Retrieved from: http://ezproxy.help.edu.my:2057/eds/pdfviewer/pdfviewer?vid=5&sid=690dc86c-c8bd-4fae-8c90-9e0e677b12ec%40sessionmgr102

Giacco, D., Laxhman, N., & Priebe, S. (2017). Prevalence of and Risk Factors for Mental Disorders in Refugees. *Seminars in Cell & Developmental Biology*. doi:10.1016/j.semcdb.2017.11.030 PMID:29174456

Gonslaves, C. J. (1992). Psychological Stages of the Refugee Process: A Model for Therapeutic Interventions. *Professional Psychology, Research and Practice, 23*(5), 382–389. doi:10.1037/0735-7028.23.5.382

Goodkind, J. R., Hess, J. M., Isakson, B., LaNoue, M., Githinji, A., Roche, N., ... Parker, D. P. (2014). Reducing Refugee Mental Health Disparities: A Community Based Intervention to Address Postmigration Stressors with African Adults. *Psychological Services*, *11*(3), 333–346. doi:10.1037/a0035081 PMID:24364594

Heide, F. J. J. T., Mooren, T. M., & Kleber, R. J. (2015). Complex PTSD and Phased Treatment in Refugees: A Debate Piece. *Eurpoean Journal of Psychotraumatology, 7*(1). Retrieved From http://www.tandfonline.com/doi/full/10.3402/ejpt.v7.28687%40zept20.2016.7.issue-s1

Hijazi, A. M., Lumley, M. A., Ziadni, M. S., Haddad, L., Rapport, L. J., & Arnetz, B. B. (2014). Brief NarrativeExposure Therapy for Posttraumatic Stress in Iraqi Refugees: A Preliminary Randomized Clinical Trial. *Journal of Traumatic Stress*, *27*(3), 314–322. doi:10.1002/jts.21922 PMID:24866253

Hinton, D. E., Chhean, D., Pich, V., Safren, S. A., Hofmann, S. G., & Pollack, M. H. (2005). A Randomized Controlled Trial of Cognitive-Behavior Therapy for Cambodian Refugees with Treatment Resistant PTSD and Panic Attacks: Across-Over Design. *Journal of Traumatic Stress*, *18*(6), 617–629. doi:10.1002/jts.20070 PMID:16382423

Hinton, D. E., Rivera, E., Barlow, D. H., & Otto, M. W. (2012). Adapting CBT for Traumatized Refugees and Ethnic Minority Patients: Examples from Culturally Adapted CBT (CA- CBT). *Transcultural Psychiatry*, *49*(2), 340–365. doi:10.1177/1363461512441595 PMID:22508639

Horyniak, D., Melo, J. S., Farrell, R. M., Ojeda, V. D., & Strathdee, S. A. (2015). Epidemiology of Substance Use among Forced Migrants: A Global Systematic Review. *PLoS One*, *11*(7), 1–34. doi:10.1371/journal.pone.015913 PMID:27411086

Inter-Agency Standing Committee. (2010). *Mental Health and Psychosocial Support in Humanitarian Emergencies: What Should Humanitarian Health Actors Know?* Retrieved from: www.who.int/mental_health/emergencies/what_humanitarian_health_actors_should_ know.pdf

James, K. (2010). Domestic Violence Within Refugee Families: Intersecting Patriarchal Culture and the Refugee Experience. *ANZJFT Australian and New Zealand Journal of Family Therapy*, *31*(3), 275–284. doi:10.1375/anft.31.3.275

Kartal, D., & Kiropoulos, L. (2015). Effects of Acculturative Stress on PTSD, Depressive and Anxiety Symptoms Among Refugees Resettled in Australia and Austria. *European Journal of Psychotraumatology*, *7*, 1–11. doi:10.3402/ejpt.v7.28711 PMID:26886488

Knezevic, B., & Olson, S. (2014). Counseling People Displaced by War: Experiences of Refugees from the Former Yugoslavia. *The Professional Counselor*, *4*(4), 316–331. doi:10.15241/bkk.4.4.316

Lauritzen, C., & Sivertsen, H. (2012). Children and Families Seeking Asylum in Northern Norway: Living Conditions and Mental Health. *International Migration (Geneva, Switzerland)*, *50*(6), 195–210. doi:10.1111/j.1468-2435.2012.00774.x

Lehnung, M., Shapiro, E., Schreiber, M., & Hofmann, A. (2017). Evaluating the EMDR Group Traumatic Episode Protocol with Refugees: A Field Study. *Journal of EMDR Practice and Research*, *11*(3), 129–139. doi:10.1891/1933-3196.11.3.129

Mann, C. M., & Fazil, Q. (2006). Mental Illness in Asylum Seekers and Refuges. *Primary Care Mental Health, 4*(1), 57 – 66. Retrieved from http://ezproxy.help.edu.my:2057/ eds/pdfviewer/pdfviewer?vid=2&sid=d6f96970-d20c-4eb3-9fbf-a522f8dd2 30e%40sessionmgr103

Marzabadi, E. A., & Hashemi, S. M. (2014). The Effectiveness of Mindfulness Training in Improving the Quality of Life of the War Victims with Post Traumatic Stress Disorder (PTSD). *Iran Journal of Psychiatry, 9*(4), 228 – 236. Retrieved from http://ezproxy.help.edu.my:2057/eds/pdfviewer/pdfviewer?vid=28&sid=ef7edb83-181d-48df-8108-368ddbf3b20e%40sessionmgr104

Mirdal, G. M., Ryding, E., & Sondej, M. E. (2012). Traumatized Refugees, Their Therapists, and Their Interpreters: Three Perspectives on Psychological Treatment. *Psychology and Psychotherapy. Research and Practice, 85*, 436–455. doi:10.1111/j.2044- 8341.2011.02036.x PMID:23080532

Miremadi, S., Ganesan, S., & McKenna, M. (2011). Pilot Study of the Prevalence of Alcohol, Substance Use and Mental Disorders in a Cohort of Iraqi, Afghani and Iranian Refugees in Vancouver. *Asia-Pacific Psychiatry, 3*(3), 137–144. doi:10.1111/j.1758-5872.2011.00136.x

Moosa, A., & Koorankot, J. K. N. (2017). Solution Focused Art Therapy Among Refugee Children. *Indian Journal of Health and Wellbeing, 8*(8), 811 – 816. Retrieved from http://ezproxy.help.edu.my:2057/eds/pdfviewer/pdfviewer?vid=0&sid=3f93fbb4-6a8f-49e2-ae1f-6f940b69925e%40sessionmgr120

Nah, A. M. (2010). Refugees and Space in Urban Areas in Malaysia. *Forced Migration Review, 1*(34), 29 – 31. Retrieved from: http://ezproxy.help.edu.my:2057/ eds/pdfviewer/pdfviewer?vid=6&sid=60d55cda-e435-419d-94ce-cc2b503ff642%40sessionmgr102&hid=120

Neuner, F., Schauer, M., Klaschik, C., Karanukara, U., & Elbert, T. (2004). A Comparison of Narrative Exposure Therapy, Supportive Counseling, and Psychoeducation for Treating Posttraumatic Stress Disorder in an African Refugee Settlement. *Journal of Consulting and Clinical Psychology, 72*(4), 579–587. doi:10.1037/0022-006X.72.4.579 PMID:15301642

Nunis, A. (2017). *The Lived Experience of Refugees (Illegal Immigrants): A Malaysia Context* (Unpublished Dissertation). HELP University, Kuala Lumpur, Malaysia.

Phillips, J. (2011). *Asylum seekers and refugees: What are the facts? Background note, Parliamentary Library, Parliament of Australia, Canberra*. Retrieved from http:// www.aph.gov.au/library/pubs/BN/sp/Asylumfacts.htm

Priebe, S., Giacco, D., & El-Nagib, R. (2017). Public Health Aspects of Mental Health Among Migrants and Refugees: A Review of the Evidence of Mental Health Care for Refugees, Asylum Seekers and Irregular Migrants in the WHO European Region. *Health Evidence Network Synthesis Report, 47*. Retrieved from https://www.ncbi.nlm.nih.gov/books/NBK391045/

Robjant, K., & Fazel, M. (2010). The Emerging Evidence for Narrative Exposure Therapy: A Review. *Clinical Psychology Review, 30*(8), 1030–1039. doi:10.1016/j.cpr.2010.07.004 PMID:20832922

Rousseau, C., Pottie, K., Thombs, B. D., Munoz, M., & Jurcik, T. (2011). *Post Traumatic* Stress Disorder: Evidence Review for Newly Arriving Immigrants and Refugees. *Canadian Medical Association Journal, 11*(Appendix). Retrieved from http://www.cmaj.ca/content/suppl/2010/06/07/cmaj.090313.DC1/imm-ptsd-11-at.pdf

Sarfo-Manch, A. G. (2009). *Coping Methods and Meaning Making of Liberian Refugees in the Buduburam Refugee Camp of Ghana.* Retrieved from http://digitalcommons.uconn.edu/cgi/viewcontent.cgi?article=1113&context=srhonor _theses

Schouten, K.A., de Niet, G.J., Knipscheer, J.W., Kleber, R.J., & Hutschemaekers, G.J.M. (2014). The Effectiveness of Art Therapy in the Treatment of Traumatized Adults: A Systemic Review on Art Therapy and Trauma. *Trauma Violence and Abuse*, 1 - 9. doi:10.1177/1524838014555032

Schweitzer, R., van Wyk, S., & Muray, K. (2015). Therapeutic Practice with Refugee Clients: A Qualitative Study of Therapist Experience. *Counselling & Psychotherapy Research*, *15*(2), 109–188. doi:10.1002/capr.12018

Schweitzer, R. D., Brough, M., Vromans, L., & Asic-Kobe, M. (2011). Mental Health of Newly Arrived Burmese Refugees in Australia: Contributions of Pre-Migration and Post Migration Experience. *The Australian and New Zealand Journal of Psychiatry*, *45*(4), 299–307. doi:10.3109/00048674.2010.543412 PMID:21303193

Shakespeare-Finch, J., Schweitzer, R. D., King, J., & Brough, M. (2014). Distress, Coping and Posttraumatic Growth in Refugees from Burma. *Journal of Immigrant & Refugee Studies*, *12*(3), 311–330. doi:10.1080/15562948.2013.844876

Sourander, A. (2002). Refugee Families During Asylum Seeking. *Nordic Journal of Psychiatry*, *57*(3), 203–207. doi:10.1080/08039480310001364 PMID:12775295

Suara Rakyat Malaysia. (2014). *Malaysia Human Rights Report.* Retrieved from http://www.suaram.net/wordpress/wp-content/uploads/2015/09/HR2014-lowres.pdf

Suara Rakyat Malaysia. (2015). *Malaysia Human Rights Report.* Retrieved from http://www.suaram.net/wordpress/wp-content/uploads/2017/02/HR2015.pdf

Tappis, H., Biermann, E., Glass, N., Tileva, M., & Doocy, S. (2012). Domestic Violence Among Iraqi Refugees in Syria. *Health Care for Women International*, *33*(3), 285–297. doi:10.1080/07399332.2011.645969 PMID:22325027

Tribe, R. (2013). Mental Health of Refugees and Asylum Seekers. *Journal of Continuing Professional Development*, *8*, 240–247. doi:10.1192/apt.8.4.240

Ullmann, E., Barthel, A., Tache, S., Bornstein, A., Licino, J., & Bornstein, S. R. (2015). Emotional and Psychological Trauma in Refugees Arriving in Germany in 2015. *Molecular Psychiatry*, *20*(12), 1483–1484. doi:10.1038/mp.2015.164 PMID:26527128

United Nations High Commissioner for Refugees. (2010). *Convention and Protocol Relating to the Status of Refugees.* Retrieved from: http://www.unhcr.org/en-my/3b66c2aa10

United Nations High Commissioner for Refugees. (2016). *Global Trends Forced Displacement in 2016.* Retrieved from: http://www.unhcr.org/globaltrends2016/

United Nations High Commissioner for Refugees. (2017a). *UNHCR in Malaysia.* Retrieved from: https://www.unhcr.org.my/About_Us-@-UNHCR_in_Malaysia.aspx

United Nations High Commissioner for Refugees. (2017b). *Schools for Refugee Children*. Retrieved from: https://www.unhcr.org.my/Education-@-Schools_For_Refugee_Children.aspx

United Nations High Commissioner for Refugees. (2018a). *UNHCR Population Statistics*. Retrieved from: http://popstats.unhcr.org/en/overview#_ga=2.251604486.1844780328.1522565339-7275457.1483770482

United Nations High Commissioner for Refugees. (2018b). *Figures at a Glance in Malaysia*. Retrieved from: http://www.unhcr.org/en-my/figures-at-a-glance-in-malaysia.html

Vijayakumar, L. (2016). Suicide Amongst Refugees – A Mockery of Humanity Crisis. *Journal of Crisis Intervention and Suicide Prevention*, *37*(1), 1–4. doi:10.1027/0227-5910/a000385 PMID:27033678

Villalbla, J. A. (2009). Addressing Immigrant and Refugee Issues in Multicultural Counselor Education. *Journal of Professional Counseling: Practice, Theory and Research*, *37*(1), 1 – 12. Retrieved from http://ezproxy.help.edu.my:2057/eds/pdfviewer/pdfviewer?vid=33&sid=ef7edb83-181d-48df-8108-368ddbf3b20e%40sessionmgr104

Vogel, S. (2016). Working with People who Identify as Asylum Seekers or Refugees. *Gestalt Journal Of Australia & New Zealand*, *12*(2), 83-100. Retrieved from http://ezproxy.help.edu.my:2052/eds/pdfviewer/pdfviewer?vid=1&sid=a0d7a383-ea6a-4ec6-bd990ad8ad602574%40sessionmgr4008&hid=4205

Wessels, W. K. (2014). *The Refugee Experience: Involving Pre-Migration, In Transit, and Post Migration Issues in Social Services*. Retrieved from: http://sophia.stkate.edu/cgi/viewcontent.cgi?article=1411&context=msw_papers

Yohani, S. C. (2008). Creating An Ecology of Hope: Arts-Based Interventions with Refugee Children. *Child & Adolescent Social Work Journal*, *25*(4), 309–323. doi:10.100710560-008-0129-x

Chapter 9
Living With Cerebral Palsy in Malaysia:
Me, Myself, and Others

Rajvin Kaur Randhawa
HELP University, Malaysia

Kiirtaara Aravindhan
HELP University, Malaysia

ABSTRACT

The authors in this chapter highlights the reality of cerebral palsy in Malaysia. The chapter is a blend experiential account and factual details. The experiential fragment includes a personal case study, providing 32 years' worth of experience and first-hand details on the life of a cerebral palsy individual in Malaysia. The factual fragment provides researched information on the general reality of cerebral palsy in Malaysia, which includes regulations, existing services and support systems, ergonomics, awareness, and inclusion. This chapter also includes an interview with a fellow CP individual. The chapter ends with an interesting take-home message that aims to encourage and motivate those negatively affected.

WHAT IS CEREBRAL PALSY?

Most people are probably familiar with the term Cerebral Palsy (CP). However, not everyone is familiar with the etiological concept of CP and how an individual with CP is affected. Therefore before delving any further, let us begin by explaining what is CP all about.

Pathologically, cerebral palsy is defined as an abnormality of motor function. It refers to the inability to move and control movements or loss of muscle control due to damage on one or more parts of the brain (Richard & Malouin, 2013). Severity and the muscle affected is dependent on which part of the brain has a lesion. It is commonly acquired at the foetal or infant stage, causing issues of sensation, feeling, perception, cognition, communication, and behaviour (Richards & Malouin, 2013). Cerebral palsy is a non-progressive condition, meaning that it does not worsen or change over time.

DOI: 10.4018/978-1-5225-6073-9.ch009

Classification of Cerebral Palsy varies. MyChild at Cerebralpalsy.org (n.d.) in their website provides excellent explanation on these classifications. According to their website, some are classified according to severity, topographical distribution, motor function and based on The Gross Motor Function Classification System (GMFCS). Topographical distribution in laymen terms can be described as which part of the body is affected.

It is important to understand that there are two different terms to describe how the body is affected; Plegia, meaning paralyzed; and Paresis, meaning weakened. If just one part of the body is affected, it is monoplegia or monoparesis. Diplegia or diparesis is when the legs are affected more than the arms. Quadriplegia or quadriparesis is when all four limbs are affected. There is also hemiplegia or hemiparesis, where a vertical half of the body, meaning the arm and leg on one side of the body is affected. Paraplegia or paraparesis describes the lower half of the body, which includes both legs affected (MyChild at Cerebralpalsy.org, n.d.).

Under motor functions, one can be spastic or non-spastic. Spastic CP is when there is an increase in muscle tone also known as hypertonia whereas non-spastic means muscle tonus fluctuates or decreases often referred to as hypertonia. Muscle tone is essential in contraction and relaxation of the muscles, for the muscles to work together. In spastic CP, the muscles are always contracting. Therefore, the limbs become tensed and resistant to movement. Even if there were movements, they are irregular and jerky (MyChild at Cerebralpalsy.org, n.d.).

CEREBRAL PALSY IN MALAYSIA: AN OVERVIEW

Regulations

Malaysia signed the Convention on the Rights of Persons with Disabilities (CRPD) on the 8th of April 2008 and later ratified the convention on the 19th of July 2010. The signing of the convention led to the establishment of The Persons with Disability Act 2008. The Persons with Disability Act 2008 is "an Act to provide for the registration, protection, rehabilitation, development and wellbeing of persons with disabilities, the establishment of the National Council for Persons with Disabilities (PWD), and for matters connected therewith" (Act 685, 2008). This act has since then provided the legal foundation for policies and legislations concerning disable individuals.

The act defines person with disability as "Those who have long term physical, mental, intellectual or sensory impairments which in interaction with various barriers may hinder their full and effective participation in society." (Act 685, art. 2), therefore includes those with cerebral palsy.

Services and Support System

There are various service and support systems for the disabled community in Malaysia be it governmental or non-governmental organisations.

Governmental Support

A national body, the National Council for Persons with Disabilities was formed in 200, in line with the implementation of PWD Act to oblige and oversee the policies implemented under the Act. The line

Ministry of this body is the Ministry of Women, Family and Community. The minister chairs the council, discussing issues with the disabled community alongside Secretary General of the other ministries involved.

Several ministries have the responsibility to provide for the disabled community, namely; Department of Social Welfare, Ministry of Health, Ministry of Local Government and Housing, Ministry of Rural Development, Inland Revenue Department and Ministry of Education (Special Education). These ministries have implemented policies based on the Person with Disability Act 2008 within various sectors, strictly prohibiting discrimination against the disabled.

Besides that, the government initiated the Kad OKU (Orang Kurang Upaya). Kad OKU, which translates to Card for the Disabled Individual, was issued to those who registered to the Registrar General for Persons with Disabilities. With the card, disabled individuals could enjoy special privileges which includes medical and rehabilitation benefits, occupational training, special needs education, financial support, prosthetics and support gear. These individuals will also be considered for Workers with Disabilities Allowance, care and shelter, training under NGOs, as well as job opportunities (Hussein & Yaacob, 2012). Registration is purely voluntary and eligibility criteria applies.

Non-Governmental Organisation (NGO)

Among non-governmental organisations, there are those that deal with disabilities in general also some that is specific to cerebral palsy. SI World Malaysia, is a non-governmental organisation that provides sensory integration therapy, occupational therapy, speech therapy and physiotherapy for the special needs community. There is also Community-Based Rehabilitation Centre (PDK) Malaysia, a one-stop centre for intervention, advocacy, information and training establishment for the disabled community. They have various centres all around Malaysia and they work closely with the Department of Social Welfare Malaysia.

GAPS (Gabungan Anak-Anak Palsi Serebrum), an organisation that actively provides support to children with cerebral palsy. They conduct regular social media campaigns as well as sports and inclusion activities such as Frame Football and CP Camp. They also have one-stop centres for cerebral palsy, focused on research and development, empowerment and training as well as conductive education.

These are just a fraction of the non-governmental organisations that exist in Malaysia. There is also Sarawak Cerebral Palsy Welfare Association (SCPWA), Hope2Walk, and Malaysian Care to name a few.

Ergonomics

The Malaysian environment is still not very conducive for disabled individuals despite "Accessibility" being a key area in the National Policy for PWD (2007). At most, there are elevators, wheelchair ramps and toilets for the disabled. Conventional schools, tourist hotspots among many others still lack the facilities. Nevertheless, parks in Putrajaya and Kuala Lumpur has the facilities necessary (Hussein & Yaacob, 2012).

As for public transportation, the needs of disabled individuals are still in progress. Rapid KL, a Malaysian transportation agency came up with a prototype of 100 non-step buses with flip-out ramps. But the endorsement was refused by the PWD due to poor design. Yet, the non-step buses still run in several major areas in Klang Valley. Perhaps the only accessible transportation is the LRT and MRT, with elevators available for the disable and parking spaces for the disabled.

Concession parking passes can be obtained when the disable individual shows their Kad OKU. There are several public spaces such as shopping malls and schools that provides disabled parking. However, it is often abused by civilians due to lax in enforcement. Concession fares are also encouraged by the government of Malaysia. MAS airlines offers up to 50% concession for domestic flights. Plusliner bus service also offers 50% concession for the disabled.

Despite various efforts, the existing facilities still pose a barrier to the needs of the disabled as claimed by experts. In an article entitled "Poor Facilities for the Disabled" dated 12th of May 2017 published by the STAR newspaper, Assoc Prof Sabariah Mohamad, supervisor for a study conducted by a group of students from Universiti Teknology Mara (UITM) gave her views. She mentioned that the existing infrastructure in Penang poses confusion and danger for the disabled. Tactile pathways and ramps are just not sufficient (Thevadass, 12 May 2017).

Awareness of Cerebral Palsy

In terms of advocacy for cerebral palsy, there is an organisation called Malaysian Advocates for Cerebral Palsy (MYCP). MYCP is a registered NGO which serves as an advocacy and support groups for individuals with CP and/or family members of those with CP. They also connect families of those with CP to doctors, therapists, educators and activist to reach out and share stories, experiences, views and sentiments. Their main mode of outreach is Facebook but they also conducts talks from time to time.

Some of the NGOs such as GAPS and PDK conduct talks and run campaigns from time to time. There are also blogs written by parents of children with cerebral palsy entailing their experience in efforts of advocating and educating the public. Experts also play their part in raising awareness of cerebral palsy by writing articles online. There is a website portal called MyHealth by the Ministry of Health Malaysia which discusses cerebral palsy among many other disorders.

Awareness of cerebral palsy in Malaysia is still a work in progress. It is difficult to gauge. However, there are speculations of lack of awareness among civilians. An article entitled "*Study shows that Malaysians don't understand disability*" was published on the 21st of November 2017 in the Malaysian local newspaper, STAR. The article explains that the concept of disability, which includes CP has yet to be grasped by Malaysians (Indramalar, 21 November 2017)

Inclusion

The level of awareness is also related to inclusion of the CP individuals in Malaysia. The government of Malaysia has devised policies in attempt to look after the needs of the disabled so that they would not be left out.

However, the perception of Malaysians towards the disabled community still needs to be improved. An interview with Maniam Sinnasamy, Project Manager, United Nations Development Programme (UNDP) Malaysia was conducted by Dorodi Sharma of Disability News and Information Service (2010). In the interview, Maniam mentions that the needs of the disabled are viewed as welfare services by the state and NGOs. Disabled individuals would prefer that these needs are observed as equal rights instead of a form of support (DNIS, 2010).

Reports shows that there is a lack of understanding among the general public. This lack of understanding has resulted in children affected by disabilities to remain hidden, feel isolated and often discriminated. Parents of these children are also constantly left in a dilemma (Indramalar, 21st November 2017)

CEREBRAL PALSY IN MALAYSIA: THROUGH AN EXPERIENTIAL LENS

Rajvin Kaur Randhawa has been living with cerebral palsy for the past thirty-two years. In Rajvin's case, cerebral palsy manifested in her as a neurological condition. She momentarily stopped breathing on the second day after her birth which caused a lack of oxygen to the brain. In that period, her movement, posture, motor skills and muscle tone was affected which then manifested as cerebral palsy. The author's condition is classified as spastic quadriplegia based on her topographical distribution and motor functions. Here, she provides experiential details on living with cerebral palsy in Malaysia.

Challenges Faced

The author, just like many others in Malaysia who suffer from cerebral palsy or other disabilities and in need of special care often face a lot of challenges. This includes physical, emotional, learning among many more. The most common challenge faced by cerebral palsy patients in Malaysia, which the author has experienced herself is societal perception towards CP. Arising alongside these experiences, the author also faced emotional challenges, physical challenges, lack of moral support, issues of accessibility and mobility, transportation difficulties and government/civic support. A more detailed description is illustrated as follows:

Societal Perception Towards CP

Based on the author's opinion and experience, the society sometimes look down on disabled individuals. The author recalls that whenever she goes out to a shopping mall or other places, she is often questioned by a handful of people about her condition. She feels that society should be more aware of the concept of CP by equipping themselves with the knowledge of CP and immersing themselves in the experience so that they will better understand the concept of cerebral palsy.

Those with CP patient or other disabilities are often labelled as handicapped. This leads to prejudice and discrimination, intended to insult the disabled individual. The author, just like many other disabled individual in Malaysia are often filled with fear leading to isolation. She prefers not to mingle with society.

In conclusion, the Malaysian society should take more steps and initiatives to understand the concept of CP and other disabilities specifically by changing their attitude and mind-set towards the disabled. Be positive and treat them like normal people. Cerebral palsy patients and others with disabilities in Malaysia should be accepted just the way they. They should be given equal rights and support despite their disabilities, which is no cause to be shunned in society.

Emotional Challenges

The author, and possibly other disabled individuals in Malaysia often experience emotional challenges such as depression, loneliness and anxiety. The author describes specific challenges below and how she overcame them;

- *Depression.*

Individuals with CP, like the author occasionally experienced depression. This is due to the inability to deal with daily challenges of the disability. The author had an episode of depression. In that period, she began questioning her disability, wondering why she was not normal, where she would not require aid to do things everyone else not affected could do easily.

However, the author eventually dealt with her depressive state by remaining positive. The author changed her perspective towards life, seeing herself as a CP fighter and survivor instead of a victim. She surrounded herself with happy people, which she recommends others with CP do as well. The author also found relaxation techniques to be useful when dealing with her depression. She used breathing techniques to relax herself and maintain a peace within her.

- *Loneliness.*

Loneliness is common among disabled individual due to various reasons. Some experience loneliness after their parent abandon. Some experience loneliness when their parents leave them at home alone for a short while. Negativity and bad thoughts can also cause loneliness. The author however is blessed to be always surrounded by people. However, there are some instances where her loved ones have to travel and she is left alone, experiencing loneliness at that time.

During moments of loneliness, the author coped by keeping busy and doing what she loved. She recommends that keeping busy and doing what a person enjoys doing is the most effective way to curb loneliness. She does things to keep her mind occupied. Her profession as a motivational speaker and writer has kept her company on several occasions. Surrounding yourself with the right people is also important. Whenever the author felt lonely, she would call a friend

- *Anxiety.*

Anxiety involves persistent worrying. CP individuals go through inconsistent muscle tone daily, which is cause for anxiety. Hence, anxiety is common among individuals with CP. Based on the author's personal experience, she consistently faces anxiety but she has a set of practice which helps calm her down.

The author suggests that the best way to overcome anxiety for CP patients and others with disabilities is to be thankful for what we have. She says that "Life with cerebral palsy is a blessing and not a bed full of roses despite challenges thus far" (Kaur Randhawa, 2017).

Opening yourself to making new friends also helps. The author was privileged to be able to mix with people of various age groups and backgrounds. With that, she found true friends that made her life journey more meaningful for the past thirty-two years. The proudly acknowledges that because of her loved ones and true friends, she would consider Cerebral Palsy as a blessing instead of a suffering.

Physical Challenges

Another common challenge for cerebral palsy patients like the author herself lies in the physical domain. For example, the inability to walk and move from one place to another. Hence, she relies on a wheelchair and a walker – while being assisted by another person – to travel from one place to another.

The author also often encounters muscle spasticity, common among cerebral palsy patients. Spasticity is defined as stiffness of the muscles that are often interrupts the ability to control movements. Therefore, treatments such as physiotherapy serves as an important intervention for cerebral palsy patients like the author. The author began physiotherapy at the age of one at the Kuala Lumpur General Hospital and also in 1995. She went to University Malaya Medical Centre (UM) after undergoing a surgery called Selective Dorsal Root Rhizotomy (SDRR) to reduce spasticity from tight muscles.

Initially, the author was clueless about the circumstance of the treatment and was reluctant to do exercise vigorously, due in part to the fact that she was also schooling at the time. She did not attend therapy regularly until 2013. Nevertheless, the author recognises and acknowledges the dedication and encouragement given to her by the Physiotherapist and Occupational Therapist in Rehabilitation Department recently since 2015.

In 2016, the author met her old college friend who became a trainer that changed her life. The author transformed from someone who used to hate exercising to someone who loved it. Ever since, the author's physical capabilities improved drastically and now, she can walk by herself, unassisted, with the walker.

This is evidence of the competency of physiotherapy. The author recommends it for every CP patient and others with disabilities in order to improve the quality of lives.

Learning Challenges

Learning is also a common challenge for cerebral palsy patients like the author and others with disabilities in Malaysia. As a cerebral palsy patient, the author was fortunate, blessed and privileged to receive an inclusive education from kindergarten until University which not many, suffering a similar condition would have had a chance. The author recommends that every patient with CP and others with disabilities to attend mainstream education just like she did if they are able to. Below are the main challenges the author faced from kindergarten up until University level:

- **Acceptance in Society:** In kindergarten, the author had difficulty finding a proper friend that would accept her for her condition. She thanks her beloved mum who had to accompany her in the class the whole day. Nevertheless, she never gave up hope and this helped inculcate the fighting spirit she still has until today. The author had to be given extra time to complete task and examinations such as during public exams and college exams and she passed all these examinations reasonably well. Currently, the author is a motivational speaker and blogger and writer. The author elaborates more on this in the next topic
- **Discrimination:** In primary school, the author was transferred to the slow learners' class, but her parents insisted for her to be in the normal education stream. Eventually she did well and proved everyone wrong and performed better than most other normal children.
- **Unfairness in Society:** In secondary school, the author was given a class on the second floor and she could not walk up the stairs. Hence, her parents had to ask the Parent Teacher Association to

intervene and relocate the class to the ground floor. Many were angry with this decision but eventually relented and agreed to the class relocation.

- **Extra Time to Complete Tasks and Examination:** The author had to be given extra time to complete tasks and examinations especially during UPSR, PMR AND SPM. As much of a hassle it was, she made it through and passed all examinations reasonably well, landing herself in college.

Financial Constraints

The author personally did not go through financial constraint but based on her observation, many individuals with CP faced financial constraints as a challenge. According to a study conducted by UNICEF, some did not have access to special need education and required facilities due to the lack of funds. This applies to both rural and urban communities.

As a CP patient, the author was fortunate to have supportive parents and family who educated her and made sure she graduated with a second class honours degree from Help University. However, she realises that many parents cannot afford to do the same for their disabled child as many work double or triple jobs. Some parents also face difficulties in enrolling their child in a proper school or college.

Personal Support Structure

Having good support structure and moral support is also another integral factor. As a cerebral palsy patient, the author was fortunate enough to get a good support structure that consists of her friends and family who made it possible for her to achieve her dreams of becoming the person she is today.

The author believes that moral support is essential for the achievement of every individuals with disabilities just like herself. In the author's opinion, moral support is defined as emotional or psychological backing as opposed to material help. For example some parents of CP patients are not supportive enough to encourage them to live their dreams despite their challenges. The author was very fortunate to have supportive parents, family and friends who were supportive of her till University level, but there were one or two challenges along the way and even at present such as uncontrollable emotions.

- **Ego:** The author felt like some of her family members felt sorry for the way she was living, especially when she was in primary school. But, the author took it as reason to prove everyone wrong by putting in extra effort to be the person she is today. Her family finally started treating her equally.
- **Anger:** The author is sometimes angry for being the way she is. She gets angry at the fact that it had to be her with cerebral palsy. But, she would then start to reflect on how blessed she was. She had good friends and family around her who constantly tried to put a smile on her face.
- **Resentment:** There are moments where the author was filled with resentment towards God. The author, being a religious often questioned why God is unfair and why God made her the way she is. But, she overcomes the resentment by praying.

Caregivers also play an important role in the lives of cerebral palsy patients and others with disabilities in Malaysia. Based on personal experience, the author is blessed to have good caregivers to take care of her. However, there were a handful of them who didn't treat her well as they didn't know how to handle a CP patient. Therefore, she recommends that cerebral palsy patients and others with disabilities in Malaysia should have good caregivers to take care of them.

Government and Civic Support

The author believes that government and civic support is essential for cerebral palsy patients just like every other disabilities. Government support refers to the initiative and measures taken by the government of Malaysia whereas civic support refers to measures and solutions taken as a collective effort by the people of the community to make the society a conducive environment for the disabled.

Accessibility

Accessibility is the most common challenge faced by cerebral palsy patients like herself and others with disabilities in Malaysia. Some disabled individuals face difficulties finding ramps, lifts and toilets in schools, colleges and other public domains. A lot of work has to be done in some places by the government authorities in Malaysia to make it more disabled friendly. The author personally experiences challenges in public places such as in school or college days or even in shopping malls.

Transportation

Mobility and transportation are the two main challenges faced by cerebral palsy patients like herself and others with disabilities in Malaysia. Most patients like herself find mobility and transportation a great challenge when they have to travel from one place to another using wheelchairs, walkers and taxis. There are many instances where taxis do not want to accept people with special needs. It is something the author personally experienced having been refused many times. A lot of work needs to be done to make travelling easier for persons with disabilities like so that they can manoeuvre themselves easily using public transport.

Therapeutic Staff Support

Therapeutic staff support is essential for those with cerebral palsy and other disabilities. In the author's opinion, therapeutic support refers to workers serving as a team to help disable individuals who have serious emotional problems leading to inappropriate behaviour.

Sometimes a patient with cerebral palsy like the author in Malaysia might act disrupted in schools, home or other public places. Therapeutic staff support professionals play an important role to follow treatment plans advised by other mental health care expert to intervene and change negative actions. Among useful therapeutic staff support based on the author's experience in Malaysia for cerebral palsy patients and others such as follows:

- Counselling and Behaviour therapy
- Writing thoughts in journals
- Calling friends
- Thinking positively

The Role of Counselling

Based on the author's experience, counselling has helped her in numerous ways such as;

Problem-Solving

From her experience, counselling has been the most successful technique in developing self-awareness. Whenever a current problem appears to be at a dead end, she will be able to look at the present instead of the past. Doing so helps her think of solutions.

Positivity

Counselling has made her a positive person despite life's challenges. The author used to be an angry and negative person due to her condition. However, counselling helped her get past her condition and she is not better at managing her emotions.

Stress Management

Through counselling, the author has learnt more effective ways to deal with her stress. She came to understand that by talking to someone, she not only feel relaxed but she is better able to regulate her emotions. Today she finds that she is much happier, which has manifested in her career as a motivational speaker, blogger and writer.

Self-Control

Counselling has helped the author to learn self-control. From her experience counselling has changed her life in a way that she is more in control of the things happening to her.

Communication

Apart from that, counselling has helped her to connect and communicate better with associates, family and true friends and caregivers. Counselling has helped her a lot to become a changed person from the person she was then till the person she is today.

Perseverance Will Prevail

On the 27th of April 2014 the author, Rajvin was among the 1216 candidates to graduate at the Help University's 26th convocation at the Shangri-La Hotel Kuala Lumpur. The author confesses that was the biggest moment in her life. Special thanks to friendly lecturers and helpful best friends who made it easier for her to accomplish her dreams of graduating with a Bachelor of Communications Honours degree majoring in Public Relations. Currently she is a motivational speaker and blogger as well as a writer. The author is so thankful to her family and true friends for making this happen.

Cerebral palsy did not hinder the author from participating in social events and become the person she is today, a motivational speaker. Your condition should not hinder you or others with cerebral palsy and others with disabilities in Malaysia from becoming what they want to be.

The author first started motivational speaking in August 2014 in Bakti Mind where she had to present her thoughts and experiences of being an individual with cerebral palsy in an inclusive society. It was an amazing experience where she dealt with people from all walks of life. It thought her that she wasn't the only one who had problems and to count her blessing. It was an amazing experience as she went up of stage for the first time in front of a large crowd although she was a bit nervous.

The second experience was being appointed as a Good Will Ambassador back in 2014 for My Mobile University and even at present. It is an online learning portal for people with or without disabilities where they can learn for free just about for anything that they are curious to know. It was also an amazing experience where she was asked to talk about various issues that are currently happening among people with disabilities like herself and others in Malaysia. She learnt a lot from there.

One of her recent motivational speaking engagements was in June 2017 among others that were given this year. It was very memorable for her as she had to work with young children aged 9-12 years for the first time where she had to give them tips on how she achieved her small step of success with cerebral palsy at one of the religious centers near where she lived. It was one of the blessed moment as she received a gift from them, the children were so happy that they learnt a lot from her.

Apart from motivational speaking the author is also a writer and a blogger. Among her recent writing engagements was to write about cerebral palsy awareness and many other topics in a magazine called Challenges in conjunction with cerebral palsy awareness month for the whole of October, through writing she learnt how to express herself more and she feels that every cerebral palsy patients and others with disabilities should do the same if they are able to just like herself. In conclusion motivational speaking, blogging and writing has taught the author two important life lessons and she hope others with cerebral palsy and others with disabilities will adopt it too. The life lessons that she learnt through motivational speaking, blogging and writing are such as follows:

1. *To be more confident of yourself when faced with challenges.* To be more confident when dealing with people in a small or large crowd and to carry yourself well in front of others.
2. *Never give up in life no matter what.* Speaking, blogging and writing taught the author an important lesson to not give up hope and have faith in God when faced with happy or sad times.
3. *To be more fluent in speaking, blogging and writing.* Speaking, blogging and writing has taught her to be fluent through practice.

In conclusion, persons with cerebral palsy and others with special needs in Malaysia should be given equal opportunities regardless of the challenges to achieve success just like the author. They deserve to be given unconditional love to have a productive life. As the author mentioned through this case study, cerebral palsy did not and will not ever hinder her from achieving her life goals or her small step of success. She believes in the saying that when" one door shuts another opens." The strength is to make the decisions and move forward. The author's advice to other CP individuals like herself and others is: "Every tomorrow starts with today not yesterday. So keep calm and carry on!"

Her future aspiration is to be more mobile and a successful motivational speaker blogger and writer despite her obstacles under the guidance of her beautiful family, true friends and caregiver.

MENTAL HEALTH CARE RECOMMENDATIONS FOR CEREBRAL PALSY

Mental healthcare is essential for individuals with cerebral palsy. There are different forms on intervention in Malaysia catering to mental needs of those with cerebral palsy, among other disabilities. The recommendation below encompasses the author's opinion of existing interventions, which has proven useful and may be useful to others.

Counselling Therapy

Living with disability can be a taxing experience, mentally and emotionally. Counselling therapy addresses the issues a person with disability may face and helps with the coping process (Stuntzner & Hartley, 2014). There are various notable counselling centres in Malaysia that caters to the mental needs of disabled individuals. Among them includes Malaysian Care, Malaysian Mental Health Association, Enrich Counselling and Therapy Centre.

Based on the author's experience, counselling played a positive role in her journey as an individual with cerebral palsy. It changed her life for the better, in terms of her behavior and outlook towards life. She became more positive and believes that counselling could work wonders for other disabled individuals in Malaysia.

Massage Therapy

Massage therapy is a common complementary form intervention for cerebral palsy. It involves soft tissue manipulation through direct contact manipulation to soothe aching joints and muscles (MyChild at CerebralPalsy.org, n.d.). However, treatment emphasised based on the type of cerebral palsy. For example, in individuals with spastic CP, the emphasis is placed on relaxing tight muscles due to the muscle rigidity and contracture (Gialelis, 2016).

The author has underwent massage therapy. According to her, massage therapy besides being a form of rehabilitation also helped her relax and remain positive. Her movement was also a lot smoother. In Malaysia, there are several massage therapy services provided to kids by organisations such as Tasputra. For adults, there are centres such as Joe's Massage Therapy and Training and the Montaine Centre of Health and Wellness among many others. You can also visit your local chiropractor, hospital or complementary therapists for treatment. However, it is worth recceing to ensure that the massage therapy is conducted by a certified and experienced therapist.

Stress Reduction Techniques

There are a number of stress reduction techniques which includes progressive relaxation, biofeedback, guided imagery, self-hypnosis and deep breathing exercises (National Center for Complementary and Integrative Health, 2016). Stress reduction techniques such as relaxation and breathing techniques has been tried and tested by the author. When she practices relaxation and breathing techniques, she had a clearer viewpoint of situations. She claims that it has helped her calm herself down in countless occasions. Therefore, the author believes that stress reduction techniques will be a useful technique for CP individuals.

Social Therapy

Social anxiety is common among those with cerebral palsy. People with cerebral palsy are often socially awkward and may have trouble mingling with the community. Therefore, social therapy is an intervention that aims to promote positive interaction within social groups. It is a group based intervention, which is based on the needs of a group and the role of the individual in that group. (MyChild at CerebralPalsy.org, n.d.).

The author strongly recommends that individuals CP whom may be facing troubles socially should go for social therapy. Based on the author's experience, CP clients get to interact with people with or without disabilities to gain confidence. She personally found happiness when interacting and felt more confident when she was exchanging thoughts and ideas with individuals with or without disabilities. Every Thursday, the author goes to a gathering known as Sikh Woman Awareness Network, where she could comfortably mingle with others. Thanks to Social Therapy, she is able to have fun and exercise in a group setting.

AN INTERVIEW WITH A FELLOW CP FIGHTER

A short email interview was conducted on the 28th of October 2017 with a young talented women with CP. The respondent was sent a list of well-prepared questions that she had to answer and revert via email. Answers were received on the 3rd of November 2017. The outcome of the interview is as follows;

Question 1

How Well Do You Understand the Concept of Cerebral Palsy?

Respondent believes she understands CP to an extent. She is aware of the different types of CP which relates to the different parts of the brain. Trauma and injury to the certain part of the brain results in impairment of motor functions. The three main types are spastic, ataxic and athethoid. The classification also being more specific based on areas and number of limbs affected. Respondent personally believes that therapies have helped immensely to improve her condition from the way she was before. For her current diagnosis, she is aware she has spastic diplegic cerebral palsy, which mainly affects her lower limbs with minor effect on her upper limbs.

Question 2

Do You Experience Prejudice, Discrimination, Fear and Isolation on a Daily Basis Due to Your Condition?

Respondent admits that prejudice and discrimination is something she can't avoid as it happens on a regular basis. Isolation is very common but she wouldn't let fear dictate her. Because of her condition, the respondent was bullied, rejected, made fun of and disrespected for years. However, she is trying her best to stay positive and move forward while chasing her dreams.

Despite bad experience growing up, respondent's family and close friends were wither entirely to support and provide encouragement. Many of her teachers and lecturers for example has been very supportive as well. Respondent always tried her best to look at the positive regardless of how challenging the situation may be, as advised by her parents. Respondent believes her parent's approach has a lot to do with her positive outlook.

Question 3

Do You Encounter Emotional Challenges in Your Daily Life Such as Depression, Loneliness and Anxiety?

The respondent believes everybody has their own set of emotional challenges but she believes she was not was depressed. She gets stressed and cried when she was frustrated but never allowed herself to stray too far from being positive. The respondent rarely got lonely as her time was occupied with work, study, family, friends and hobbies. She swim and does physiotherapy to keep fit. These things also keep her anxiety at bay. The respondent said that she focused on the things that she does and remained happy.

Question 4

What Kind of Physical Challenges Do You Encounter in Your Daily Life?

Respondent claims that if she had to choose a physical challenge, it would be muscle overstretch or overuse as she walks long distance. Climbing stairs is also a challenge as her ability to balance is not very good. Her poor balancing abilities also prevents her from passing the roadside curbs, especially the high structured ones. She also faces difficulties crossing the ditch-drain, which usually become more challenging on a regular basis.

Performing fine coordination activities has been a challenge to the respondent. It takes her a long time to complete tasks such as typing, writing, sewing, tying shoe laces among many others. This is the reason why she always start her tasks early in the day just so she can complete them. Life has not been easy for her but she is trying to adapt and improvise.

Question 5

How Supportive Is Your Support Structure? What Are the Issues Faced by Your Family and Friends?

The respondent firmly states that support is crucial when you are challenged with a disability. For her, her family and friends are her rock. Her family especially, has sacrificed a lot for her in terms of their time and effort, to make sure that all her physical goals are met on a daily basis. They put so much work and dedication to make sure the therapies sessions happened on schedule and all appointments are one time and went well. School and work can be rough but my friends and colleagues make the coping process bearable

That's why my family and friends are important although there are other people question them for helping me out or be friends with me. They sometimes face isolation themselves but it seems that don't bother them as much every time I have discussions with them about.

Question 6

Do You Experience Any Accessibility Mobility and Transportation Issues Regularly?

According to the respondent, yes, because she usually does not drive long distances. Public transportation sometimes presents their own issues towards disabled people. She just usually relies on family and friends to travel long distances.

Question 7

Do You Receive Any Therapeutic Support?

The respondent does horse riding and swimming. She believes it is therapeutic and keeps her fit.

Question 8

Do You Have Any Final Message to Share With Fellow Individuals With Cerebral Palsy?

Be brave to try something new every day. Small milestones bring small victories. Many small victories build up bigger ones. Smile, dream and believe

ACKNOWLEDGEMENT

Rajvin Kaur Rhandawa

My journey has and will continue to be bumpy, winding and strewn with obstacles on my life's pavement but I am determined to ride on as a CP survivor, motivational speaker, blogger and writer. Rajvin Kaur Randhawa

It is with greatest and deepest gratitude that the author, as a physically challenged individual have made her mantra in the writings of this chapter. The author has so many to thank that the list is endless. God has blessed the author with a very supportive family that is her mum, dad and her siblings as well as her true friends and caregivers. They have been the pillar of strength for her and catered for her needs day in and day out from the first day of school till now and throughout her journey as a CP survivor. Ultimately making her the person she has become today; a motivational speaker, blogger and writer.

Heaven sent is her counsellor and friend, senior lecturer and head of program Associate Professor Dr. Anasuya Jegathevi Jegathesan who has gone out of her way to not only help the author but accommodate all her short comings. She appreciates her continuous encouragement and suggestions to keep her on track to complete her chapter- Living with cerebral palsy in Malaysia. Me, myself and others. She also would like to thank her dad and caregivers for their guidance and see her through her depths of despair when she was stress in the process of writing this chapter. She would like to thank her one and only respondents of the short interview she conducted while email Mastura Binti Mahammad who gave her, her valuable input, time and their cooperation for this effort. Her caregiver for fulfilling all her needs during the process of writing this chapter and always.

A very special vote of thanks to all her true friends who has supported her and always being there for her. Special thanks also to her lifetime best friend and sister Jesvin Kaur who motivated her till today and soldiered her and always especially during the process of doing this chapter. There are many others who have inspired her but the list is too long so, she thanks all of you from the bottom of her heart.

Kiirtaara Aravindhan

Being a Bachelors of Psychology (Hons) graduate and standing at the cross-road of young adulthood, the co-author has been attempting to do something substantial for the society. Therefore when presented with the opportunity to work on this chapter, the co-author felt that it would be a great opportunity to create awareness among society at the same time highlight the struggles of those living with disabilities. The co-author would therefore like to thank beloved mentor, Dr Anasuya Jegathevi Jegathesan for this opportunity and Rajvin Kaur Rhandawa for agreeing to work hand-in-hand. The co-author would also like express gratitude to her beloved family and the handful of friends whom has been nothing short of amazing in terms of encouragement and support.

This chapter is the co-author's first and most exciting works so far. The days spent researching the reality of cerebral palsy in Malaysia and trying to convey the author's experience in a way that sounds experiential yet academic was challenging but insightful. Living with a disorder in Malaysia is definitely not an easy experience but working alongside the author made the co-author realise just how strong of an individual the author truly is. May this chapter serve an influential role in society.

REFERENCES

Alias, R., Alias, N. A., Ibrahim, A. B., Attan, H., & Kadir, A. L. (2013). What do the disabled students need? A study on the needs of the special educational needs (SEN) learners in Malaysian public universities. *The European Journal of Social & Behavioural Sciences*, 603-623.

Disability News and Information Service. (2010). *The needs of disabled persons in Malaysia are still seen largely as a welfare function, Maniam Sinnasamy*. Retrieved from http://www.dnis.org/interview.php?issue_id=6&volume_id=7&interview_id=150

Gialelis, J. (2016). *Massage improves quality of life for the cerebral palsy patients.* Retrieved from https://www.massagemag.com/massage-improves-quality-of-life-for-the-cerebral-palsy-patient-40731/

Hussein, H., & Yaacob, N. M. (2012). Development of accessible design in Malaysia. *Procedia: Social and Behavioral Sciences*, *68*, 121–133. doi:10.1016/j.sbspro.2012.12.212

Indramalar, S. (2017, November 21). Study shows that Malaysians don't understand disability. *The Star Online*. Retrieved from https://www.star2.com/people/2017/11/21/disability-prejudice-malaysia/

Lee, M. N., Abdullah, Y., & Mey, S. C. (2011). Employment of People with Disabilities in Malaysia: Drivers and Inhibitors. *International Journal of Special Education*, *26*(1), 112–124.

Lim, V. W. L., & Staines, A. (2007). Pathways to Services for Children with Cerebral Palsy in Selangor and the Federal Territory, Kuala Lumpur. *The Medical Journal of Malaysia*, *62*(5), 398. PMID:18705475

Malaysia, R. (n.d.). *Persons with disabilities act 2008.* Retrieved from https://relate.com.my/persons-with-disabilities-act-2008/

Malaysiancare.org. (2018). *Service Directory for People with Disabilities.* Retrieved from https://www.malaysiancare.org/pwd_list?pg=8

Mustafa, L. (2017, June 27). Doing more for disabilities. *News Straits Times*. Retrieved from https://www.nst.com.my/news/2017/03/155019/doing-more-disabilities

MyChild at CerebralpPalsy.org. (n.d.). *Massage Therapy*. Retrieved from http://www.cerebralpalsy.org/about-cerebral-palsy/treatment/therapy/massage-therapy

MyChild at CerebralpPalsy.org. (n.d.). *Social Therapy*. Retrieved from http://www.cerebralpalsy.org/about-cerebral-palsy/treatment/therapy/social-therapy

National Center for Complementary and Integrative Health. (2016). *Relaxation Techniques for Health*. Retrieved from https://nccih.nih.gov/health/stress/relaxation.htm

Ong, L. C., Afifah, I., Sofiah, A., & Lye, M. S. (1998). Parenting stress among mothers of Malaysian children with cerebral palsy: Predictors of child-and parent-related stress. *Annals of Tropical Paediatrics*, *18*(4), 301–307. doi:10.1080/02724936.1998.11747964 PMID:9924586

Persons with Disabilities Act. (2008). (Act 685). Retrieved from http://ilo.org/dyn/natlex/docs/ELECTRONIC/86297/97318/F1567227890/MYS86297.pdf

Richards, C. L., & Malouin, F. (2013). Cerebral palsy: Definition, assessment and rehabilitation. *Handbook of Clinical Neurology*, *111*, 183–195. doi:10.1016/B978-0-444-52891-9.00018-X PMID:23622163

RoketKini.Com. (2013). *DAP mohon kerajaan sediakan pendidikan khusus kanak-kanak lumpuh otak atau Cerebral Palsy.* Retrieved from https://www.roketkini.com/2013/10/03/sediakan-pendidikan-cerebral-palsy/

Shen, L. (2014). *Culture and stigma: Social exclusion of families of children with cerebral palsy in China.* Retrieved from https://www.researchgate.net/publication/266784978_Culture_and_stigma_Social_exclusion_of_families_of_children_with_cerebral_palsy_in_China

Sman, C. (2017, April 16). SPWCA seeks greater awareness on CP. *Borneo Post Online*. Retrieved from http://www.theborneopost.com/2017/04/16/scpwa-seeks-greater-awareness-on-cp/

Stuntzner, S., & Hartley, M. (2014). Disability and the counseling relationship: What counselors need to know. *Ideas and research you can use: VISTAS 2014*. Retrieved from https://www.counseling.org/docs/default-source/vistas/article_09.pdf?sfvrsn=157ccf7c_12

Thevadass, L. (2017, May 12). Poor facilities for the disabled. *The Star Online*. Retrieved from https://www.thestar.com.my/metro/community/2017/05/12/poor-facilities-for-the-disabled-study-infrastructure-at-terminals-pose-danger-and-confusion/

Tin, C. S. (2013). *Children with disabilities in Malaysia: Mapping the policies, programmes, interventions and stakeholders*. Family Health Development Division, Ministry of Health Malaysia.

Chapter 10
Developing Multicultural Counselling in an Australian University:
Applying Hinduism to Counselling

Carl Vadivella Belle
Independent Researcher, Australia

ABSTRACT

Lifetime experiences have equipped the author with a broad and diverse background in approaching counselling and problem resolution. This has ranged from grief counselling to management of rural financial counselling and spiritual counselling. In 2004, the author was appointed Inaugural Hindu Chaplain at the Flinders University of South Australia, a position held until late 2007 (although his counselling role has continued until this day). The chaplaincy to which he was appointed was one of several that collectively comprised a multi-faith chaplaincy involving a team approach. The concept was one in which chaplains of different faiths would respect each other's traditions, would eschew proselytization, and would work cooperatively to mount joint educational and community interest projects. However, at the more fundamental level, his role consisted of providing chaplaincy services to Hindu students and staff studying or employed at Flinders University. (Increasingly this role extended to members of the other two universities based in Adelaide, neither of which possessed a Hindu chaplain.)

INTRODUCTION

In January 2004 the Hindu Society of South Australia nominated me to become Hindu Chaplain to the Flinders University of South Australia, a university containing an enrolment of 25,000 students and located in Adelaide's southern suburbs. This appointment was subsequently ratified by the University Council and I commenced duties in late February. I was the first Hindu Chaplain to be appointed to any Australian University.

DOI: 10.4018/978-1-5225-6073-9.ch010

BACKGROUND

Although I was new to chaplaincy I was familiar with the concept of counselling. Between 1976 and 1979 I had been posted to the Australian High Commission, Kuala Lumpur, where the bulk of my work had consisted of organising the placement in Australia of trainees nominated by the Malaysian Government under the auspices of Australian funded aid programs. These ranged from an annual intake of senior secondary school students and undergraduates to postgraduates and specialist ad hoc trainees (many of whom occupied prominent positions in management and business). Prior to my posting I had been provided with a series of briefings which were designed to familiarize me with the political and cultural realities of Malaysian life. I rapidly discovered that these had left me ill-prepared for the complexities of my appointment, or to decipher the myriad of ethnic, religious, socio-economic, educational and linguistic issues which dominated Malaysian political discourse. I quickly learned that within Malaysia culture and religious beliefs were intertwined far more comprehensively that was the case in deeply secular Australia, and that if I hoped to understand those with whom I was dealing, I would need to acquire a working knowledge of all the major religions practiced in Malaysia. I also learned the importance of, as far as possible, providing advice to students within the context of the cultural framework with which they were acquainted.

Some years later (1992-2004) I chaired the Barossa, Hills and Plains Rural Counselling Service Incorporated. In addition I served for two years as the State Secretary of the South Australian Association of Rural Counselling, and several more years on the State Executive. Both organisations were jointly funded by the Australian and South Australian Governments. In addition the Barossa body received support, mainly in-kind, from local government and various community groups. The Service was dedicated to providing financial counselling and where appropriate advisory options to rural producers and associated business organisations. At this point Australian rural producers were subject to a series of challenges. These included unstable commodity demand, fluctuating prices, and comprehensive industry restructuring. These issues were complicated by seasonal problems such as drought, bushfires and mouse plagues. We were also required to respond to financial crises resulting from emergencies, mainly devastation resulting from bushfires and floods. Our region incorporated a wide array of enterprises which not only included broad acre farming but also horticulture, viticulture, livestock, poultry production, and market gardening. Market gardening engaged a considerable number of recent migrant families, mainly of Vietnamese, Cambodian and Indian background, and the Service was required to devise new and innovative approaches to ensure that all potential clientele were aware of the range of counselling that we offered, that such counselling was free and confidential, that we operated entirely independently of the government, and that there was no shame or stigma in requesting our assistance.

During those years I acted as a sounding board for several counsellors for a strategy known as "de-briefing". This involved counsellors discussing in some detail the more stressful cases with which they had been dealing (without, of course, breaching confidentiality). The management of Rural Counselling Services throughout South Australia believed that regular de-briefing was an essential means of avoiding emotional fatigue (or "burn-out") among counselling staff. Financial stress often produces a range of subsidiary conditions which, if left unchecked, may actually prove life threatening. These conditions include depression, alcohol and substance abuse, domestic violence, feelings of alienation, inadequacy and helplessness, serious eating disorders, and in extreme cases, suicide. Moreover rural producers forced to sell properties due to financial pressures, especially those which had been held by the same family for several generations, often considered themselves failures and frequently suffered feelings of grief and guilt. Debriefing often assisted counsellors to manage caseloads which might otherwise have proven exhausting and perhaps even overwhelming.

THE MULTI-FAITH CHAPLAINCY

Flinders University, founded in 1966, established a dedicated Religious Centre on campus in the early 1970s. This followed recognition of the need to provide for the spiritual welfare of its staff and students. The university anticipated that religions on campus would cooperate with outside religious bodies and that these bodies would provide support to chaplains (as a consequence the university would not recognise self-appointed chaplains; chaplains would need to be nominated by the peak bodies of specific religious traditions). The University Charter stipulated that religious activities would be directed toward the overall development of a "university community based on mutual respect and understanding, and on social cohesion." It followed that the university would not assist religious groups which acted against the interest of other students, nor would it provide space or facilities for the activities of any such groups. In its early years the Religious Centre had operated as a largely Christian establishment, but other religions had appointed chaplains in the years immediately prior to my arrival.

The chaplaincy at Flinders was multi-faith, a concept which at that stage was unique within Australian universities. My chaplaincy would thus operate on two levels. Although my primary function would be to provide support to Hindu students studying at Flinders University, I would also work in conjunction with other chaplains to provide a safe and harmonious environment for students and university staff of all religions. The concept of a multi-faith centre working both jointly and singularly had been and was largely promoted through the vision and energy of Mr Geoff Boyce, a Uniting Church Chaplain. It contained chaplains drawn from Christian, Muslim, Buddhist and Pagan faiths and with my appointment a Hindu representative. From time to time we welcomed visiting chaplains, most notably those representing Lutheran, Jewish, Baha'i and Mormon faiths. Our working covenant included the provisions that we would make no attempt to convert any visitor to our religion, that we would not pass critical comments on other religions represented within the centre, and that in speaking at community forums, while we would clearly enunciate the perspectives that our religious tradition took on particular doctrinal and philosophical issues, we would not seek to censure other beliefs.

One significant religious body on campus, an evangelical Christian group, declined to join the Flinders Religious Centre, as the coordinators felt that they could not subscribe to the no-conversion/no criticism ideal that we adhered to.

But the concept of a multi-faith chaplaincy embraced much more than religious tolerance. It was expected that chaplains would:

1. Mount joint projects to promote the goal of inter-faith harmony and goodwill. Thus, for example, we planned and convened a public forum on Religion and Violence, which featured distinguished speakers representing different faiths, and which was designed to highlight the dangers of religious fanaticism.
2. Offer support to religious bodies and communities in times of need, especially when we felt that specific religions were the target of unfair and unwarranted pressures. Thus in response to sustained political criticism and indeed acrimony directed against Muslim refugees fleeing violence

in Afghanistan, (criticism which led to many Muslims believing that their entire community was under attack), the combined chaplaincy compiled a statement condemning all religious prejudice and assuring Muslim students and staff of their welcome on campus. This was jointly presented and read to Muslim staff and students during Friday prayers.

3. To conduct, where appropriate, multi-faith services. These often marked significant occasions. Thus one such service was held on the fortieth anniversary of the university's founding.
4. To address various community forums designed to promote general religious education, and in particular to outline the fundamental beliefs, practices and philosophies of various religious traditions. This involved visits to schools and to public meetings arranged by religious and community organisations. Our joint presentations, the sight of faiths working together, often came as a surprise to an Australian public conditioned to the concept of intrinsic hostility between different religions.

The educational aspect of the multi-faith chaplaincy sometimes manifested in unexpected ways. One morning, a young Somali woman, a recently enrolled postgraduate student, appeared in my office and asked me whether I would talk to her about the fundamentals of Hinduism. Registering my surprise, she quickly added that she wasn't contemplating *becoming* a Hindu. She explained that the imam had informed the community that while in Somalia they had known only Islam, Australia was a multi-faith society. In order to become responsible citizens, and to interact better with their fellow Australians, they should learn something of the beliefs of other religious traditions. In consulting me, she was merely following her imam's advice.

ESTABLISHING A HINDU CHAPLAINCY

Because I was the first Hindu chaplain appointed to any Australian university, I had no role models from whom I could seek advice in constructing a working and responsive chaplaincy. I devised a schedule of basic tasks which could be pursued sequentially and to some extent concurrently.

The most basic requirement was to gauge the potential size of my clientele to whom I was required to minister; that is, the number of Hindu students enrolled at Flinders University. The University kept no statistics of the religious beliefs of the general student enrolment. However, I was aware that while there was a small minority of Australian born Hindus, (born of migratory parents), most were overseas students who were temporary residents and in Australia on student visas. The largest groups were from India, Malaysia, Singapore, Sri Lanka and Fiji. Because I was the only Hindu chaplain in any Adelaide-based University I also found that I attracted approaches from students enrolled in the two other local universities, namely the University of Adelaide and the University of South Australia (my profile at the former was established after I delivered a eulogy at a special service convened by the Medical Department to commemorate those who had donated their bodies to medical science, perhaps one of my more unusual roles as chaplain.)

However my main initial task was that of publicity; to make students and staff aware of my presence. My appointment had been announced in the Hindu Temple in Adelaide (the Shri Ganesha Temple), and a feature article included in the temple's newsletter. I also placed a sign in the main window of the Religious Centre which advised of the days and times I would be available on campus. This also furnished my home phone number and email address. This notice made it clear that I was happy to receive visitors on any level ranging from purely social calls to more involved personal matters. I made a point of each week meeting with different key figures within the administration and governing bodies of the University not only to advise them of my appointment, but also to seek ways as to how I might be of assistance to them. One obvious way was to contact lecturers in social sciences and related disciplines to inform that, upon request I would be able to arrange for suitable experts to provide specialist Hindu perspectives on a swathe of topics. (The Hindu community is among the best educated religious communities in Australia.) While I was occasionally invited to lecture on Hindu ethics and *puranic* mythology, over time I arranged the visits of Hindu experts to lecture on specialised subjects such as Women's Studies, History, Education, and Grief Management.

Experience has taught me that counselling, whether on financial or personal issues, is often a cooperative exercise, and that a counsellor does not exist in isolation. While there was a range of matters, (e.g. accommodation, culturally sensitive medical assistance), which could usually be resolved by a single referral, other more complex cases, (for example, deep seated psychological problems), might require specialist counselling which a chaplain was not necessarily equipped to provide. I thus made it a priority to establish a network of contacts, both within the University and in the wider community. The latter included agencies such as police, legal aid, emergency services, etc. A couple of these bodies actually invited me talk to their employees as part of their scheduled cultural awareness programs. Finally I compiled a list of consular contacts within the embassies and consulates representing the home countries from which the vast majority of Hindu students originated. This array of connections covered nearly all conceivable fall-back contingencies which I would experience as a chaplain, and was to prove invaluable.

One of the central roles in a university chaplaincy is that of public education. This reaches beyond discussions on the function of religions and the spiritual disciplines which sustain it. The chaplain should aim to increase public knowledge of the central doctrines, philosophies and rituals of the religious tradition to which he/she belongs. This was especially important in the case of Hinduism. Although Indian Hindus were members of the First Fleet which attended the colonisation of Australia, arriving in Botany Bay on 26 January 1788, the positioning of Hinduism as a mainstream religion in Australia is a comparatively recent development. As a result general Australian understanding of Hinduism is often limited, and indeed remains shaped by outdated stereotypes, many of which have been bequeathed from colonial commentaries. Thus one of Australia's most acclaimed historians, drawing on an 1891 source, in explaining the failure of Hindus to colonise Australia, could write:

The Hindu religion...prohibited sea voyages, as well as contact with foreigners, and a queer 'geography' supplemented the teaching of religion. For the Hindu believed the world was flat and triangular, that it was composed of seven different habitations, each surrounded by its own peculiar seas; that one sea was of milk, another of sugar, another of butter, another of wine, and so on; that the whole of this world was supported on the heads of elephants... (Clark, 1981, p 6)

I thus advertised my preparedness to speak on Hindu philosophical traditions and general belief structures to any group which issued an invitation.

As a Caucasian received into Hinduism, I had some concerns as to how I might be accepted by students and staff with whom I would be required to deal. However, my profile as repeated pilgrim to the major Hindu festival of Thaipusam, both in Malaysia and in South India, my former role as Australian correspondent to the international journal *Hinduism Today*, as an acknowledged speaker and writer on Hinduism, and my position as Vice President of the Hindu Society of South Australia, seemed to reassure all with whom I came in contact.[1]

PRACTICAL CHAPLAINCY

Ultimately the core responsibility of a Chaplain is to provide spiritual, social and emotional support to those who subscribe to the religious tradition he/she represents. This role may incorporate general guidance through resolution of personal problems and life crises, discussing ethical issues, taking up cases of alleged or actual discrimination with the relevant authorities (fortunately comparatively rare in Australian universities), and assuming, where necessary, an advocacy role on behalf of a student or a group of students. (One of the latter interventions was to request the university catering staff to provide a greater range of vegetarian dishes for Hindu students. It was necessary to point out that Islam and Judaism were not the only religions which observed dietary restrictions and that a significant percentage of Hindus (and Buddhists) were vegetarians.)

The Hindu theory of creation holds that all substances are unique and that each person is an individual in the deepest sense. Thus each human on the planet has his/her own pathway to the Divine. Hinduism incorporates an extraordinary collocation of belief structures, deities and behavioural patterns which include regional and sub-regional variations as well as clan-related cultural practices which are often specific to sub-groups. Accordingly each person who presents for spiritual advice and support comes with a mental framework influenced and often moulded largely by the specific cultural-religious background to which he/she has been habituated. This must be explored from the outset, especially in more complex cases, so that firm points of engagement and mutual understanding can be established.

However, there are a number of basic tenets upon which most Hindu systems of belief converge. These are as follows:

1. The major Hindu texts are divided into *sruti* ("those [texts] which are heard", that is, revealed scriptures), and *smriti* ("that which is remembered"), the latter shaping the various philosophical schools of Hinduism. *Sruti* include the Vedas, the Upanishads, and the *Agamas* (Literally "that which has come down"; that is, revealed sacred texts), while *smriti* include the *Puranas* (mythological texts, which explicate the deeds of the gods and provide philosophical perspectives, belief structures, and guidelines for both ethical conduct and the enactment of rituals). *Sruti* and *smriti* collectively provide the scriptural and related authority which underpins the *Sanatana Dharma*, the eternal religion which has neither beginning nor end.
2. Although Hinduism has many gods and goddesses, all are regarded as manifestations of One Supreme Being, a deity who is both imminent and transcendent, both Creator and Manifest Reality, both taking form (*Saguna*) and existing beyond form (*Nirguna*). All of the gods/goddesses, ranging from guardian/village deities ("little" gods or godlings), through to the great deities within the received Hindu pantheon, are emanations of this Supreme Being and all worship is, at base, worship of this essential Oneness.
3. Hindus believe in the concept of *karma*, the doctrine of cause and effect, so that the individual, by his/her thoughts, words and deeds, controls his/her own destiny. All actions, whether good or bad, entail consequences which will rebound, either sooner or later, upon the individual.
4. Each individual has his/her own *dharma* to fulfil within a given lifespan. This rather abstruse concept refers to one's inherent nature, the individual pattern one should observe through life. This intrinsic quality is largely determined by the totality of past karmas, but is also moulded by a myriad of other factors including familial structure, social status, bodily and intellectual capabilities, the culture and locality into which one is born, etc.

5. Hindus believe in the concept of reincarnation, that the soul will transmigrate through a succession of births and deaths until all karmas are resolved and the soul reaches *moksha* (illumination/enlightenment). Hinduism follows a logic of inner direction; that is, movement from the world of flux, shapes and forms toward the stillness, bliss and Oneness of Divine Transcendence. All souls are destined to reach this state.
6. The vast majority of Hindus regard worship within a temple as a necessary concomitant of a healthy spiritual life, and view the observation and fulfilment of appropriate temple rituals as essential for advancing communication with, and knowledge of, the Divine. However a minority of Hindus construct their spiritual lives around personal disciplines including advanced yogic practices and deep meditation.
7. Hindus believe that the pathway to true spiritual unfoldment is best accomplished under the tutelage of a recognized Guru, a realised individual who will direct the *sishya* (disciple) in matters relating to personal conduct and spiritual disciplines.
8. Hindus hold as an ideal the doctrine of *ahimsa* (non-violence) which moves beyond passivity to embrace an active reverence for life. This leads many Hindus to become vegetarian.
9. Hindus believe that even though the pathways to illumination are many and varied, all religions contain and seek truth and thus should be respected.

As previously stated, these beliefs will often be deeply influenced by a raft of other factors ranging from the specific tradition to which the individual belongs, the region of origin, through to family circumstances, practices and expectations.

After a slow start to my chaplaincy I found that on an average day I would be visited by four or five students (generally I attended my office twice weekly). In addition I received several phone calls each week.[2] In following up issues related to student/staff visits, this resulted in an average weekly workload of between 24- 30 hours.

Prior experience in the field of counselling had taught me that in assuming my chaplaincy there were certain guidelines I should be constantly aware of. These were:

1. Certain matters may be regarded as "insoluble". Thus, for example, the death of a partner, the suicide of a relative, a personal tragedy, are events that had occurred and cannot be reversed. But in such situations the Chaplain has a vital role to fulfil. This not only includes that of journeying with the subject; that is, of being a "constant" in a time of turmoil, but offering practical advice, helping to explore and manage emotional responses, and offering spiritual solace.
2. Accepting that counselling is highly unlikely to succeed with certain individuals, including those with pronounced personality disorders, (for example, psychopathy, deep-seated narcissism, conflicted neurosis etc.) Counselling may also have limited success with those of extreme or obsessive dispositions whose ideological or rigid convictions form an emotional barrier to acceptance of even the most basic lines of alternative thought.
3. Chaplains must also guard against "ownership" of a particular client. There may be cases where he/she needs to operate in tandem with other authorities. In such cases and where possible the chaplain should ensure that the advice the subject is receiving is consistent. Insistence on exclusive "ownership" of a particular subject may prove deleterious to the welfare of that subject.

4. The Chaplain must recognise where his/her role ends and that of other professionals begins. Thus some clients may require specialist medical or psychiatric assistance which falls beyond the purview of therapeutic counselling.
5. The Chaplain should guard against emotional burn-out, and must develop strategies to counter this. The constant pressures of others' problems can and often does create a psychic burden which may prove impossible to sustain. (I had a close and confidential source to whom I could debrief. This proved invaluable.)

In the remainder of this chapter I have outlined some generic instances of my workload, as well as specific case studies which exemplify the overall deployment of these guidelines in the practical role of chaplaincy.

Homesickness

Homesickness affects nearly all students who enroll from another country, and can be exacerbated by loneliness, and exposure to a new way of life which embraces nearly every aspect of daily existence from diet to interpersonal relations. A student plunged into a totally new environment, and without the reassuring backdrop of family, relatives, friends, the cultural prompts of home, can often find the challenge of adjustment intimidating. The advent of modern forms of communication such as email, mobile phones and apps such as Skype, have allowed students much more regular and consistent access to home, but in some cases this may actually increase feelings of isolation – the knowledge that life in the home environment goes on without them can inculcate a sense of displacement. Irruptions of homesickness may be especially acute on significant dates; for example, birthdays, anniversaries, religious festivals. Homesickness and culture shock may be temporarily disorienting but after an initial period most students manage to settle into their new way of life. General encouragement, the reminder that other students before them have managed to adapt, (and often in more difficult circumstances), and introduction to other newcomers can help to ease the transition. However chronic homesickness/culture shock can prove totally incapacitating and may not only vitiate an individual's ability to study but may also lead to a range of increasingly serious conditions including depression, despair, uncharacteristic behaviour, and in extreme cases, self-harm and paranoia[3]. During my chaplaincy I dealt with one such case, a nursing student who had come to believe that the staff and other students were conspiring to destroy her reputation and to humiliate her. With the University's assistance she was placed in a class which contained other Hindu students from her home country with whom she was not previously acquainted. Her condition showed marked improvement within a couple of weeks after this move.

Sexual Harassment

During my period as Chaplain I dealt with two separate cases of young women alleging sexual harassment by university authorities. The first was easily dealt with; it was an instance of misinterpretation of Australian vernacular combined with the unanticipated exuberance of the tutor; exuberance which this young woman found highly intimidating. I subsequently telephoned the tutor and explained how his comments might have been received by a young Hindu woman only recently arrived in Australia. He in turn contacted the young woman, informed her as to the meaning he had intended to convey, and offered an apology.

The second case was far more consequential. "A", a young Sikh woman, presented with claims of repeated sexual harassment by her lecturer who also doubled as her tutor. This had involved a series of risqué and increasingly sexually loaded comments culminating in a suggestion that A should trade sexual favours in return for guaranteed high grades. These were serious allegations, and with "A's" agreement I arranged an early meeting with one of the University's Equal Opportunity Officers. A subsequent investigation substantiated "A's" allegations, and the lecturer/tutor was issued with a formal warning. "A" was placed in a fresh tutorial group, and was assured that her assignments would be independently assessed. There remained a residue of personal guilt. "A" worried that something in her demeanour may have provoked the supervisor to act in the way he did. I informed her that research had shown that many victims of sexual harassment were made to feel at least partially responsible for the actions of the predator. Over a couple of sessions we discussed in some detail the potential power relationship between a lecturer and his/her students and how an unscrupulous individual might exploit this. "A" was finally reassured only after receipt of a letter of unqualified apology, a letter that the University administration had dictated that the lecturer write.

SPECIFIC CASE STUDIES

Case Study 1

A male aged 25, "M", a postgraduate Masters candidate, based in a South Australian University, presented with a case of confused sexual identity. He informed me that he was strongly attracted to men, had no sexual interest in women, and was deeply worried that he might be a "girly-man". Over a prolonged discussion we went through all of the major touchstones that would assist in determining his sexual orientation – his upbringing, his relationship with parents and family, recollections of his feelings on entering adolescence, his subsequent sexual predilections. These conversations left me in no doubt that this man was gay, both in inclination and in practice.

However, a chaplain is not necessarily a psychologist, and before reaching a definitive conclusion I felt it necessary to refer "M" to a specialist counsellor whose judgement and cultural sensitivities I felt that I could trust, and who would respect "M's" particular religious beliefs. As with all cases involving referral, I held a discussion with the counsellor prior to M's appointment. The psychologist's report confirmed both "M's" concerns and my own judgement. There thus remained the need to reconcile what he felt was a dichotomy between his perceptions of what his religion taught and his confirmed sexual identity. Personally "M" felt a sense of great relief that his sexual confusion was now at an end, and he knew (in a sense) who he really was. But he was repulsed by notion of effeminacy that the word "gay" seemed to connote, and was appalled by what he perceived as the "stridency" and "intolerance" of Australian, (and indeed Western,) gay activism. Over time we were able to establish that there was no need to conform to any received public stereotype of the gay male, and that he should chart his own course. With regard to a Hindu outlook on human sexuality, I was able to convince him that the religion had traditionally displayed great latitude in the matter of sexual orientation, and that there were both *puranic* and textual sources which pointed to a "third sex" which existed beyond heterosexual mores. I stated that I knew of gay couples who were in stable, loyal and enduring relationships, and who were anything but the flighty, promiscuous creations of popular imagination.

But there remained a further major issue which was cultural rather than religious. "M" was the only son of parents whom he described as "very traditional". They had anticipated that their son would marry and be the father of descendants, thus maintaining the family lineage. "M" was concerned that his father would react badly to news that his son was gay and might even disown him. On the other hand an arranged marriage might provide a cover for his homosexuality, but would prove an "empty shell" devoid of both fulfilment and emotional support.

In response I pointed out that Hinduism encouraged the pursuit of truth, a concept which embraced personal authenticity. Hinduism also emphasised avoidance of harming others. To illustrate this I referred to a case that had previously come to my attention. A prominent surgeon in a Southeast Asian country sent his elder son to study Medicine in the United Kingdom. At first all went well. The son completed the first two years of his studies and gained high grades. Then the father discovered, (though information provided by an anonymous source), that the son had been involved in a homosexual liaison. The father terminated the son's studies, and brought him home in disgrace. The son suffered an immediate nervous breakdown from which he took some months to recover. The father thought that marriage would provide a "cure" for the son's condition and imported a young woman from India as a bride for his son. After eighteen months the young woman, who was well educated, sued for the divorce on the ground of non-consummation of the marriage. A second marriage followed with the same result. When last consulted the father was contemplating a third bride from India in an attempt to find the "right girl" who would "bring my son to his senses". (He even approached me to ask whether I might find a suitable bride in Australia.)

This case showed the consequences of the father's failure or inability to face or confront the reality of the son's homosexuality. All parties involved in this saga had suffered varying degrees of needless harm. The son's medical studies had been curtailed, thus denying him the possibility of a career in Medicine. This, and his "disgrace", had led to a nervous collapse. Two young women had had years of their young lives squandered, and had been used as mere instruments to try to satisfy the father's delusion that the son's sexual orientation would be "cured" by marriage. I opined that I felt it incumbent upon "M" to eschew such a scenario.

"M" ultimately decided to place his trust in a close family friend. Both "M" and I exchanged several emails with this man. "M's" choice was apt. His Indian confidante, an aged man, had a scholarly grasp of Hinduism, was of wise and benevolent disposition, and had long suspected that "M" was gay, even before his departure for Australia. He agreed to discuss the matter with "M's" parents. The explosive reaction that "M" had feared did not eventuate. Both parents accepted that the son was gay, that there was no "cure", and that he was and always would remain their son.

Case Study 2

One evening, at about ten p.m., I received a call from the South Australian Police advising me that a Hindu postgraduate student, aged about 28, had been killed in a road accident in an Adelaide suburb. His widow was too distraught to offer any instructions regarding funerary arrangements, and had collapsed following formal identification of the body. A social worker was with the widow, and the Indian High Commission had been notified and would advise the deceased's family in India. The police wished to know whether I would be willing to act as a liaison point in oversighting funerary arrangements.

The young man's father contacted me the following morning. He wanted his son's body to be repatriated to India for cremation and asked whether I would ensure that the remains were consigned to an undertaker familiar with Hindu ritual who could arrange this. I pointed out that cremation in Australia and the return of ashes would be considerably cheaper, but he assured me that the financial costs were not an issue. Once I had organised the return of the son's body I should contact him and he would settle all costs. The widow should be booked to return home on the next available flight.

There were two major considerations. The first, and more immediate, was to contact the temple to acquire the name of a funeral director who would be familiar with the requisite procedures in managing Hindu funerary rites. This was relatively straightforward. Appropriate pre-funerary prayers were arranged, and an undertaker, nominated by contacts within the temple, advised me that the remains could be prepared for despatch from Adelaide within twenty-four hours. Because I was the nominated liaison point I was required to sign several regulatory and customs authorisations relating to this process. I then contacted the family in India so that financial matters could be settled, and bookings confirmed.

The second was the welfare of the young widow, (who had been married for less than two years). I made an appointment to see her and explained the arrangements that had been made for the repatriation of her husband's remains, and that funerary rites would be conducted in his ancestral village. I advised her of the details of her flights back to India. She advised that female friends, the wives of two of her husband's colleagues, would take her to the airport. I therefore arranged for the airline tickets to be made available at the Adelaide Airport, and requested that a volunteer be assigned to assist her through the initial stages of departure.

Case Study 3

Very early one morning I was telephoned by student "C", a nineteen year old Arts undergraduate, who advised me that the military had visited the family compound in central Sri Lanka, and had taken her two brothers and a cousin away for questioning. She informed me that she had no relations in Australia. I advised her that I would visit within the hour.

When I arrived I discovered a young woman who was in a state of emotional meltdown. Her parents had not contacted her since the brothers' and cousin's disappearance and she feared the worst. There was no authority in her home district that she could contact, and she knew from past experience that the Sri Lankan High Commission in Canberra would refuse to take her call.

Prior to the visit I had rung a medical doctor, a person I knew was an active member of the Ceylonese Tamil Association in Adelaide. He told me that I should take "C" to the temple and he would meet both of us there. He would get her particulars and make his own enquiries among members of the Tamil community who had hailed from her district of origin.

About ten minutes after reaching the temple, and while awaiting the arrival of the doctor, "C" received a telephone call from her parents advising her that her brothers and cousin had been returned, unharmed, to the family home. Although the military provided no explanation for the detention, the parents had concluded that they had been arrested either as a case of mistaken identity, or (as they suspected), as a result of false information sent anonymously to the authorities. The doctor arrived five minutes later. I apologised that he had been called to the temple on a matter that had now apparently been resolved. Although he had an extremely full schedule, he sat with me and the temple priest for thirty minutes while we all comforted "C" who was shaking uncontrollably, and who had dissolved in floods of tears. It was obvious that she was in no fit condition to attend university, and I offered to ring her tutors. The doctor advised "C" that she was suffering severe shock, and that she should allow herself several days to recover. "C" later visited me on a couple of occasions to talk through this incident and to analyse her reactions.

Case Study 4

The final case study provided in this chapter was perhaps the most unusual of my chaplaincy. This involved a mature woman, "D", who worked on contract as a lecturer in science at a South Australian university. "D" had arrived in Australia with her husband, who had been nominated for a doctoral program, several years previously. The marriage had been unhappy; her husband had been both violent and unfaithful, and finally returned to India to take up residence with a woman whom he had known prior to their departure to Australia. During their time in Adelaide, their son, aged ten, had become terminally ill with cancer. "D" had been converted to Catholicism by a Goanese friend and had become a member of the small Goanese Catholic community in Adelaide. When her son died he had been interred in a Catholic cemetery.

"D" informed me that she had nothing to return to in India. Both her parents were dead, and her only sibling, an elder sister to whom she had never been close, had rejected her following her separation from her husband. She had been a member of an orthodox and "very traditional" Brahmin community which would look unfavourably on a woman who had separated from her husband. Neither the Brahmin community to which she had belonged, nor the Catholic community of which she was now a member, recognised divorce, and unless her husband died she could never consider remarriage. In any case she was now beyond the age of childbearing. While there was nothing for her in India, Adelaide offered her continuing and active membership of a small and close-knit religious community, and access to her son's grave, which she visited regularly. In addition the university in which she was employed was prepared to offer her an extended contract should she succeed in gaining Permanent Resident status.

"D" had made initial approaches to the Department of Immigration offices in Adelaide, but felt that she had been treated poorly and with considerable suspicion; indeed she had been appalled at what she had interpreted as the "racism" of the officers of whom she had made enquiries. There was no Catholic chaplain at any South Australian university but I had been recommended by a Hindu friend who felt that with my knowledge of Indian society, and my diplomatic background, I might be able to assist her.

I responded that I would need to conduct some enquiries, and that we should meet again in a fortnight's time to discuss possible courses of action. Although I was convinced of "D's" sincerity I telephoned Immigration to discuss the state of her application and to ascertain whether there were any anomalies in her case. I also phoned the Dean of her university department, and the Catholic priest who ministered to the Goanese community. Both attested to the depth of "D's" character, her scrupulous honesty, and the warmth with which she was regarded by her colleagues, her students, and the religious community to which she belonged. The priest also advised me that "D's" visits to her son's grave, and her conviction that the earth in which he was interred was sacred, underpinned both her faith and her emotional integrity, and that deprivation of access, (that is, deportation to India) might well result in severe personal dislocation. Following our next meeting I prepared a submission to the Department of Immigration. This not only outlined "D's" personal circumstances, but also emphasised the contribution she was making to education in Australia and the further contributions she could potentially offer. In forwarding this I warned "D" that the review process might well be both complicated and prolonged, and that if the initial application was rejected we might need to proceed to appeal. Both the University and the Church prepared letters of recommendation on "D's" behalf.

I was telephoned a fortnight later by a senior Immigration officer who discussed "D's" application and the supporting documentation at some length. At the conclusion of our conversation he advised me that he intended to recommend that "D" be offered Permanent Resident status, and this was likely to be finalised within the next few weeks. However, it was several months before "D" received her formal approval. (I was advised at the same time of the success of her application.) During this time "D" and I kept in touch through a fortnightly phone call. Past experience had revealed the emotional strain that applicants for Permanent Residence can feel, and the need to provide appropriate networks of support.

A FINAL OBSERVATION

When I left the chaplaincy I felt that the office had comes a worthwhile and indeed vital point of reference for Hindu students and staff upon the Flinders University campus, and to some extent upon those of other university campuses in Adelaide. There was no doubt of the need for the chaplaincy; during my occupancy I had met with numerous students and staff and spoke to many more at public functions and lectures. For several years after my departure from Adelaide I continued to receive phone calls and emails from students requesting my assistance on a variety of issues, some of them serious.

However, I considered that there were measures, which if implemented, might have made the chaplaincy more effective. A chaplaincy relates to its peak religious body and draws much of its strength and resilience from the support provided by that body. While requests to the Hindu Society for specialist advice were always honoured, I was deeply concerned that there was no undergraduate or university based association to meet the religious, cultural or social needs of the large number of Hindu students and staff in Adelaide tertiary institutions, or which served to mitigate the high levels of personal anxiety I felt I had discerned among many Hindu students. Although an attempt had been made to inaugurate a youth body, this had faltered and had not been revived. (Nor was there an established regime of religious education for children and adolescents; a void which deeply worried several members of the Executive Committee of the Hindu Society.) Institutions which provide for these needs are integral to ensure the successful transplantation and dynamism of religious and spiritual needs of both migratory and transient communities, and were generally well entrenched in other religious communities. Their absence and the pressing need to rectify this situation, were constant themes in my regular chaplaincy reports.

REFERENCES

Armstrong, K. (2009). *The Case for God: What Religion Really Means*. London: The Bodley Head.

Belle, C. V. (1992). *Towards Truth: An Australian Spiritual Journey*. Kuala Lumpur: Pacific Press.

Belle, C. V. (1998, May). *Consultative Report: The Future Directions of Rural Counselling in South Australia*. Prepared for the Hon. Rob Kerin, Minister for Primary Industries, Natural Resources and Regional Development, South Australia, Adelaide, Australia.

Belle, C. V. (2005). *Evaluation Report: Funding for AIDS in Rural South Australia*. Adelaide: South Australian Farmers' Federation.

Belle, C. V. (2012). *Keynote Address: Religious Minorities in Australia: Past and Present*. Adelaide: Tertiary Ministries Conference of Australia.

Bowker, J. (2015). *Why Religions Matter*. Cambridge, UK: Cambridge University Press. doi:10.1017/CBO9781316048023

Chelliah,. K. (2012). *Hinduism: A Brief Study of It's* (sic) *Origins, Traditions and Practice*. Bukit Berunding: Kandiah Chelliah.

Clark, C. M. H. (1962). *A History of Australia: From the Earliest Times to the Age of Macquarie*. London: Cambridge University Press.

Eastman, R. (Ed.). (1993). *The Ways of Religion: An Introduction to the Major Traditions* (2nd ed.). New York: Oxford University Press.

Flood, G. (2012). *The Importance of Religion: Meaning and Action in Our Strange World*. Chichester, UK: Wiley Blackwell.

Rural Youth of South Australia. (2001). *A Practical Counsellor's Handbook*. Gawler: Rural Alliance Network.

Stocker,, M. (1996). *Valuing Emotions*. New York: Cambridge University Press.

Subramuniyswami, S. (1993). *Dancing with Siva: Hinduism's Contemporary Catechism* (4th ed.). Himalayan Academy.

ENDNOTES

1 Indeed, the only rejection I received came from an unlikely source. In 2006 I submitted the abstract of a paper I proposed delivering at a world-wide chaplain conference which was to be held in Helsinki, Finland. I received no response to my submission and later emails drew one non-committal response and then no further correspondence at all. I later discovered that the organisers felt it vaguely troubling that a Caucasian with traceable Scandinavian ancestry should identify as a Hindu, and as a response, my abstract should be quietly forgotten.

2 The most unusual – and brazen – phone call was from a Christian missionary who wanted me to nominate a Telegu speaker from the temple to teach missionaries how to speak the language so that they could travel to Andhra Pradesh to convert Hindus! I reminded him that I was a practising Hindu ministering to other Hindus.

3 During my posting to the Australian High Commission, Kuala Lumpur, I was required to deal with one such extreme case. A young man, "J", aged about twenty-five, had been posted, under a non-government Australian aid scheme, to teach secondary school students in Malaysia. He was allocated a post in a prominent school in the state of Negri Sembilan, south of Kuala Lumpur. About a fortnight after "J" commenced duty I received a rather alarming phone call from one of his colleagues. He informed me that "J" was behaving rather strangely and had become both temperamental and emotional. I responded that I would be visiting the area the following week, and I would arrange to drop in at the school. However, before I could do so I was phoned by a medical doctor who reported that "J" had used a hockey stick to attack a man walking past his house, and being of small and slight build had come off second best. I was told that he was now recovering from his injuries in Seremban General Hospital. I arranged to visit "J" the following day. During

our interview it was obvious that "J" was completely disoriented, emotionally fragile, and exhibiting symptoms of paranoia. At one point, in response to my questioning, he proclaimed, "You don't seem to understand. There are *Asians* walking past my house every day." Given his mental state it was obvious that repatriation was the only realistic option. His home organisation arranged his departure to coincide with his discharge from hospital. Upon return home "J's" recovery was both rapid and complete.

Chapter 11
Buddhist Approaches to Counselling and Psychotherapy:
Exploratory Discussions From Different Traditions

Alvin Lai Oon Ng
Sunway University, Malaysia

Ee Mun Hon
HELP University, Malaysia

Ming Tik Chia
HELP University, Malaysia

ABSTRACT

Three authors from differing Buddhist backgrounds share their approaches to using Buddhism in psychotherapy. The authors argue that Buddhism itself is fundamentally a psychotherapy approach because it is essentially a prescription to end discontent and misery. This chapter provides basic points on how Buddhism can be used in counselling by discussing how different Buddhist traditions might approach counselling. This chapter also brings up reflections on how practice may differ according to experience in the fields of counselling and clinical psychology. Overall, the chapter is subdivided into six parts: (1) introduction; (2) basic tenets of Buddhism relevant to psychotherapy; (3) case study illustrations of applied Buddhism in counselling and psychotherapy; (4) discussion on reconciling differing Buddhist schools of thought in the practice of counselling and psychotherapy; (5) discussion on compatibility of Buddhist principles with applied Western philosophies and therapeutic approaches; and (6) suggestions of future directions given the current research literature patterns.

DOI: 10.4018/978-1-5225-6073-9.ch011

INTRODUCTION

This chapter looks at the application of Buddhist principles within the practice of counselling and psychotherapy. The three authors who contributed this chapter are mental health workers with different backgrounds and approaches to Buddhist practice as well as upbringing. The main angle of this paper is to discuss the applications of Buddhist principles in the helping professions of counselling and psychotherapy by exploring and discussing illustrated examples from each individual author's journey as mental health workers.

The chapter begins with a general introduction to the chapter coupled with personal introductions of the three authors as a primer for the later discussion of case studies using Buddhist approaches to counselling. These introductions aim to provide some familiarity to the reader concerning the authors' backgrounds to be able to relate better to the case studies being brought up in the middle of the chapter. This introduction also touches on how religious aspects of psychotherapy has the potential for a wider reach into the larger community, especially for lower socio-economic status groups who tend to have less access and exposure to professional mental health providers.

The introduction would then lead to a brief discussion of basic Buddhism that underlies the use of its principles within the practice of counselling and psychotherapy. Given the presence of both Theravada and Mahayana traditions in this chapter, Pali, and Sanskrit terms will be used to explain certain Buddhist concepts. A short background into the spiritual development triad (*Silā-Samādhi-Pañña* / Morality-Mind Cultivation-Wisdom) within Buddhism sets the stage for concepts discussed in this section. Main concepts to be introduced are the Four Noble Truths which includes the Eightfold Noble Path; the Five Precepts of lay Buddhist practice; the concept of the Four *Brahma Viharas* (Divine Dwellings), the concept of the Three Evils – *Lobha, Dosa, Moha* (Greed, Hatred and Delusion) and lastly, the concept of *Paticca Samupada* (Dependent Origination). These Buddhist concepts are central to the practice of Buddhism that are, in turn, applied directly in attitude, behavior and observation for the improvement of individual well-being though conduct, reflection and meditation practice, regardless of cultural traditions. The mechanisms of how these concepts help with gaining insight and wisdom for better well-being will be summarized.

The brief introduction into the tenets of Buddhism will be followed by a note on Buddhism in Malaysia, describing a short history and context to which this chapter can be better understood, especially with regards to the very diverse understanding and practice of Buddhism in the country (i.e. cultural, linguistic, historical and education level). References to articles of interest will be given so as to maintain the scope of this chapter without having to digress to other discussions on the development and practice of Buddhism in Malaysia.

Following from the description of Buddhist concepts are three case studies using Buddhist principles within counselling and psychotherapeutic practice by the three authors respectively. Given their diverse backgrounds and Buddhist practice, the authors will discuss their approaches from the Buddhist traditions of Mahayana, Vajrayana and the Theravada schools of thought. These cases that are discussed come from each authors' personal experiences and are based on multiple cases combined to mask any identifiable information to protect the identity of the clients.

After the case studies, the chapter compares Buddhist principles to similar concepts within Western philosophy such as Stoicism, and contemporary applied therapeutic practices such as Acceptance and Commitment Therapy (ACT), Reality Therapy (RT) and Rational Emotive Behavior Therapy (REBT).

This comparison would spell out the compatibility of using Buddhist thought within Western counselling practice given the similarities in approach to the improvement of mental well-being.

This chapter ends with a very brief review of current trends in research literature to point towards suggestions of future directions in the development of applied Buddhist practice in the field of counselling and psychotherapy. A rehash of the discussion on using Buddhist principles in methods of psychotherapeutic intervention within the larger communities will be added in to reinforce the relevance of applied philosophy for social well-being.

PERSONAL BACKGROUNDS

Overview

The three authors of this chapter have different beginnings from which they developed their understanding of Buddhism. AN comes from an English-speaking background Theravada tradition, while EM and MC are Chinese-literate and lean towards the Mahayana traditions of Buddhism. This background presentation serves to provide a frame of sort towards the understanding of the approaches to counselling and psychotherapy cases later in the chapter.

AN

AN is a clinical psychologist by training with a professional doctorate in clinical psychology from Murdoch University, Western Australia. He practiced as a clinical psychologist and a postgraduate trainer in clinical psychology for 11 years at Universiti Kebangsaan Malaysia (National University of Malaysia) before moving on to focus more on teaching and research at Sunway University where he is at the time of publication. He currently does not provide clinical consultations per se but is still much into the field of clinical psychology through research and his role as the Vice President of the Malaysian Society of Clinical Psychology (MSCP) which he founded in 2010 as the Founding President. He was also a consultant psychologist, appearing weekly on a breakfast radio show to provide discussions on mental health topics and to answer public questions about mental health issues for two years from 2015 to 2017. AN is also a sought-after speaker and consultant for various issues pertaining to mental health management.

With regards to Buddhism, AN credits his meditation practice and study of Buddhism as part of his work principles in applying clinical methods in helping people solve personal problems. AN attended Buddhist Sunday school at the Buddhist Maha Vihara in Kuala Lumpur since the age of 10. He attended a Buddhist monk novitiate program there when he was 16, under the tutelage of Venerable M. Mahinda and his preceptor, Venerable K. Sri Dhammananda Maha Thera. Growing up with Buddhism primed his venturing into meditation classes while he was on his clinical internship at a hospital in Perth, Western Australia. He met a renowned meditation teacher, Venerable Ajahn Brahmavamso then, and continued to practice meditation, occasionally joining meditation retreats in the Theravadin tradition of Buddhism.

To AN, Buddhism should be used as practical wisdom that is relatable to the general public. The practice of Buddhism personally is more to philosophy of the good life that is principle-based rather than something that is religious or spiritual. He believes that spirituality is a personal thing. Therefore, when it comes to applying Buddhist principles in therapy or counselling, he approaches it from the pragmatic perspective that is through experiential learning, which is to extract out the knowledge and answers from the client in providing insights to problems. This approach also encourages the client to learn as a teacher, rather than as a student. The empowerment that comes from realizing something useful, that can be taught or shared with others is more likely to be sustainable, compared to just a personalized learning. A wider perspective is obtained in that clients are better able to realize they belong to a system that is interconnected, and that there are many factors at play that contribute to their well-being in relation to others. In terms of philosophical leanings, AN also applies Taoist principles of balance and flow, as well as Stoic principles of acceptance. Both philosophies have much in common with Buddhist practice.

EM

EM is a registered counsellor, with a Master's degree in Counselling, and Bachelor degree in psychology from HELP University. Her foray into counselling began as a psychology intern at Universiti Malaya Medical Centre where she spent two years and then two more years as an intern counsellor at a number of centers including private universities, government hospital, vocational boarding center, primary schools and a refugee center. EM is currently practicing in a mental health specialist clinic, providing therapy sessions to individual clients. She is certified in Choice Theory and Reality Therapy (CTRT), which she actively uses in her practice. When working with clients, EM stresses the importance in exploring their strengths and resources in supporting their needs, by incorporating and applying different techniques and tools in helping them solve problems.

EM's approach to helping her clients in counselling is inspired by her yoga practice and meditation as well as her study of Buddhism. She was exposed to formal Buddhism at a tender age of 5 where she attended Buddhist Sunday School at the Jetavana Monastery in Kuala Lumpur led by abbot Venerable Zheng Kong. As a teenager, she became more active in engaged Buddhism where she attended a Buddhist youth camp when she was 13 years old and a Dharma camp when she was 15 years old, organized by Blia Yad Malaysia Subdivisions, under the tutelage of Venerable Hui Xian. Since then, she has been an active volunteer at Buddhist camps for children and youth. EM encountered mindfulness practice while she was on internship at a hospital, which inspired her to join Hatha yoga classes. She practices weekly meditation and Hatha yoga, with a yoga teacher whose spiritual approach is within the Mahayana Buddhist tradition.

To EM, Buddhist teaching is daily wisdom and a philosophy of life, where it's learning progresses a person towards a better self and a better life. The practice of Buddhism is through experiential learning that varies according to individuals, depending on their understanding of and connection with Buddhism. When it comes to actively applying Buddhist principles and ideas into therapy sessions, it is important to firstly understand the client's cultural background as well as their perspective of Buddhism. This would help facilitate knowledge and insights from Buddhist practice to help the client gain further understanding and new learnings about their situations in order to help him/her manage their challenges. These gains are usually internalized and help empower the client to become more adaptive in life, especially when acting according to the understanding of systemic consequences of one's action that is dynamic and constantly interacting with many other factors around them. Self-awareness of this continuous interaction could bring clients more contentment in their lives. EM also incorporates Taoist philosophy in her approach. She believes in the balance between Yin (energy of being) and Yang (energy of doing). Individuals proportionally have more energy of doing to conduct activities and roles on daily basis, it is equally important to have some time and space to nourish their energy of being for manifestation of emotional, physical and psychological health.

MC

MC is currently pursuing a Master's degree in counselling and practicing as an intern counsellor at a Buddhist temple and also at a Christian church. At the temple, he provides individual counselling and play therapy services, while also acting as a trainer / facilitator for children and youth at Buddhist camps and as well as a trainer for the social workers. At the church, he assists the pastor in running separate groups for grief support, and special children. He also helps out in mission work. MC applies Person-centered, Satir Model and Mindfulness-Based Stress Reduction (MBSR) in his counselling sessions. He believes that clients are better able to explore their strengths and work out solutions by themselves, when their emotions are stabilized.

In terms of Buddhism, MC is an active practitioner and derives his methods from his regular meditation to help his clients to create self-awareness and relaxation through guided meditation and mindfulness-based intervention. Born into a Taoist family, MC used to participate in Taoism temple activities and is exposed to many types of Taoism ceremonies.

MC became a Buddhist at the age of 18 after participating in a Buddhist monks' novitiate program at Fo Guang Shan Centre, Malaysia. Since then, he participated in Buddhist monk novitiate programs in different countries and under different Buddhism traditions. As such, he has a wide exposure to the diversity of Buddhist traditions. He studied and practiced Mahayana Buddhism under Venerable Hui Nian from Singapore for three years and Theravada Buddhism under Venerable Uttamasara from Myanmar as well as meditation under Venerable Kassapa from Sri Lanka. MC explored Christianity for one year before continuing his spiritual journey in Vajrayana Buddhism. He practices Vajrayana prostrations daily and abides by the practices under Venerable Nubpa Rinpoche from Nepal.

To MC, the teachings in Buddhism helps improve self-awareness and provides guidance in improving daily life. One concept from Buddhism that MC relies on heavily is the concept of impermanence. He contends that the truth of impermanence helps us to be more aware of personal attachments that lead to problems, and that it is important to realize the need for letting go or detachment.

Relevance to the Community

The three authors may be from different backgrounds but the type of approaches they use from Buddhism are pragmatic and directly relevant in addressing challenges in daily life. While there are generic approaches that are easily applicable to the general public, some may be more suitable for individuals who actually believe in more Buddhist-centric thoughts and rituals. These will be expounded in the later sections of this chapter.

BASICS TENETS OF BUDDHISM RELEVANT TO PSYCHOTHERAPY

Buddhism originated from the search to end suffering. As such its philosophy and teachings are already aligned with well-being. Siddhartha Gautama's insights to his emotional troubles as a pampered prince led him to renounce the worldly life and seek methods to end his sufferings once and for all. His success in finding the answers to his questions about the eternal cessation of suffering resulted in him being called the Buddha, or "the Awakened / Enlightened One". Buddhism is basically the teachings of the Buddha Gautama that provides practitioners with the methods to manage and ultimately stop suffering.

The Four Noble Truths

The main teachings of the Buddha are summarized into what is commonly called the Four Noble Truths. These truths provide the way in which suffering can be better understood so that it can be conquered. The First Noble Truth makes the acknowledgement that suffering exists. The Second Noble Truth states that there are causes of suffering. The Third Nobel Truth states that there is an end to suffering. This leads to the Fourth Noble Truth that provides the means to end suffering, which is also commonly known as the Middle Way, or the Noble Eightfold Path.

The Middle Way / Noble Eightfold Path

While the first three Noble Truths state that there is suffering, causes of suffering and the end of suffering, the Fourth Noble Truth details the way to end suffering with a prescription of eight qualities to develop as a practitioner. These eight qualities are:

1. Skillful thought
2. Skillful speech
3. Skillful action
4. Skillful livelihood
5. Skillful effort
6. Skillful mindfulness
7. Skillful stillness
8. Skillful understanding

The concept of skillfulness within this prescription is whatever that brings adaptation in beneficial ways and that avoids harm, while maintaining peace. It is taught in Buddhism that when one has skillful understanding of their circumstances, cognitions and behaviors, one is also likely to be skillful thus amounting to adaptive daily discipline that in the long run, reduces suffering. So Buddhist practitioners are constantly reminded to refer to this basic teaching to calibrate their attitudes and behaviors towards a balanced lifestyle where extremes are avoided while wisdom is cultivated via mindful practices such as meditation and following precepts.

The guidelines for the reduction of suffering as suggested in the Noble Eightfold Path can be divided into a triad of sort that is to be observed for spiritual development in Buddhism. This is commonly known as *Silā-Samādhi-Paññā* (Morality-Mind Cultivation-Wisdom) where moral attitudes and behaviors (e.g. speech, action, livelihood, and effort) would facilitate the cultivation of mental faculties (e.g. mindfulness, and stillness) that result in wisdom (e.g. understanding, and thought). The wisdom that is mentioned here refers primarily to the realizations that help stop suffering.

The morality part of practice in Buddhism is also known as *silā,* which is set out as daily precepts for lay Buddhist practice for personal training in the cultivation of moral qualities of the Middle Way (e.g. speech, action, and livelihood, effort). For lay Buddhist, five precepts are prescribed for daily practice as the most basic qualities to cultivate in pursuing the goal of Buddhism. These five precepts are:

1. To abstain from killing
2. To abstain from stealing

3. To abstain from sexual misconduct
4. To abstain from false and unskillful speech
5. To abstain from intoxicating substances

The idea of observing these precepts is to provide the practitioner with a regulation in daily life that improves overall morality, which is in line with the Noble Eightfold Path. Abstaining from the five immoral actions prevents one from a lot of trouble, shame and guilt, which would hinder personal practices of mindfulness and observing peace, thus increasing suffering. The other side of these five precepts is that while abstaining from unskillful behaviors, the practitioner is also encouraged to engage in behaviors of the opposite, which are:

1. To promote kindness and compassion
2. To promote generosity
3. To promote trustworthiness and responsibility
4. To promote honesty and pleasantness
5. To promote health and well-being

The above five prescriptions to promote goodness are likely to result in well-being in others as well as the individual who does them. These plus the abstention from the listed five immoral behaviors would reduce suffering and improve well-being. So the basics of Buddhist practice are fundamentally designed for well-being and to minimize any suffering – similar to "the Good Life" preached by ancient Greek philosophers such as the Epicureans and Aristotle.

The mind cultivation part of practice in Buddhism is termed as *samādhi,* which is usually translated into English as "concentration". However, being practitioners and amateur scholars in Buddhism, we are more inclined to use the term "stillness" because meditation requires the individual to be still and to observe the processes that occur in the mind without adding any other efforts to it. "Concentration" seems too forceful a word to use to describe an activity that is meant to be relaxing and natural.

Nevertheless, the concept of *samādhi* is, in essence, the training of the mind to be able to perceive with strong awareness, the natural processes that arise and dissipate within it. The reason for this training is to develop a level of awareness within the self in relation to the interactions with one's senses to the point of understanding perspectives in life that can help to manage daily challenges that typically bring not just dissatisfaction, but a whole gamut of emotions that disturbs the peace of stillness.

The practice of meditation is said to be the exercise for the mind, which is somewhat parallel to what physical exercise does to the body. There is no such thing as good or bad meditation because every effort to remain still and observe processes within and without strengthens the individuals mind to be better able to be clear and sharp in perceiving information. Without any disturbance that is brought about by the results of immoral activities, the meditator is better able to remain still and have a strong awareness of the processes in the present moment. A strong mind built from meditation is better able to obtain the wisdom to understand perspectives that can help solve problems of discontentment and misery.

As such, moral practices provide the foundation to a light heart that allows the mind to be clear for wisdom to arise from effortful meditation practice. This is how the triad of spiritual development is connected. One has to practice a moral code, in order to improve mindfulness practice which then results in wisdom that can help overcome suffering.

Divine Dwelling (*Brahma Vihārā*)

The concept of *brahma vihārā* (divine dwelling) is usually used as a metaphor for good qualities that are to be cultivated by the Buddhist practitioner to facilitate better *samādhi* practice. These qualities are *mettā* (loving-kindness), *karunā* (compassion), *muditā* (sympathetic joy) and *upekkhā* (equanimity). The idea of developing these qualities comes from the immediate effect of having them, which is a general feeling of well-being, that aids cognitive and affective functioning for meditative practice.

These qualities are called Divine Dwelling because they reflect how a divine being would be and are goals that a practitioner should seek to achieve. Given that these are highly revered qualities, having them would also improve one's social standing, which then provides a more nurturing environment for the practitioner thus, reducing the likelihood of any suffering which may arise.

For example, a person who has developed loving-kindness well would come across as very warm and friendly, therefore putting people at ease, and having strong compassion would also improve empathy and care towards others. These two qualities are significant enough to be very attractive and therefore are protected from harm. Sympathetic joy is also known as vicarious joy where one rejoices with others when something skillful is demonstrated. Having such quality would give someone the impression of being supportive and nurturing. Equanimity is usually expressed as calmness and nonthreatening. So, in terms of well-being, these four qualities when cultivated exude an attractive resonance that also affects others positively.

Three Evils

While there is encouragement to develop qualities of divine dwelling as described above, Buddhists also put effort into avoiding the Three Evils, which as *lobha* (greed), *dosa* (hatred) and *moha* (delusion). Greed is expecting from the world what it cannot give you, thus increasing discontentment and hence suffering. Hatred is a strong dislike for something or someone that is usually brought on by rumination, thus increasing suffering. Delusion refers to the tendency for people to expect permanence when the truth is that every conditioned thing is impermanent. This is tied to greed where expectations of the impossible brings about suffering. Therefore, to reduce suffering is to live with less greed and hatred and to have better ability to embrace impermanence (*anicca*).

Dependent Origination

Simply speaking, the concept of dependent origination (*paticca samupada*) is the law of how suffering is caused and how it is ended, by a chain of causes. The key to the end of suffering is to be able to identify the causes that lead to suffering and to systematically stop them. Through insight that is usually facilitated by regular meditation practice and reflections of observed processes, the individual is able to detect the causes and conditions that bring about suffering, and so learns from it to prevent any further future suffering by the same causes and conditions. These causes and conditions are basically what the Three Evils are about. The law of dependent originations reminds the practitioner of the consequences of actions that occur from chains of previous actions. The insight from this law can help the practitioner decide on making changes to stop suffering and improve well-being.

While karma (or *kamma*, in Pali) is a large part of Buddhist belief, it is not necessarily beneficial to be accepting of current miseries as purely karma and to resign by nothing but just suffer. One of the reasons why meditation practice is important in Buddhist practice is that it internalizes the scholarly points of its teachings through practical realization, rather than an intellectualization of knowledge. Meditation is about being in the present and observing the rise and fall of phenomena occurring in the mind, and to some extent, the physical body. The basics of dependent origination applies where any addition to a chain of actions would lead to more natural consequences of whatever was added. For example, if there is already misery, and guilt is added – the misery becomes worse. In this case, guilt itself causes bad karma – propagating the cycle of shame and guilt. Therefore, to change from discontentment to contentment, there has to be a start to a chain of actions that leads to contentment. Therapy would then focus on working towards encouraging more skillful and beneficial actions to bring about better circumstances for well-being, and the cessation of suffering.

Basic Tenets but Different Traditions

These are the basic tenets of Buddhist teaching that form the bases of practice towards personal and communal well-being. Nevertheless, they may not be known or practiced by people who declare themselves to be Buddhists in Malaysia. This is due to the diversity of traditions and practices that come under the name of Buddhism, given its historical development and cultural assimilation throughout the centuries since its founding. The next section briefly discusses the context within which Buddhism is practiced in Malaysia.

Before that, it is important to name the main traditions of Buddhism. There is Theravada, Mahayana, Vajrayana and Zen of Ch'an. Some would argue that there are only two divisions where Vajrayana and Ch'an are forms of Mahayana. Nonetheless, this chapter will not make any arguments as to which division is more precise. The authors will contend with just talking from the perspectives of Theravada, Mahayana and Vajrayana. In short, the Theravada tradition, which is also called the Hinayana tradition is the predominant school of thought for Buddhism in India, Sri Lanka, Myanmar, Laos, Cambodia and Thailand. The Mahayana tradition is found in China, Vietnam, and South Korea. The Vajrayana tradition has many similarities with Mahayana practices and in some cases, are the same but only differentiated by the former being of Tibetan origins. Zen or Ch'an is usually found in Japan and Vietnam. While traditions may differ in customs and rituals, all of them are based on the basic Buddhist teaching, or *Dhamma* (*Dharma* in Sanskrit) as described above.

BUDDHISM IN MALAYSIA

Buddhism has had a long history in the South East Asian region. There are archaeological sites in the north parts of Malaysia identified as belonging to Hindu-Buddhist communities dating back to the fifth century. Currently, Buddhism is the second most prevalently declared religion in Malaysia, after Islam. Majority of people who consider themselves Buddhist in the country are ethnic Chinese and they tend to follow the Mahayana Buddhist school of thought. A smaller segment of Buddhists is from the Theravada tradition – these tend to be the English-speaking ethnic Chinese, the ethnic Thais, Sinhalese, Indians, and Burmese (Myanmar) communities. Among the ethnic Chinese in Malaysia, many practice a combination of Taoism, Buddhism, and Confucianism but would consider themselves Buddhist when asked what their religion is. More recently, in the past 20 years, the Vajrayana tradition has been growing with new centers opening around the country.

Generally, Buddhist devotees from all traditions in Malaysia have established many centers for missionary and scholarly activities, with many coordinating multiple charity organizations and community welfare centers. Some of the Mahayana based centers are branches of very established global Buddhist organizations from Taiwan. These centers also respond to natural disasters such as floods. Some of these centers also provide mental health services. Few of these centers, usually temples and hermitage focus on the development of Buddhist monastics. As such, Buddhism is a very established religion with many organizations that work to develop its practice within the community at many different levels, from lay devotees, to intellectual scholars to monastics. Malaysia is a hub for Buddhist scholars of diverse denominations and languages in South East Asia given the number of publications that have been churned out over the years.

Given the diversity of beliefs and practices of Buddhism in Malaysia, we should be careful in applying personal understanding of the tenets or impose the more streamlined and basic teachings of Buddhism on whoever who calls themselves Buddhist. Much of Buddhist practice in the lay community are infused with rituals and supernatural beliefs, that are not necessarily the intellectual teachings of Buddhism but have many pragmatic benefits to the believers. As such the next section illustrates how diversity is acknowledged in the approaches to using Buddhism in counselling and psychotherapy.

CASE STUDIES USING BUDDHIST APPROACHES IN COUNSELLING

The Theravada Buddhist approach to practice is typically based on personal efforts in self-development in the cultivation of mind towards the cessation of suffering and ultimate enlightenment. Self-reliance is a main focus of the Theravadin practitioner. However, this differs from the Mahayana Buddhist school of thought where spiritual development is more of a systemic effort that usually involves the belief that wellness is a mutual communal concept. Therefore, approaches in counselling between the two schools of thought in Buddhism can be simplified into independent (Theravada) and interdependent (Mahayana). In the case studies below some are presented in a more individualistic approach to personal practice towards well-being while another case highlights a more relational approach to applying Buddhist principles. There are also hints of practice that are relevant to individuals who believe in supernatural powers of rituals. Without any declaration from the authors in terms of who contributed to which case, it is virtually impossible to tell which one is leaning towards Mahayana or Theravada approach. Nevertheless, it should be noted that regardless of tradition, the approaches used in psychotherapy are not identified as Theravada or Mahayana because there is no qualitative demarcation between the two traditions in their applications.

Case 1: Mr B

Mr. B was a 39-year-old corporate lawyer who was recently divorced after three years of marriage. He was the one who initiated the divorce after finding out that on top of being emotionally abused on a daily basis by his former wife, she was also cheating on him with another man. Mr. B presented as depressed with the tendency for self-blame for his situation. He was a devoted husband although he received verbal and emotional abuse from his wife who, according to him, kept insisting that he was never good enough. He felt trapped in his relationship but after realizing that his former wife was also cheating on him, he decided to call it quits and somehow reluctantly asked for a divorce. He had, in his mind, the perception that a good husband should stick with his wife through thick and thin, regardless of how he is being treated because he should practice compassion at all times. So, he viewed himself as a failure in being a husband as well as being someone to uphold the Buddhist qualities such as loving-kindness and compassion. This led him to feel a lot of guilt and shame with the thought that if only he did a bit more, she might have accepted him better.

Mr. B kept saying that he must have had bad karma from his past lives that led to how he was treated by his former wife. He had concepts of karma where his guilt and thoughts of being punished led to depression. He expressed the need to perform some kind of ritual cleansing to rid himself of the so-called curse due to bad karma. While Mr. B tried performing some cleansing rituals and blessings with the aid of a familiar monk, his relief was short-lived as he still kept ruminating about how silly he was to allow his wife to manipulate him and that he had lost his confidence in being a lawyer.

The therapist discussed Mr. B's understanding of Buddhism where the misconceptions of punishment and sin in the law of karma had helped him understand that all these while he was adding on the "bad karma" to himself by ruminating. Applying the concepts of the three evils – guilt itself is a form of hatred (*dosa*) towards the self which is also latched on to the idea of permanence (a delusion) – once there is understanding that there is impermanence and that there is no greater punishment than what we do to ourselves. Furthermore, he also realized that his wife was no longer with him and therefore there was no longer any manipulation. He realized that he was still living in the past. When given some guided meditation instructions on the present moment, Mr. B's regular practice helped him let go of the guilt and shame and move on to a more adaptive mindset. This included his realization that his attachment to the past was what made his misery somewhat permanent, when in actual fact, it was not. While there were still frequent relapses towards self-blame and guilt, the improved mindfulness in Mr. B helped him to be better able to gently reframe his automatic reactions to a more beneficial set of beliefs so he could move on from his mistakes.

Case 2: Madam T

Madam T was a 60 year old retired Chinese woman, who was referred by her psychiatrist for follow up treatment for depression. She had been on anti-depressant for three years prior to her visit. At the initial presentation, the client seemed to attribute her depression to hardships in the past. She acknowledged that she was not ready to let go of past troubles as well as her current ones. For this, she was brought through the discussions of the four Brahma Vihara (Divine Dwellings) of loving-kindness, compassion, sympathetic joy and equanimity, by the counsellor. After relating these qualities towards herself and her situation, Madam T was better able to be kinder to herself, and to rejoice in her own efforts through the years, as well as the efforts from her children and grandchildren. By doing this, she formed better relationships with her family members and improved in her overall emotional well-being.

As the therapeutic relationship strengthened, Madam T eventually disclosed a traumatic and miserable memory from her past. She shared that she was nearly molested by her biological father in her formative years as an adolescent, and she had a troubled marriage to her abusive husband who used her past as a threat throughout their marriage. Nevertheless, she worked hard to financially support her family of origin as well as her own family. The couple only owned their own home late in their lives. Over the years, she has lost siblings and parents-in-laws whom she was close to. Madam T was involved in family conflicts over the selling of their previous family home as coerced by her husband and spent more time in her children's homes. This led to relationship difficulties with her children and grandchildren.

Madam T was conflicted because her Buddhist perspective sees devotion to family in her multiple roles as wife, mother and grandmother as very important in maintaining harmony in her life, but she was not able to cater to everyone's needs. At the time Madam T broke down in the session and spoke about her emotional pressure for the first time. She was very ashamed of sharing this part of her struggles and was anxious that her personal disdain towards her roles might go against her Buddhist beliefs. She believed that she was depressed because she had not done well enough in her roles and responsibilities, and she was being punished for that reason.

Similar to the other sessions discussion on loving kindness, compassion, sympathetic joy and equanimity, Socratic dialogues and discussions related to Buddhist principles helped Madam T feel that she can begin to love herself more compassionately prior to taking care of others. She was better able to gently validate and affirm her own feelings, actions and thoughts, which led to better self-acceptance and reduced depressive feelings. The therapist encouraged Madam T to reflect on how she felt about being unconditionally accepted in the therapy session, and this helped her to be more accepting of who she was and helped her believe she had an active choice to make changes for the better. Madam T had been desperately seeking reciprocal love from others that made her feel overwhelmed and confused whenever her family members did not seem to appreciate her love and care. When Madam T obtained the insight that the only person's behavior she could control was herself, she was able to let go of her expectations and practice the qualities of the four Brahma Viharas, and thus had much less blame and anger. Eventually, Madam T found some closure for her past in that she recognized it was the best she could have done then, but in the present, she has the power to make the changes she wants. She regained the sense of self-confidence and motivation to be more involved in the activities that she enjoys in her daily life, while also spending quality affectionate moments with her children and grandchildren in their house while maintaining healthy boundaries with them.

A Side Note to Case 2: Mahayana Buddhist Application of the *Brahma Viharas* (Divine Dwellings)

Following from the above case study under a Mahayana approach. This subsection explains how the *Brahma Viharas* would have been related to Madam T above. As mentioned under the basic tenets of Buddhism, the four sublime states of mind called *Brahma Vihara* (Divine Dwelling) are ideal individual practice. The *Brahma Viharas* provide guidance for challenging situations, and help individuals to regain a sense of peace, heal emotional wounds and revive joy in their lives. These four states of mind are incompatible with the negative emotion of hate. Individuals have the seed of Brahma Viharas that comes from nature rooted in their mind and heart. However, individuals do not easily discover the seed when they are shaded by the surface of what is happening and are occupied with hatred, anger, jealousy, and dissatisfaction. Through repetitive mindful self-awareness and practice, individuals can cultivate more energy to develop these sublime states of mind as a dominant perspective of mind, which is close to Brahma-like (boundless-like) state of mind. The core ideology of Brahma Viharas in Buddhist scripture of "*Āgama Sutra*" is based on continuous practice of self-purification in loving-kindness, compassion, empathetic joy and equanimity apparent to significant immediate environment to selfless immeasurable pervading of loving-kindness, compassion, empathetic joy and equanimity towards living and non-living beings in the universe (Liao Tuo, 2014).

Loving-kindness (*mettā*) describes an unconditional love that includes caring, acceptance and forgiveness towards every creature in the universe. In the Mahayana Buddhist perspective, because of one's own desires and confusion-driven behaviors, they become trapped in the life and death cycle of suffering. With this profound, gentle and kind of love to embrace all these beings, individuals deliver a deeper blessing by hoping that all living creatures will achieve a true sense of happiness and well-being. The ultimate meaning of love is love without possession. Absent from the idea of having, the act of showing and giving loving-kindness is a happiness and comfortable existence.

Compassion (*karuṇā*) describes a willingness to open one's eyes and heart to experience the emotions that bring pain and an intention to soothe the suffering. All beings are afflicted by emotions, confusion and suffering from birth, old age, sickness and death. Feeling of pain, sadness and distress can be overwhelming. Little did individuals realize that the suffering and sorrow they experience arise from their minds. With a little more kindness and compassion, individuals could be better at distinguishing themselves (solely as a person existed in the world) from the suffering and emotions. With a rich sense of experiencing suffering, compassion reconciles individuals to their life, to appreciate what they have, to have strengths to overcome life challenges, and to contribute whenever they could to others. A peaceful mind is the best way to eradicate misery and achieve liberation.

Sympathetic joy (*muditā*) describes the joy that individuals feel towards achievement of others (and also themselves). This joy empowers them to be freed from perceived hardships in life. When something happens according to individuals' wish, they feel happy and satisfied. At other times when others achieve certain accomplishments or have done good deeds, rejoicing with them and encouraging further accomplishment brings up good feelings in the one rejoicing, even when it was not them who directly contributed to the success. This type of joy brings a serene calmness that leads individuals to a contemplative state of mind (equanimity). Study has shown that a human brain tends to activate different processes when they feel different emotions (Etkin, Egner & Kalisch, 2011). A mind that is serene and peacefully aware can eventually allow individuals to obtain wisdom to be freed from afflictions and achieve true happiness by avoiding the causes of suffering. This is very much related to the next *Brahma Vihara.*

Equanimity (*upekkhā*) describes the abandonment of own desires, expectations and confusions in order to experience peace and stillness of mind. Life is two-sided, the end of birth is disintegration, and the end of gathering is separation. When experiencing life's journey which moves between contrasts of rise and fall, success and failure, loss and gain, individuals can feel how they respond with hope and fear, happiness and sorrow, satisfaction and disappointment. Mahayana Buddhist perspective encourages the concept of moderation. When individuals practice equanimity, they gradually give up the idea of possession, the thought of "mine". Individuals who has a mind of equanimity can empathize and accept more with who or what that stands out differently contrary to the pictures in their mind as they thought. When individuals demonstrate the invaluable good and accumulation of innumerable merits in generosity of the Brahma Viharas, the art of practicing loving-kindness, compassion, empathetic joy and equanimity is fulfilling and truly happy in itself. Followers of Buddhism believe that the evil actions will fall into the hell realm and the virtuous actions will lead to the good path and higher realms eventually.

Case 3: Mr. H

Mr. H was a 33-year old man who presented as depressed due to financial hardship and relationship issues with his family members. He had volatile emotions, which made him easily agitated, and had trouble sleeping for a few months prior to seeing the therapist. After an intake session, the therapist had an agreement with Mr. H that there was a pressing need to help him calm down and to get enough sleep given his presenting symptoms. Managing his relationship issues were secondary at that time. So, the therapist helped by teaching Mr. H some mindfulness activities, including relaxation exercises to practice for better skills in improving his ability to be calmer. One of the mindfulness activities, was to recite "Om Mani Padme Hung" repeatedly. In Tibetan Buddhism or Vajrayana tradition, this recitation also helps to produce good karma, on top of bringing calmness and focus. These mindfulness activities helped Mr. H to be calmer, and as a result, become more aware of his feelings and thoughts. Once he was better at noticing his feelings and thoughts, the therapist went through sessions of guided breathing technique and body scan to help the client to reduce his anxiety and tension. Mr. H was taught to be aware without passing judgement to the sensations of his body that arise and fall. Regular practice of these techniques helped Mr. H become more aware of his immediate thoughts and feelings. Once this was achieved, the therapist discussed the concept of impermanence with Mr. H and related it to his thoughts and feelings. This discussion helped Mr. H realize that the sensations he feels are constantly changing and are not permanent. This helped him understand that he does not have to be attached to his feelings – be it pleasant or unpleasant. He learnt to treasure the pleasant ones and sit out the unpleasant ones until they went away. This realization of letting go of control helped Mr. H reduce his agitation and he slept much better. This became his preparation to work on his relationship problems with his family members.

Reconciling Different Traditions in Buddhism on Psychotherapy Approaches

While there are tendencies of both schools of thought – Theravada and Mahayana Buddhist traditions to have generally different approaches in their counselling methods, the essence of both traditions originates from the basic teachings of Gautama Buddha, called the *Dhamma* (or in Sanskrit, *Dharma*). The Mahayana Buddhists, being more communal in practice, employs concepts of the *Bodhisatta* (*Bodhisattva* in Sanskrit, e.g. *Kuan Yin*, *Maitreya* and *Manjushri*) and a pantheon of lesser gods and goddesses, saints as well as spiritual protectors of the Dharma for spiritual practices. So, it seems as though it is more complicated with various sutras to be read and rituals to be carried out for a better well-being outcome in practice. Similar traditional rituals and beliefs, though not as elaborate, can be seen in Theravada traditions depending on which country they are practiced in. Theravadins do not highlight the practices related to Bodhisattas and the extended pantheon that is seen in the Mahayana tradition, but focuses more on ritualistic chanting for protection, precept-observing behaviors as basic customs for lay Buddhists.

Both traditions teach meditation as mental cultivations towards better wisdom in dealing with life and death. However, the means by which meditation is taught may also differ between traditions, with Mahayana Buddhist more likely to refer to their sutras and koans, while the Theravadins have *vipassanā* (insight) and *samatha* (calmness) meditations based in the *Satipattanā Sutta* (the Buddha's purported manual on meditation). Either way, both traditions recognize meditation as part of the spiritual practice, on top of observing moral precepts, to achieve wisdom.

Though it is beyond the scope of this chapter to discuss the origins of these practices, it should be noted that these concepts are pragmatic methods for engaging individuals in spiritual practice at different levels of understanding. Ultimately, the basic tenets of Buddhism are reflected in these practices that have long histories of development to suit the needs of the cultures they are assimilated into.

With regards to the examples above, it would have been very easy for either tradition of Buddhism to employ each other's approaches e.g. Theravada using *Brahma Vihara* focus and Mahayana using *paticca samupāda* focus in psychotherapy. So, in essence, there is nothing actually to reconcile. Much of the practice, in the authors' opinion, is in the language of therapy, which can be very diverse.

Given the age of rapid globalization, there has been many instances of cross-overs between Buddhist traditions in practice, especially in the West, where different denominations of Buddhist practitioners have been exchanging notes and developing mutual practices based on the scriptures, and applying them to modern day challenges in pragmatic ways. Therefore, in this case, reconciliation of traditions is automatically happening already in spiritual and intellectual practice. What is important also is how traditional Buddhist approaches are compatible with mainstream Western psychotherapy methods. This will be briefly discussed in the next section.

THE COMPATIBILITY BETWEEN BUDDHIST APPROACHES AND WESTERN TECHNIQUES OF COUNSELLING AND PSYCHOTHERAPY?

From the case studies given, there are many parallels to what we know as cognitive therapies. Much have been written about these parallels with many authors arguing for the compatibility between Buddhism and Western Psychotherapy. In some cases, to the point of duplicity of Eastern and Western philosophies in their applied approaches to improving mental health.

In terms of Western psychotherapy, the end of the millennium has seen a boom in mindfulness-based intervention that originated from Buddhist meditation practices. The treatment of borderline personality disorder (BPD) also highlighted the importance of insight and mindfulness that stem from Buddhist teaching. Older concepts of therapy such as Rational Emotive Behavior Therapy (REBT) has very close reasoning to Buddhist tenets. The more current "Third Wave" therapies are very much "Buddhistic" in nature – i.e. Acceptance and Commitment Therapy (ACT) and Self-Compassion Movement.

To illustrate an example of parallels, we compare Buddhist approaches with Choice Theory / Reality Therapy (CTRT). One aspect of the Buddhist approach in psychotherapy is to return the sense of choice to the individual. There is much encouragement in Buddhism to look inwards for a deeper understanding of self and its habits, and then make an informed choice to make changes for betterment. These steps are guided by the precepts and Eightfold Noble Path. Nevertheless, the main point is that the individual has to "walk the path themselves" in order to reach their goal. This is in line with CTRT where the main believe is that the only person's behavior they can control is their own. What individuals perceive from the external world is merely information and they decide what and how they want to respond to it, as said by Glasser (2011, p.5), "Nothing we do is caused by what happens outside us. If we believe that what we do is caused by forces outside us, we are acting like a dead machine, not living people." Also in line with the Noble Eightfold Path of Skillful Understanding, CTRT posits that once you have an understanding of how suffering happens, you can choose to prevent it, by also acting in ways that leads to preferred outcomes. Skilled practitioners know how to replace unskillful actions with more skillful ones. In CTRT, the awareness is active and it leads to more adaptive behavior.

Given that the *Dhamma* is meant to reflect the universal truth, it is not surprising that there are many parallels in approaches from Western psychology towards the management of personal suffering. Ancient Greek philosophies, especially Stoicism has many instances where their reasoning resembles that of Buddhism. Given that Western Psychology originated mostly from Greek and European philosophies, there is much compatibility between it and Buddhist approaches. Some scholars even argue that these philosophies have come full circle, or at least they have traveled all around between India and Greece during ancient times where the nature of exchanges made it difficult to tell of their origins.

There are more discussions to be had and descriptions of parallels between Buddhism and Western psychotherapy but it would be beyond the scope of this chapter. These can be found in many literatures already. The idea of mentioning parallels here is so that there is some acknowledgement of how relevant Buddhist teachings are in promoting mental well-being within the psychotherapy situation.

THE (MIDDLE) WAY FORWARD: FUTURE DIRECTIONS FOR BUDDHISM IN COUNSELLING AND PSYCHOTHERAPY

This chapter so far has touched on Buddhist approaches in counselling and psychotherapy in general. Much more has to be studied systematically with regards to methodology and outcomes before more comparisons can be made with more established Western cognitive therapies. However, this can be a very difficult task given the limited research to being with that show specifically Buddhism-based approaches are scientifically efficacious. Furthermore, there are many overlaps between techniques in Buddhism and Western psychotherapy. The whole idea of technique itself may be a questionable concept or term that may require its own investigation. It is difficult to ascertain how a Buddhist approach might look like minus the Western formula of psychotherapy. What this chapter has demonstrated so far was the use of Buddhist concepts within Westernized psychotherapy settings. Perhaps investigations should also look into situational difference of the Buddhist approach. For example, how would monastics members of the Buddhist clergy use their teachings as means of directly propagating well-being in troubled individuals who go to them for help. This would be relevant especially when individual insecurities revolve around afterlife, supernatural beliefs and religious intellectual confusion.

Many evidence have been largely anecdotal rather than based on rigorous randomized control trial-type research. Much of the studies that are related to Buddhist approaches have been largely on mindfulness-based cognitive therapy (MBCT). These researches have established MBCT's efficacy as part of the "Third Wave" of psychotherapies. Nevertheless, there has been recent criticisms towards MBCT as being misapplied outside of the overall context where the morality aspects of behavioral change have not necessarily been applied. These criticisms come from how mindfulness was extracted from Buddhist practice of *samādhi* for its strong effect on improving focus and self-understanding but had neglected the *silā* or morality side, coupled with respect for cultural customs that facilitates the practice of mindfulness. Therefore, more research beyond just mindfulness-based interventions are needed, partly also to address the criticisms towards MBIs as missing the context for mindfulness, which is part of the spiritual development triad – which needs moral development as well.

CONCLUSION

This chapter has presented a basic view of Buddhism in relation to how its teachings can form part of the psychotherapeutic process in helping individuals improve their mental health. Much of the Buddhist approach is cognitive in nature and can easily be intellectualized without actual realization. However, when delivered in a more experiential manner, the tenets of Buddhism can be applied to daily challenges in life that are rife with personal attachments, inaccurate assumptions of permanence and aversive events. The main teachings of Buddhism serve to help individuals understand the nature of suffering or discontentment and how, by understanding the nature, taking steps to stop the causes and conditions that bring about the misery that suffering and discontentment lead to. Given that Buddhism is in essence a manual for freedom from suffering, it is argued by the authors that it is basically a psychotherapy practice. While Western psychotherapy uses organized techniques developed over the last two centuries by psychiatrists and psychologists, Buddhism is largely infused into social lifestyle as a religion or spiritual practice, which has overshadowed its value as a mental health system of knowledge. Much of the practice of Buddhism has been demonstrated by ritualistic activities than actual internalization of its basic teachings that are meant for personal betterment. This is not to say that the rituals are not beneficial, but the deeper understanding of the basic underpinnings of what the Buddha taught can be very effective and practical in promoting mental health. It is hoped that this chapter highlights Buddhist philosophy as something more than just a spiritual identity but also a tool for overall well-being.

REFERENCES

Etkin, A., Egner, T., & Kalisch, R. (2011). Emotional processing in anterior cingulate and medial prefrontal cortex. *Trends in Cognitive Sciences*, *15*(2), 85–93. doi:10.1016/j.tics.2010.11.004 PMID:21167765

Glasser, W. (2011). *Take charge of your life: How to get what you need with Choice Theory psychology*. Bloomington, IN: iUniverse.

Pochelli, M. (2015). *This is what happens to your brain when you experience happiness*. Retrieved from http://reset.me/story/this-is-what-happens-to-your-brain-when-you-experience-happiness/

Tuo, L. (2014). 慈悲喜舍的意义与修习方法. Retrieved from http://www.liaotuo.org/fjrw/jsrw/zxjs/66904.html

ADDITIONAL READING

Brazier, C. (2003). *Buddhism on the couch: From analysis to awakening using Buddhist psychology*. Ulysses Press.

Dhammananda, K. S. (2001). *Why worry?* Singapore Buddhist Meditation Centre.

Hanh, T. N. (2008). *The heart of Buddha's teaching*. Random House.

Murguia, E., & Díaz, K. (2015). The philosophical foundations of cognitive behavioral therapy: Stoicism, Buddhism, Taoism, and Existentialism. *Journal of Evidence-Based Psychotherapies*, *15*(1), 37.

Thera, V. N. (2017). *Buddha and his Teachings*. Pariyatti Publishing.

Chapter 12
Psychotherapy and Christianity: Methods and Challenges

Jeremy Lim
HELP University, Malaysia

Ke Hui Chuah
HELP University, Malaysia

ABSTRACT

Christianity is counted as one of the biggest religious groups in the world, numbering at over 2 billion individuals who identify themselves with this religion. As of the 2010 census, the Department of Statistics Malaysia Official Portal reported that an estimated 9.2% of the population in Malaysia identified themselves as Christians. In numerical terms, this equates to approximately 3 million individuals spread out all over the Malaysian peninsular as well as Sabah and Sarawak who consider themselves part of the Christian church. This chapter intends to do four things: 1) provide a brief history of the church and Christianity, 2) acquaint the reader with basic Christian beliefs, 3) provide insight into the methods and challenges of working with the population in Malaysia drawing from both local as well as international literature, and 4) provide the implications of the methods and challenges of working with the Christian population.

INTRODUCTION

He answered, "'Love the Lord your God with all your heart and with all your soul and with all your strength and with all your mind'; and, 'Love your neighbor as yourself.'" - Luke 10:27, NIV

Worldwide, Christianity (including Protestants, Roman Catholics, and others) is counted as one of the biggest religious groups in the world, numbering at over 2,000,000,000 individuals who identify themselves with this religion (BBC, 2011). As of the 2010 census, the Department of Statistics Malaysia Official Portal (2010) reported that there is an estimated 9.2% of the population in Malaysia identified themselves as Christians. In numerical terms, this equates to approximately 3,000,000 individuals spread out all over the Malaysian peninsular as well as Sabah and Sarawak who consider themselves part of the Christian church. This essay intends to do 4 things: 1) provide a brief history of the church and

DOI: 10.4018/978-1-5225-6073-9.ch012

Christianity, 2) acquaint the reader with basic Christian beliefs, 3) provide insight into the methods and challenges of working with the population in Malaysia drawing from both local as well as international literature, and 4) provide the implications of the methods and challenges of working with the Christian Protestant population.

BRIEF HISTORY OF THE CHURCH

For many people, Christianity is synonymous from its founder from whom the name derives from – Jesus Christ. The following contains a short exposition on both the story of Jesus Christ and the history of the church as a means to provide the reader a basis for which to approach clients. This approach is presented from a Protestant point of view.

The Bible, Christianity's holy book, teaches that Jesus Christ (which means Yeshua the Messiah i.e. the Savior) was born in Bethlehem, Israel, to a virgin called Mary. Christians believe that Mary was pregnant not by human or physical means but by direct divine action through the Holy Spirit (BBC, 2009a). Jesus himself represented the fulfillment of prophecies of other parts of the Bible and was believed to have been born over 2000 years ago (approximately 4-7 BC) (BBC, 2009a; Robinson, 2008). The Bible covers Jesus' early life in brief and Jesus' public influence in detail in the books of Matthew, Mark, Luke, and John, reputed eyewitness accounts of Jesus' life (BBC, 2009a). During this period in the public sphere, Jesus gathered many followers, foremost of whom were the 12 disciples who later went on to lead the early church (BBC, 2009a). The climax of Jesus' story is when the religious leaders, critical of Jesus and believing him to proclaim falsehoods, apprehended and crucified Jesus (crucifixion is an ancient Roman means of execution, where the condemned is nailed to a cross and left to hang until he/she suffocates) (BBC, 2009a). However, the Bible teaches that three days after Jesus' death by crucifixion, Jesus was raised to life again by the power of God whereupon he was taken up to heaven a few days later after having spent time with many eyewitnesses (BBC, 2009a).

Jesus' ascension to heaven marked the beginning of the church where Jesus' disciples and followers spread His message throughout the Roman Empire (BBC, 2011). This was also when the term Christians (literally, Christ-followers) began to be used to refer to Christ's followers (Acts 11:26, New International Version). This early movement faced many troubles such as condemnation, torture, and execution by Roman emperors such as Nero, Domitian, and Diocletian who believed the religion to be heretical (BBC, 2009a). However, Christianity became more accepted under the rule of Constantine whose efforts resulted in the codification of Christian doctrine (BBC, 2009a). Over the centuries, various divides such as the Great Schism in 1054 and the Protestant reformation resulted in different ways of understanding Christianity (e.g. the Roman-Catholics versus the Protestants versus the Orthodox church) (Encyclopedia Britannica, 2017).

The verse from the Bible at the opening of this chapter is Jesus' summary of the teachings of the Bible which have been handed down throughout the centuries. Differences in doctrine and interpretation of teachings have also resulted in the various denominations today (e.g. the Methodists, the Anglicans, the Presbyterians, the Baptists, the Jehovah Witnesses, etc). However, it is beyond the scope of this chapter to cover the differences between denominations in detail and interested readers would do well to consult other sources. Regardless, most Christian denominations today believing these commands are thus motivated to be able to better the lives of others. While some efforts in the distant past were extremely misguided (e.g. the Great Crusades), in the present day, the Christian church's main efforts outside of the church are in helping those who need assistance wherever they can in different capacities (e.g. building schools and hospitals, working among the poor and needy, caring for the outcasts in society) (Velarde, 2009). Unfortunately, efforts in the mental health field have been slower as various disorders were seen as spiritual issues and religion itself seemed to be vilified by early mental health practitioners (CT Editors, 2018). However, today, there is more understanding and acceptance of differences between spiritual and mental disorders and the Catholic church has even included a catechism which states that before an exorcism is performed, it must be ascertained that it is not a psychological illness causing a certain behaviour (Catholic Church, n.d.; CT Editors, 2018).

In Malaysia, Christianity first landed on these shores via the arrival of the Portuguese as early as early as the 1500s, the Dutch in the 1600s, and subsequently the British which brought Roman Catholicism into the country (Roxborogh, 1989). Through the subsequent years of various colonial attempts, World War Two, as well as Malaysia's independence, the churches in Malaysia continued to expand resulting in a growing Christian movement especially among those from Sabah and Sarawak (Roxborogh, 1989). Today, the churches in Malaysia face various challenges including continuing to integrate into a multi-ethnic and multireligious society (Roxborogh, 1989).

Individual Christian denominations in Malaysia generally subscribe to a higher council (e.g. the National Evangelical Christian Fellowship) (Christian Federation of Malaysia, 2018). These federations and councils come together under the banner off the Christian Federation of Malaysia which unites the Catholic Bishops' Conference of Malaysia, the Council of Churches Malaysia (i.e. Anglicans, Lutherans, Methodists, Orthodox, Presbyterians and others), and the abovementioned National Evangelical Christian Fellowship (i.e Assemblies of God, Baptists, Brethrens, independent and free churches, and others) thus accounting for the majority of Christians in Malaysia (See Christian Federation of Malaysia, 2018 for the full list). Other churches include the Mormon Church (i.e. the Church of Jesus Christ of Latter-day Saints) and the Jehovah's Witnesses. It is important to note that evangelical parties (i.e. mainstream denominations) may not consider either of these two denominations as fully "Christian" as they subscribe to teachings that do not conform to the traditionally espoused doctrines of the church (McDermott, 2016). Interested readers can consult other sources for a more in-depth exposition.

In terms of mental health related work, there exist seminaries and higher learning institutions that provide courses related to the mental health field such as pastoral counselling (e.g. the Alpha Omega International College) or a variety of certificate and diploma level Christian counselling courses at places such as Seminari Teoloji Malaysia, Bible College Malaysia, and others. Christian counsellors and therapists in Malaysia also have the option of connecting with others through the National Association of Christian Counsellors which was founded in 2011 and aims to provide ethical mental health services to the Christian community (National Association of Christian Counsellors, 2018).

The Basics: Tenets of the Faith

To begin the work of therapy with Christians, it would be of great use to examine some basic Christian beliefs in order to begin understanding how Christians make sense of their faith and its relation to the world. For Christians who identify as Protestants (any mainstream Christian denominations such as Methodists, Baptists, and so on), the basic Christian beliefs can be summed up in five Solas. A Sola is a Latin word meaning "alone". The five Solas are as follows:

- Sola Scriptura. The meaning of this phrase is "Scripture alone" and points to the belief that the Bible alone is the highest authority as the word of God. This phrase does not mean that truth is only found in the Bible but the Bible informs Christians about God's message and all other truth should be interpreted in light of the Bible (Holcomb, n.d.).
- Sola Fide. This phrase means "faith alone", and points to the belief that Christians are saved and justified as righteous in God's eyes only by their faith in Jesus Christ, his divinity, and his message (Holcomb, n.d.). This phrase reminds Christians that this salvation is not a result of any righteous or "good" actions that the individual may undertake or do. Essentially, this phrase states that one cannot "earn" one's salvation through good works.
- Sola Gratia. This particular phrase means "grace alone". Christians believe that they possibly match God's perfection and holiness and it is only through His grace alone that they are offered the opportunity for salvation, not our own goodness and regardless of our sin (Holcomb, n.d.).
- Solus Christus. This phrase means "Christ alone" and points to the belief that Jesus Christ is the revelation and incarnation of God in the flesh and only His death could redeem Christians from their sin (Holcomb, n.d.).
- Soli Deo Gloria. Meaning "to the glory of God alone", this belief helps the Christian put him or herself into the proper perspective, that all glory belongs to God alone and that God's glory is the primary motivator and purpose for the life of the Christian. However, this also reminds Christians that God is good, and that His purpose for the Christian is the enjoyment and improvement of life for themselves and others (not necessarily physical or material improvement) (Holcomb, n.d.).

These five phrases sum up some of the core Christian beliefs about God and His purposes for humanity as Christians believe is revealed in the Bible. Another often used method of expressing the basic doctrines of Christianity were codified in the creeds spoken in churches around the world as a reminder and proclamation of what the church and each Christian believes. One of the oldest declarations of the basics of Christian faith is the Apostles' Creed which is usually given as:

I believe in God the Father Almighty, Maker of heaven and earth, And in Jesus Christ his only Son our Lord, Who was conceived by the Holy Ghost, Born of the Virgin Mary, Suffered under Pontius Pilate, Was crucified, dead, and buried. He descended into hell; The third day He rose again from the dead; He ascended into heaven, And sitteth on the right hand of God the Father Almighty; From thence he shall come to judge the quick and the dead. I believe in the Holy Ghost; The Holy catholic Church, the Communion of Saints; The Forgiveness of sins; The Resurrection of the body, And the Life everlasting. Amen. (Billy Graham Evangelistic Association, 2004).

Some key points to note are that the beliefs espoused in this creed are ecumenical, key doctrines of the Christian faith that cut across all denominations and traditions (Tang, 2004). Another is that the term "catholic" (note the small "c") in this creed means universal and does not refer to the Roman Catholic church as a group (Billy Graham Evangelistic Association, 2004). Creeds were used as answers to perceived false teachings of that time and were used to present a summary of key teachings (Tang, 2004). Most creeds (including this one; others include the Roman Creed and the Nicene Creed) covers the basics of salvation, the understanding of God, the divinity and physical incarnation of Jesus, the crucifixion and resurrection of Christ, and the doctrine of grace (Tang, 2004).

A further elaboration of basic Christian beliefs include but are not limited to:

- Monotheism; A belief in one God but present in three forms, elements, or aspects (the Trinity): the Father, the Son (Jesus Christ), and the Holy Spirit (BBC, 2009b).
- God's love: Christians believe that God is a personal God and loves all humanity unconditionally (BBC, 2009b). However, to receive salvation, the individual who desires must obey certain conditions as stipulated in the Bible (BBC, 2009b).
- Jesus' teachings can be summarized into two commands which Jesus himself proclaimed: Love God with all of oneself and, the second, love one's neighbour as one loves one's self (BBC, 2009b). This provides a point of entry for the therapist to discuss self-care in the Christian context.
- Christians believe in life after physical death, the spirit as eternal, and most believe in some conception of heaven and hell (BBC, 2009b).
- Prayer is the method of communication with God. Christians believe that the Bible gave a model of prayer from Jesus in the New Testament and are told to address God as Father (BBC, 2009b). Prayers can be both rituals or spontaneous (BBC, 2009b). Some groups believe that prayers should be directed through other individuals such as saints or Mary, the mother of Jesus (BBC, 2009b). Some groups believe in "praying in tongues", a form of prayer where the person praying utters sounds that do not appear to resemble any known language as empowered by the Holy Spirit (Got Questions.org, 2017).
- Baptism (i.e. the submerging and reemergence of the person's body) in water, whether as an infant or an adult (depending on the group) as an outward symbol of commitment to Christ and His teachings (BBC, 2009b).
- Communion or the Eucharist: A Greek word meaning thanksgiving, Christians believe that the Communion meal, consisting of bread and wine, are an emulation of the last meal (the Last Supper) of Christ before His crucifixion who commanded His disciples to continue the tradition in memory of Him (BBC, 2009b). Disagreement has arisen in between different denominations due to different understanding and interpretation of Christ's teaching on the Communion (BBC, 2009b).
- A personal relationship with God: Christians believe that God is active and in communication with the church as a whole and individual believers (Piper, 2008). God speaks to Christians through the Bible, through the Holy Spirit, through other believers, and through circumstances (Piper, 2008).

While these summarize most of the basic doctrines of Christian faith, it is also worth noting that there exist differences between different groups of Christians (e.g. Protestant versus Catholics) and between denominations (e.g. Methodist versus Baptist). Thus, it would be a worthwhile exercise for the therapist to explore the specific interpretations and beliefs of the Christian client's belief system while keeping in mind these basics to better grasp the religious and spiritual context of the client. Readers interested to delve into the differences between such denominations are encouraged to consult other definitive sources.

The Lay of the Land: Christians and Psychotherapy

It is undeniable that psychotherapies have been shown to be effective in treating relational and emotional issues but yet remain as one of the most controversial discussions in the church in this day and age (Christian Research Institute, 2009). Bob and Gretchen Passantino from the apologetics discipleship organization, *Answers In Action* illustrated that some members of the Christian community perceives psychology as a rival religion that challenges their Christian faith (Christian Research Institute, 2009).

Christians were found to be more likely to attribute spiritual causes to psychological disorders (Choi, 2013) and amongst the difficulties of working with Christians, one of the main concerns was the idea that therapists were against religious establishments (Beck, 1997). However, in the 1960s and 1970s, there was a growing understanding that the usual spiritual methods in the church were not effective at treating relationship and emotionally-related issues (Esau, 1998). This coupled with the fact that psychotherapists are more likely to identify as "spiritual but not religious" (Post & Wade, 2009) all potentially contributed to the rift between Christianity and psychotherapy.

Some other debates surrounding the controversies of Psychology in the Christian community include the different views of Psychology vs. Christianity in topics such as personal suffering, self-love, and the sufficiency of recovery through biblical scriptures and Psychology being a "worldly wisdom":

- Personal suffering.

Barnes (2014) argued that modern psychology strived to remove all forms of personal suffering whether through the removal of guilt, or self-esteem improvements; while the Christian doctrine contended that personal suffering served the purpose of drawing Christians closer to God, builds character, and that Jesus Christ also suffered for a purpose (Philippians 3:10, Hebrews 5:8-9, 1 Peter 5:10, New International Version). Such Christians might not desire to eliminate personal life suffering but to learn how to live with it and adapt accordingly. For the therapist working with such a client, this means that being aware of such a mentality could change the approach that the therapist takes with his or her client e.g. working with them to accept their suffering instead of striving to remove it completely.

- Self-love.

Barnes (2014) also argued that some modern psychology approaches were intended to help an individual begin to develop love and acceptance of himself or herself to recover from self-destructive behaviours; whereas, the Bible teaches that Christians should learn to deny themselves, turn away from making themselves the most important person in their lives, and follow Jesus (Matthew 16:24-25). Biblical teachings also condemned the mentality of being a lover of oneself (2 Timothy 3:1-2). However, closer examination appears to reveal that the self-love espoused by Psychology has been taken out of context and equated to narcissism and the Scriptures themselves have been taken out of context by the arguments above. The first Scripture appeared to revolve more around the theme of learning to place God first before oneself; while the second Scripture seemed to put forth the proposition to focus more upon being mindful of not falling into self-absorption rather than condemning self-love.

- Sufficiency of recovery through biblical scriptures and Psychology being a "worldly wisdom".

Cole (1993) explained that the Bible provided warnings about succumbing to worldly wisdom as it opposed God's wisdom (Psalm 1:1-2; Isa. 55:8-11; Jer. 2:13; 1 Cor. 1:18-2:16, New International Version). He also argued that instead of depending on psychology which is a form of worldly wisdom, Christians should be depending solely on God and the scripture for wisdom and support in the trials and difficulties of life (Psalms 19:7-11; 32:6-11; 33:6-22; 119). Furthermore, Cole (1993) also proposed that as Christians learn to depend on God and the scriptures as their source of healing and strength, the glory of recovery goes to God as the only true God; whereas, if Christians rely on secular psychology for healing, it would contribute to psychology receiving said glory. This in turn goes against the Christian teaching of God being the all-sufficient One who understands our deepest needs and is able to meet them.

However, despite the controversies surrounding Psychology for the Christian community, Bob and Gretchen Passantino also acknowledged that amongst the Christian community, psychotherapy has indeed became enormously popular and sought after (Christian Research Institute, 2009). They explained that many Christians have often focused their attention on criticising psychotherapy and urge other Christians to go back to the Word of God as a form of solutions to their struggles and problems, but argued that although such approach has its merit, it is also an inaccurate generalisation (Christian Research Institute, 2009). Instead, they believe that the limitations of current practice and the lack of emphasis on biblical counselling was a far more critical concern to the endeavours and efforts of the church and is the main cause of Christians who are suffering from mental disorders or emotional struggles turning away from biblical scripture to psychotherapy as a form of healing (Christian Research Institute, 2009). This is illustrated in their article where stories were reported about certain churches who refused to embrace "the repentant alcoholic, the parent with the troubled teen, or those emotionally bruised by sinful behaviour", churches who fail to support, nurture, and fulfil a church's responsibilities and obligation towards the their community, whether Christian or not. The Passantinos also contended that when these hurting Christians do not feel nurtured, protected, admonished, and matured by the Church, they will look elsewhere for help and in this case, they found healing through more secular psychotherapy instead (Christian Research Institute, 2009).

Jones and Butman (2011) suggested that in order to provide optimal assistance to the recovery journey of hurting individuals, it is vital to have an explicit and comprehensive understanding of human behaviour through psychology. However, they also argued in their analysis of psychotherapy theories that different theories and/or models have their own compatibilities and incompatibilities with Christian and biblical faith alongside with its strength and weaknesses, insights and inconsistencies. So where exactly does psychotherapy and its associated theories stand in the Christian community and vice versa? This chapter posits that while biblical Scripture does govern the fundamental practices and beliefs of Christians, "Scripture does not provide all that we need in order to understand human beings fully", which is similar to Jones and Butman's (2011) perspectives. Therefore, it would be of great importance for Christian psychologists and counsellors to remain flexible and explore an integration of their Christian belief with the evidence based psychological findings, theories, and models to provide psychotherapy that could be most effective in assisting individuals struggling with mental health and/or life struggles. In fact, Jones and Butman (2011) also contended that neither is there one definitive model that exists nor would such a perfect model ever exist, thereby supporting the suggestion that integrated models would be the most efficient way of conceptualizing this apparent dichotomy.

IMPLICATIONS AND RECOMMENDATIONS

In discussing how Christians view psychotherapy, it cannot be denied that as more awareness is created, the need to work effectively with this population continues to increase. The effective multicultural therapist would begin to examine how a client's faith could be turned into support or even direct intervention in order to better assist a client instead of simply brushing this valuable resource aside. Thus, it would also be helpful to examine practical steps that therapists can take to begin to work more effectively with Christian (and other similarly religious) clients.

Post and Wade (2009) in a review paper describe the methods of clinicians who were deemed to work effectively with spiritual and/or religious clients. They describe these clinicians as approaching clients with an openness and appreciation of different religious and/or spiritual traditions and were also cautious not to place their own religious values on clients (Post & Wade, 2009). To facilitate greater spiritual and religious self-awareness and become more aware of their values, therapists were recommended to generate a spiritual autobiography as a means of self-reflection (Wiggins, 2008, as cited in Post & Wade, 2009). This openness was supported by a proposition by Esau (1998) that therapists who were effective at working with Christians must be willing to explore the client's religious life and be aware of their own potential for countertransference. To facilitate such exploration with clients, Post and Wade (2009) recommend an explicit statement or discussion facilitation outlining therapists' openness and commitment to explore such issues with their clients. Post and Wade (2009) also recommend that while understanding the basic tenets of religion was helpful, what was more important was therapists' attitude and openness towards understanding and exploring the client's religion. Furthermore, as illustrated earlier in the essay, Jones and Butman (2011) also stepped forth and suggested for therapists and counselors who are working with the Christian community to familiarise oneself with the Christian teaching and constructively integrate these teaching with the fundamental psychological findings.

Other important points to note for therapists included being acquainted with non-mainstream religious traditions as they had a great likelihood of assigning psychopathology to non-mainstream traditions (O'Connor & Vandenberg, 2005) and assessing religious commitment as a correlate with client willingness to share about religious or spiritual issues (Walker, Worthington, Gartner, Gorsuch, & Hanshew, 2011). Therapists should also be aware that despite being open to discussing religious issues, clients may not want therapists to view their religion as part of their presenting problem (Walker, Worthington, Gartner, Gorsuch, & Hanshew, 2011). Highly religious clients may experience difficulty discussing their faith with secular therapists as they might be uncertain about the therapists' reactions (Cragun & Friedlander, 2012). As already espoused above, secular therapists who were open and allowed clients the autonomy to decide when and how much to share facilitated more positive psychotherapeutic experiences for their clients (Cragun & Friedlander, 2012). In contrast, religious clients with secular therapists who articulated opposing religious perspectives or even avoided discussing spiritual and/or religious issues experienced greater negative psychotherapeutic experiences (Cragun & Friedlander, 2012).

On top of that, highly religious clients may expect and request spiritual integration in their psychotherapy process (i.e. discussing Scripture or praying with them) (Walker, Worthington, Gartner, Gorsuch, & Hanshew, 2011). This was found to be the case among Orthodox Christians where there was an emphasis placed on using faith, prayer, meditation, teachings from the Bible, and Christian counselling in the therapeutic process (Gass, 1984). This was further supported among conservative Christian adults who stated a preference for both explicitly Christian and secular therapists to engage with them using a greater emphasis on religiously oriented interventions (Bellaire & Young, 2005). However, therapists should be careful not to assume and take caution in assessing a client's needs and desires for more religiously-oriented intervention techniques and should make it a practice to obtain informed consent before attempting any interventions (Post & Wade, 2009). In cases with client agreement, there is some research to show that religious or spiritual interventions were more effective for these clients than more secular interventions and that despite therapists' own religious commitment, effectiveness was mediated more by correlation with clients' own religious commitment (Post & Wade, 2009).

CONCLUSION

At the end of the day, there is a place for both biblical counselling and more secular psychotherapies especially when working with a Christian client. A person may draw strength, hope and even healing from biblical scriptures or biblical counselling, while psychotherapy could come in handy to facilitate the Christian client to re-evaluate dysfunctional, irrational, and/or unhealthy beliefs that perpetuates the Christian client's mental struggles. Nonetheless, as with all therapy, it is also crucial for the therapist to be flexible when working with different individuals. As this chapter has illustrated some of the different controversies of psychology to Christians, and discussed some of the limitations of solely biblical counselling, an integration of psychology with a client's Christian beliefs could help achieve a balance and a mode of recovery that would be more optimal for Christians who are wary about secular psychotherapies. In conclusion, the effective multicultural therapist should consider both the person's faith as well as the modality of application, in this case, for the Christian community.

REFERENCES

Barnes, J. (2014). *Christianity vs. modern psychology: Centered ministry or problem centered counseling?* Retrieved October 19, 2017, from http://www.the-gospel.org/stdy_psych/christ-centered.php

BBC. (2009b, August 14). *Religions - Christianity: The basics of Christian beliefs*. Retrieved October 19, 2017, from http://www.bbc.co.uk/religion/religions/christianity/beliefs/basics_1.shtml

BBC. (2011b, June 30). *Religions - Christianity: Christianity at a glance*. Retrieved October 19, 2017, from http://www.bbc.co.uk/religion/religions/christianity/ataglance/glance.shtml

Beck, J. R. (1997). Value tensions between evangelical Christians and Christian counseling. *Counseling and Values*, *41*(2), 107–116. doi:10.1002/j.2161-007X.1997.tb00393.x

Bellaire, C., & Young, J. S. (2005). Inclusion of religious behaviors and attitudes in counseling expectations of conservative Christians. *Counseling and Values*, *49*(2), 82–94. doi:10.1002/j.2161-007X.2005.tb00255.x

Billy Graham Evangelistic Association. (2004). *What is the Apostles' Creed?* Retrieved October 19, 2017, from https://billygraham.org/answer/what-is-the-apostles-creed/

Choi, F. H. (2013). *The Faithful and the Distressed: How Likely are Christians to Seek Psychotherapy Treatment for Psychological Distress?* (Doctoral dissertation).

Christian Federation of Malaysia. (n.d.). *Christian Federation of Malaysia*. Retrieved from http://cfmsia.org/

Christian Research Institute. (2009). *Psychology and the church (part one)*. Retrieved October 19, 2017, from: http://www.equip.org/article/psychology-and-the-church-part-one/

Cole. (1993). *Christians and psychology: Some common questions answered*. Retrieved October 19, 2017, from: https://bible.org/article/christians-and-psychology-some-common-questions-answered

Cragun, C. L., & Friedlander, M. L. (2012). Experiences of Christian clients in secular psychotherapy: A mixed-methods investigation. *Journal of Counseling Psychology*, *59*(3), 379–391. doi:10.1037/a0028283 PMID:22563669

Department of Statistics Malaysia Official Portal. (2011, July 29). Retrieved October 19, 2017, from https://www.dosm.gov.my/v1/index.php?r=column/cthemeByCat&cat=117&bul_id=MDMxdHZjWTk1SjFzTzNkRXYzcVZjdz09&menu_id=L0pheU43NWJwRWVSZklWdzQ4TlhUUT09

Editors, C. T. (2018). *What Made Mental Illness a 'Sin'? Paganism.* Retrieved from https://www.christianitytoday.com/ct/2018/february-web-only/mental-illness-sin.html

Encyclopædia Britannica. (2017, February 15). *Reformation*. Retrieved October 19, 2017, from https://www.britannica.com/event/Reformation

Esau, T. G. (1998). The evangelical Christian in psychotherapy. *American Journal of Psychotherapy*, *52*(1), 28–36. doi:10.1176/appi.psychotherapy.1998.52.1.28 PMID:9553638

Gass, C. S. (1984). Orthodox Christian values related to psychotherapy and mental health. *Journal of Psychology and Theology*, *12*(3), 230–237. doi:10.1177/009164718401200308

gotquestions.org. (2017, January 4). *What is praying in tongues? Is praying in tongues a prayer language between a believer and God?* Retrieved October 20, 2017, from https://www.gotquestions.org/praying-in-tongues.html

Holcomb, J. (n.d.). *The Five Solas - Points from the Past that Should Matter to You*. Retrieved October 19, 2017, from http://www.christianity.com/church/church-history/the-five-solas-of-the-protestant-reformation.html

McDermott, G. (2016). *Mormons and Christians: So Close, Yet So Far Away*. Retrieved from https://www.christianitytoday.com/ct/2016/june-web-only/mormons-and-christians-so-close-yet-so-far-away.html

National Association of Christian Counsellors. (n.d.). *National Association of Christian Counsellors*. Retrieved from https://www.nacc-malaysia.org/

O'Connor, S., & Vandenberg, B. (2005). Psychosis or faith? Clinicians' assessment of religious beliefs. *Journal of Consulting and Clinical Psychology*, *73*(4), 610–616. doi:10.1037/0022-006X.73.4.610 PMID:16173848

Piper, J. (2008, February 13). *What does it mean to have a relationship with God?* Retrieved October 19, 2017, from https://www.desiringgod.org/interviews/what-does-it-mean-to-have-a-relationship-with-god

Post, B. C., & Wade, N. G. (2009). Religion and spirituality in psychotherapy: A practice-friendly review of research. *Journal of Clinical Psychology*, *65*(2), 131–146. doi:10.1002/jclp.20563 PMID:19132737

Religions - Christianity. The basics of Christian history. (2009a, June 08). Retrieved October 19, 2017, from http://www.bbc.co.uk/religion/religions/christianity/history/history_1.shtml

Religions-Christianity. Paul. (2011a, June 21). Retrieved October 19, 2017, from http://www.bbc.co.uk/religion/religions/christianity/history/paul_1.shtml

Robinson, B. A. (2008). *Christianity: A brief history*. Retrieved October 19, 2017, from http://www.religioustolerance.org/chr_intr1.htm

Roxborogh, J. (1989). *A Short Introduction to Malaysian Church History: A Guide to the Story of Christianity in Malaysia and How to Go About Discovering the History of Your Church* (2nd rev. Ed.). Seremban: Seminari Theoloji Malaysia.

Stewart, D. (n.d.). *What Precautions Were Taken to Keep the Tomb of Jesus Secure?* Retrieved October 19, 2017, from https://www.blueletterbible.org/faq/don_stewart/don_stewart_247.cfm

Tang, A. (2004). *Understanding the Apostles' Creed.* Retrieved October 19, 2017 from http://www.kairos2.com/Apostles_Creed.pdf

Velarde, R. (2009). *What Is the Church?* Retrieved May 31, 2018, from https://www.focusonthefamily.com/faith/the-study-of-god/why-study-god/what-is-the-church

Walker, D. F., Worthington, E. L. Jr, Gartner, A. L., Gorsuch, R. L., & Hanshew, E. R. (2011). Religious commitment and expectations about psychotherapy among Christian clients. *Psychology of Religion and Spirituality*, *3*(2), 98–114. doi:10.1037/a0021604

Chapter 13
Hinduism and Counseling:
Karma, Women Empowerment, Grief and Death, Anger Management, Bhagavad Gita, and Psychotherapies

Devi Venashinee Muruges
HELP University, Malaysia

ABSTRACT

Indian psychology lays enormous importance on the research of religious experiences and the expansion of approaches by which to accomplish them. In addition to that, it also provides understanding of the different states of consciousness. Hence, it is undeniable that Indian psychology will be able to make a definite therapeutic contribution to many psychological problems. For mental health practitioners dealing with Hinduism, there are teachings within various texts that directly strengthen counseling and mental services. Some of the examples include perceiving the conscious and the unconsciousness aspects of the mind, utilizing meditation to support people with mental health issues, yoga exercises to curb anxiety and stress, and many others. Therefore, this chapter intends to elucidate the application of Hinduism in therapy.

INTRODUCTION

Hinduism is one of the five largest practiced religions in the World. There are so many books and beliefs that are part of Hindu practices that some see Hinduism as more a way of life rather than a dogmatic religion. While Hinduism is seen as pantheistic religion, that are practitioners of Hinduism that are monotheistic and even atheist believing in the concepts rather than the ritualistic practices of the religion. Conceptually however there are concepts that guide Hindu, this article looks at the beliefs of Hindus that has an impact on counselling and therapeutic practices.

DOI: 10.4018/978-1-5225-6073-9.ch013

Our basic philosophy is trinity. Trinity means we believe there are three basic things: matter, soul and God. God to us is all pervading. It is not something that is static and sitting on one place. It is matter through which this world came out of. And the third thing is soul. Regarding soul we believe in transmigration: the circle of life and death. And that circle is according to our Karma. Our deeds become our destiny.

(Quoted from a Hindu participant for Research Karma, reincarnation, and medicine: Hindu perspectives on biomedical research, Sharp &Hutchinson, 2008).

What Is Karma?

Many Indian religions such as Buddhism, Jainism, and Sikhism share karma as their core concept (Berkeley, 2017). Despite that, their specific views on karma vary. Before talking about Karma, I think it's crucial to talk about the atman, (the real self). In Hinduisme, the atman (the soul/ real self) is distinct from both the body and the mind. The atman refers to the self beyond gender, race, species, religion, and nationality.

Karma is a concept in Hinduism which dominantly elucidates causality in which good actions, words, thoughts, and commands directs to favorable repercussion for a person or vice versa (Berkeley, 2017). Hindus more often than not believe that good or bad fortune encountered in life may be the consequence of good or bad actions carried out in a past life. These effects may not necessarily be instantaneous as it can be visited upon a soul in future lives through reincarnation. Unfortunately the misconception here is Karma dictates what to do. As a matter of practice Karma creates situations, how one chose to behave is based on their freewill. One's choice of action determines either they will be accumulating positive karma or negative karma. For instance if you had been wrong by an individual in the past, Karma will put you in a situation where you can continue the negative relationship, forgive and cut the karmic ties or simply just walk away. The choice of what to do is that individuals.

Transmission of a Soul

Transmission of soul is believed to be facilitated by one's karma. One's accumulation of good and bad karma unfolds to determine one's destiny. The family you are born in is Karmic, you have the choice to rise above or sink in the situation that you are born in. Since Hindus believe in transmission of the soul, the focus of Hindu philosophy is on the development of the soul in relation to the body. The driver in the vehicle analogy can be used in further comprehending the soul or atman concept. A body will never function without a soul just like how a car can never move without the driver. Just like how many drivers form attachment with their cars and get concerned about the car's needs, most people without the proper enlightenment may begin identifying with the body and it's needs without finding and acknowledging the soul within it. Failure in acknowledging the soul within may lead to one being trapped, a broken and ignored car however will not be able to move the driver effectively. Therefore the individual while focusing on the soul must ensure the health and safety of the car, which has led to the development of Ayurveda, Yoga and breathing practices which are strongly rooted in Hinduism.

In the nutshell, Karma entails the notion that we are all responsible for our own lives. As such, all therapies that address freedom of choice can utilize the concept of Karma in empowering their client.

Karma entails the notion that karma creates circumstances yet how we choose to react depends on our choice. Therapist can utilize this understanding in empowering clients to make up the right choices. Besides that, Karma in a way suggests the notion that one can only control one's own behavior which would lead to accumulation of karma.

Besides that, the concept of Karma can also be incorporated in behavioral Psychology. In behavioral Psychology, more often than not reinforcements are used to influence probability of an action. Positive reinforcements like rewards enhance the occurrence of an event while negative reinforcements like punishments reduces the occurrence of the event. However, often time negative reinforcements like scolding, yelling and punishing could cause negative repercussions to the psychological well-being of a person. Desired behavior is probably attained using this technique yet it causes adverse effects on social relationships which will lead to accumulation of bad karma. Positive reinforcements on the other hand amplify self-contentment and happiness. As such, they accumulate good karma. On one hand with this, when people use ignorance technique while being confronted by situations that they don't like, they avoid accumulation of bad karma.

Women Empowerment

Sakthi (Divine Feminine Energy)

The significance of women is so intense in Hinduism to the extent it cannot be comprehended in just one distinct way. According to Hindus, the Supreme Being is ultimately believed to be the divine output of the entire universe. As such, Hindus also believe the Shakthi (divine feminine energy) is pertinent for the existence of the Supreme Being to exist. Essentially, Sakthi means "power". In the words of Kolluru, (2011), energy of divinity manifests itself in many forms. Kolluru further described this by categorizing energy manifestation in the masculine form as a male and feminine form as female.As a matter of fact, Hinduism worships the Supreme Being as a divine mother in the form of Shakthi because just like how mothers are accountable for birth, Shakti is accountable for creation (Johnson, 2017).

The Main Goddesses and Their Roles

The only major religion of the world with both God and Goddess is Hinduism. Prominently, most major male Gods have Goddess as their partners. Lord Shiva has goddess Parvati, Lord Vishnu has Goddess Lakshmi, and Lord Brahma has Goddess Saraswati. Ultimately, Hinduism implies the notion that all living beings are fraction of the similar great consciousness which is the almighty. The Almighty is neither male nor female. Within manifest creation, a balance of male and female energy is vital.The goddess in Hinduism displays various roles and freedom of choices.

Ultimately, the goddess portrays the universal truth that all woman are entitled to have their own choice whether to get married, have children, pursue higher education, or stay single. For example, Goddess Parvati is married to Lord Shiva and has children; Lord Ganesha and Lord Muruga. Goddess Lakshmi is married and does not have any children. She is on her mission which is to protect the universe along her husband, Lord Vishnu. However unlike the regular superstitious whereby married woman with no children are considered as inauspicious, Goddess Lakshmi is seen as the symbol of auspiciousness and happiness. On the other hand, Goddess Saraswathi is never seen in any pictures with her husband.

Goddess Sarawathi is known as the goddess of knowledge of wisdom and art. Lord Saraswathi is more career oriented as she is mostly pictured with her veenai and books. On one hand with this, fierce and protective Kali Ma, doesn't have a male counterpart.

Navarathri

Navarathiri is celebrated as the divine feminine element of Shakthi. This is a nine day celebration whereby the divine form of Shakthi in its' nine different form: Durga, Bhadrakali, Amba Devi, Annapoorna Devi, Sarvamanagal Devi, Bhairavi Devi, Chandika Devi, Saraswathi Devi, Bhavani Devi, are worshipped. Each forms illustrates on the different portrayals of Shakthi. Durga is depicted as the invincible mother, Bhadrakali refers to the mother of fortune and wealth while Amba Devi refers the mother of the universe. Annapoorna Devi mother of Anna (rice) and is responsible to provide food. Sarvamangala Devi is the divine mother that brings peace and joy to the world. Bhairavi Devi on the other hand is the divine mother of good who does goodness to good people and evil for bad people who demolishes the negative energies in the Universe. Chandika Devi is the fierce goddess who is the Supreme one. Saraswati Devi and Bhavani Devi are depicted as the Goddess of beauty and the Goddess of mercy respectively.

By close inspection of this nine day celebration, it can be clearly noted that this celebration was devoted to celebrate the different traits and qualities in woman. The different forms of shakthi have simply elaborated the equality of man and woman. Women are as capable of man in fighting against injustice. In session, these stories can be used to bring woman to a sense of awareness of their situations and awaken the power within them in fighting against discrimination.

Hindu Stories of Strong Roles Portrayed by Female Figures

So while the Hindu Goddess themselves empower women, historically and culturally male dominance has been practiced the significance of the goddesses themselves lost in translation. Essentially, most women are expected to portray traits like compassionate, forgiveness, compassion, and tolerance of others' misbehavior. Women that comply with the cultural norms are accepted while women that attempts to portray independence and assertiveness are seen as destructive and as a disgrace to family reputation. Women are forbidden from expressing their opinions and views boldly. The actual pantheon of Hinduism, the concept of Shakti can be used to empower women in fighting against patriarchy. In Hinduism, women are acknowledged as the vessels of shakti with both creative and destructive power (Kolluru, 2011). Ultimately, each forms of Shakthi portray different roles of a woman .While Shakthi is mostly seen as the gentle and loving Uma, Shakthi is also portrayed as the fierce Kali and warrior Durga .

Apart from that, equality was also strongly emphasized in Hinduism. The form of Ardhanarishvara, which is the merging of Lord Siva and Goddess Parvati represents the union of the masculine and feminine energies (Kolluru, 2011). Ardhanarishvara is evidential in demonstrating the fact that female element (Goddess Parvati) is inseparable from the male element of God (Lord Shiva) .With respect to the Ardhanarishvara form, it can be clearly noted that Hinduism also shatters all questions with regards to its' perspectives on homosexuality.

A look at the Hindu puranic stories will further illustrate the freedoms and the unique roles played by women. For instance, Goddess Dhurga is depicted as a courageous battle queen with many arms, with each carrying a weapon. Draupathi was known as the heroine of Mahabharata who has stood strong despite going through many trials. As a matter of fact, Draupathi was married to five different husbands (the Pandavas) at the same time. As such, it definitely demanded lots of skills and responsibilities to be the wife of the Pandavas. Draupathi had to spend one year with each husband. Her other husbands were forbidden from having any sexual contact with her while she spends one year with each husband. Draupadi was adored for being compassionate and humble to good people and was volcanic to her enemies. In addition to this, Draupadi was also well-known for her firmness and for having a unbreakable will.

On the other hand, Kannagi was known for her bravery. Kannagi took revenge on the great Pandyan King of Madurai for wrongfully putting her husband to death. Kannagi's curse burned the whole town of Madurai. Besides that, Avvayar was a famous female poet whose poems and stories are widely used to educate young children till today. These stories have depicted some of the bold roles played by women of those days who did not comply to the expectations and norms of the society, these stories can be used in sessions to help women break away from oppressive situations.

Grief and Death

Perceptions About Death

For sure is the death of all that comes to birth, sure is the birth of all that dies. So in a matter that no one can prevent thou hast no cause to grieve. (Mascaro, 1962, chapter 2, verse 27)

Maya (an illusion) is termed in the Hinduism as an attempt to find permanent happiness in this world (BBC, 2014). A person's atman (spirit) based on the Hindus believe is eternal. Unlike the atman, the physical body is not enduring and can change. Without proper enlightenment people will get trapped in the samsaric cycle (reincarnation). As such, Hindus view death as a natural event that would facilitate the process of the atman attaining Moksha (ultimate release from rebirth).

Reincarnation

Reincarnation simply refers to life continuing after death. Referring back to the driver in the vehicle analogy, just like how people change their car once it gets old, not functioning, people will be using a new body after their death. We buy cars on the basis of what we want and what we can afford. Similarly, the nature of the new body is influenced by their desires and their respective karma. Bhagavad Gita has three main listings for human actions: Karma: those which elevate; Vikarma: those which degrade; Akarma: those which create neither good nor bad reactions. This is believed to lead towards liberation. For most Hindus, this can be an important belief that facilitates grieving process. In addition to this, funeral rituals in Hinduism are designed in such a way to facilitate grieving process. Funeral prayers help people to come out of shock and accept the reality. Longer mourning period often times give a long time frame to survivors of the deceased to come in terms with the death of their loved ones. Psychologically speaking, the hindu funeral rites and rituals are specifically targeted to help the relatives of the deceased in coping with the loss.

After-Life Beliefs

Hinduism elucidates on the four main paths that a man will follow upon his death. Devayana the first path is known as the path of the gods (Ramakrishna, n.d.). This path is taken by spiritually advanced souls who have devoted themselves to meditation yet have not succeeded in accomplishing self knowledge prior to their death. Pitriyana is known as the second path. This path is followed by ritualists and philanthropists who have done worship, charity, vows and austerity. People here enjoy immense happiness for their good will before returning back to earth as they still possess earthly desires .Hell is referred as the third course. This path is followed by those who led an impure life .Such people are born as sub-human species to expiate their evi actions before being reborn as humans. The fourth path is for those who have done extremely unpleasant actions. They are reborn as insignificant creatures like mosquitoes countless times to eliminate their evil actions before being reborn as human form (Ramakrishna, n.d.). Souls that have attained self-knowledge however do need to pass through any of these realms. Such souls attain Moksya.

Suicide and Euthanasia

Suicide in Hinduism is perceived as an act against humanity (Lakhan, 2008) as it causes pain to the family and friends of those who complete suicide. As such, suicide is deemed as a bad death which is violent, premature occurring at the wrong time and wrong place. However there are two prominent distinctions made to distinguish suicide and euthanasia. One killing him or herself for selfish reasons such as financial burden portrays one's ignorance on nature of life. Hindus believe that a person who dies by committing suicide will continue the samara cycle of birth and death. In addition to this, committing suicide will cause negative repercussions in next birth. Ultimately the point of life is to develop and attain self-knowledge. Suffering is part of life. Bliss is just an illusion, (maya). As such when one chooses suicide as an alternative path to end his sufferings, it creates negative repercussions in next birth and hence lessons have to be repeated till next birth. In the nutshell, suicide is never encouraged in Hinduism. On one hand with this, death is seen as a natural occurrence in Hinduism whereby one is karmicly bound to die in time. As such, one should not blame himself or herself when they are unable to save someone from dying. A therapist dealing with suicidal clients could use this explanation to help client understand the consequences of killing themselves. Euthanasia on the other hand is seen as an act of compassionate in case of extreme suffering and lack of consciousness. A doctor does euthanasia by injecting lethal drugs to patients. Euthanasia is not seen as a sin in Hinduism (Lakhan, 2008).

Anger Management

Perceptions on Anger

According to the Gita, desire and anger provoke a man into sinful action (Hindu Dharma, 2017). Desire is deemed as a deadly enemy as if we want something, we will get it by fair or foul. This will drive us to committing sin. As such, anger is also seen as an equally deadly enemy. Anger is caused by unfulfilled desire. The concept of throwing a ball against the wall can be used to comprehend how anger is caused by desire .Desire represents ball being thrown against the wall meanwhile anger is represented by the ball bouncing from the wall (Hindu Dharma, 2017).

While we attack people in our anger, we are hurt more than those we wanted to hurt (Hindu Dharma, 2017). Our whole body shakes when we are angry .Anger triggers pain both to the body and the mind In addition to this, we make ourselves appear ugly when we are angry (Hindu Dharma, 2017).

Sadness and anger are two different types of unreciprocated cravings (Hindu Dharma, 2017). If a person that hampers us from attaining our desire is inferior to us, we turn our anger on them . In contrast to this, if the respective person happens to be superior than us, we have no other choice than mourning by ourselves. Thus, anger is best when it is kept at a distant (Hindu Dharma, 2017).

Stories Relating to Anger

Dhritaraashtra's wrath is an example of story used to elaborate on effects of anger. Pandavas visited their uncle Dhritarasshtra after defeating his sons in the final war (Bhide, 2007). Bheem who killed Dhritaraashtra's son Duryodhana was called closer by Dhritaraashtra so that he could embrace Bheem. Krishna, holds Bheem back and placed a solid metal statue of Bheem before the blind Dhritaraashtra. The statue was reduced to rubble by the vigorous hug of the old man. Such is the intensity of the anger that burns inside him . Dhritaraashtra's Queen, Gandhari blindfolds herself since her husband is blind. When Yudhisthira bends to touch the feet of Gandhari, her partially covered vision falls on his' fingernails. As a consequent, Yudhisthira's fingernails turned black . The anger of the mother was also very profound and literally burning. These stories are significant enough in portraying the dangerous consequences of intense anger .

Focusing Emotions on God

However as humans we are prone to experience anger, so how are we to control it. Associate Professor Dr. Anasuya Jegathevi Jegathesan in her experience with dealing with adolescents and young people with anger issues from a Hindu perspective said this "Your parents, your family, your friends, they cannot take your anger. You will say words that will hurt them and that creates more Karma. So what do you do when you are angry, get angry with God. Sit in your alter scold God, express your anger to God. The Almighty can take your anger, God absorbs it, forgives it and accepts it. Anything offered to God has no Karmic backlash, like the story of Shishupala . Do not of course take your anger out on God in public places like in a temple because there your anger will upset other who does not understand and their upset will create negative Karma. But scolding God in your private space can be a huge anger management too." (Talk, Hindusim and Counselling, HELP University April 2016)

Krishna and Shishupala's Story

The story of Shishupala from the Mahabaratha is as follows he was a prince born with three eyes and four arms. It was said that a heavenly voice told Shishupala's parents that the additional eyes and arms will disappear when a certain person took the child on his lap. However, that person will be the cause of Shishupala's death. When Krishna placed Shishupala on his lap, Shishupala's third eye and additional arms vanished indicating the fact Krishna will be causing Shishupala's death. Witnessing this scene, Shishupala's mother who was Krishna's aunt requested a boon from Lord Krishna. The boon was that Lord Krishna would forgive Shishupala for 100 offences. Krishna agreed, Shishupala's father decided to save his son it was best to let him be brought up by a very powerful rival of Krishna, who instilled hate in the young man, who would openly insult Krishna. As Krishna did not retaliate, he mistook the forgiveness as cowardice, and the young was obsessed with bringing Krishna down.

Both Sushipala and Lord Krishna were invited to a ceremony at Indraprastha by the King. At that event, the King decided to credit Lord Krishna as the guest of honor. Hearing this, Sushipala got furious and insulted Lord Krishna finally exceeding the hundred pardons. A duel commenced and Krishna to the shock of everyone watching when Krishna finally killed the man, the audience witnessed a light of the soul of the man rise from his body and merge with the Krishna who is seen as an incarnation of God on earth. How could someone who had insulted Krishna merge with God?

Focusing emotions on god will help one in regulating their anger. In Hinduism, it's okay to get angry with god. We can blame god and have a conversation with God. This would give an avenue to express our anger out. When we scream or yell out of anger, it creates negative energy in the surrounding. This would then create unnecessary karma for us. The notion of taking god's name in vain is not a concept in Hinduism. Hindus believe Gods are above emotion. As such, they are non-reactive to emotions. The story of Krishna and Sushipala implies that by focusing emotions on God we are able to express those emotions without negative consequences. This is a powerful anger management practice for young Hindus.

Bhagavad-Gita and Contemporary Psychotherapies

Bhagavad Gita

Bhagavad Gita has approximately 700 verses from Hindu scriptures and is a prominent part of the famous Hindu epic known as Mahabharata. Ultimately, the Gita is based on the conversation between Lord Krishna and Arjuna during the Kurukshetra war. According to Reddy, (2012) Mahatma Gandhi was cited as declaring he would refer to the Bhagavad Gita whenever he encounters a problem as the Gita provides him with the answer and solution to his problem. Resolution of conflict and flourishing recommencement of action from a state of acute anxiety and guilt laden depression are precious case study lessons in psychotherapy for psychology students Many psychotherapeutic principles is believed to have been implemented in The Bhagavad Gita (Bhatia,Madabushi, Kolli, Bhatia, & Madaan, 2013).

The Story Line of Mahabharatha

Essentially Mahabharatha depicts on the Kurushethra war between the Kaurava and the Pandava princes. It is also seen as the longest epic in world literature comprising of 100000 of two line stanzas (Davis, 2001). As such, the Mahabharaha is seen at eight times longer than Homer's Iliad and Odyssey together as well as three times longer than the Bible .However, in the words of Naramsin only about 4000 lines recount to the main story, whereas the rest part of the Gita contains additional teachings In the nutshell, Mahabharatha bears a resemblance to a long journey with many diversions. Hence it was concluded that *"Whatever is here is found elsewhere. But whatever is not here is nowhere else."* (Davis, 2001).

Psychodynamic Psychotherapy

Conflict related to unacceptable aspects of self is the central theme of psychodynamic theories (Bhatia,Madabushi, Kolli, Bhatia, &Madaan, 2013).. Adaptation is encouraged when distress arises due to incongruence between internal dissonance and external requirement. Healthy ego defense mechanisms according to Freud's structural theory resolve the conflict between id, ego and superego (Bhatia et al., 2013). The Gita illustrates on the victorious resolution of discord confronted by Arjuna which shows similarities with id, ego and superego concept .As described in the Gita, the senses (*indriyas*) construct attractions which in turn direct to desire, and a hunger for for possession. Anger displays itself in quest to nurture and conquer that desire.

As elaborated in the id functions, attributes like *kaam* (lust), *krodh* (unadaptive anger), *lobh* (greed), *moh* (insatiable attachment) and *ahankar* (unfounded self glorification) which are are *tamsic* in nature shows significant similarities (Bhatia,Madabushi, Kolli, Bhatia, & Madaan, 2013).. On one hand with this, the Gita also has affirmed that mind is superior than senses which is in harmony with theories illustrating the relationship between ego and super ego (Bhatia et al., 2013). A stable mind is often times carried away by the stable mind. Several layers of consciousness and subconscious were illustrated in the Gita just like how it was illustrated in the Jung's idea of collective unconscious. *Tamas* also displays self-centeredness and deficiency in regard for consequences. This again shows evidential resemblance with the concept of id. On the other hand, *Rajas* and *Satwic* are in many ways analogous respectively to the ego and superego. Good thought, altruistic action and relationships are referred as *satwic* qualities. Doing an action with an expectation of reward similar to ego function refers to *Rajas* qualities Symptoms of anxiety according to the Gita are caused by conflicts among the Gunas As such, Gita advocated rising above the *Gunas* in attaining a stable and a peaceful mind .

Cognitive Behavioral Therapy

Arjuna associating guilt by visualizing the death of his relatives scene during the Kurushthra war was one of the earliest CBT documented sessions illustrated in The Gita (Bhatia,Madabushi, Kolli, Bhatia, & Madaan, 2013) . Dry mouth, tremors, dizziness and confusion were the symptoms of his anxiety (Bhatia et al., 2013). Arjuna was so distressed to the extent he wanted to withdraw from war by dropping his weapon. Arjuna was then inspired by Lord Krishna who described the laurels of a warrior and humiliation with regards to non-participation. However, this method was still inadequate. As such, Lord Krishna conveyed the Gita discourse. This was helpful for Arjuna in identifying his thought process and thus coaching him for an action. Arjuna was experiencing guilt and anxiety as a result of catastrophizing the future. With regards to this, Arjuna also demonstrated several other cognitive distortions. As a method of helping Arjuna, Lord Krishna elucidated the misery he is in transient. In harmony with that, Lord Krishna emphasized on the prominence of possessing an undistorted view of the world. This is pretty much similar to how a therapist would explain the temporary nature of anxiety following psycho-educating on how cognitive distortions affect the symptoms .

Mindfulness

A way of paying attention that is sensitive, accepting and independent of thoughts is known as "Mindfulness"(Bhatia,Madabushi, Kolli, Bhatia, & Madaan, 2013). This is a way to prevent one from being affected or attached (Bhatia et al., 2013). This principle is harmonious with the concept of Zen and Gita has several references with regards to this practice. Mindfulness in the Gita is prescribed as a way of attaining *Sthithapragna* (a state of unperturbedness) by being disconnected from the onslaught of the senses . "One should be tranquil like the ocean which is unaffected by rivers flowing into it","one should draw self away fromthe senses as a tortoise withdraws its limbs", "being similar to water drop on a lotus leaf which does not havean attachment to the leaf."are some metaphors from the Gita that will be useful in directing clients towards mindfulness . The mindfulness state can be reached using meditation. In the western concept of psychotherapy, mindfulness if often times a widely accepted concept. More models along with the proliferation of eclectic therapies are utilizing these techniques.

Notions on Mindfulness

Even as all waters flow into the ocean, but the ocean never overflows, even so the sage feels desires, but he is ever one in his infinite peace. (Mascaro, 1962, Chapter 2; Shloka 70)

Offer all thy works to god, throw off selfish bonds, and do thy work. No sin can then stain thee, even as waters do not stain the leaf of the lotus. (Mascaro, 1962, Chapter 5; Shloka 10)

When in recollection he withdraws all his senses from the attraction of pleasures of sense, even as a tortoise withdraws all its limbs, then his is serine wisdom. (Mascaro, 1962, Chapter 2; Shloka 58)

Grief Therapy

Death of our precious ones is definitely a throbbing phenomenon to accept and as such grief counseling has become an important part of therapy these days (Bhatia,Madabushi, Kolli, Bhatia, & Madaan, 2013). In Hindu Funerals, listening to a discourse on the Bhagavad Gita is seen as one cultural practice. Theory of reincarnation from the Bhagavad Gita is pertinent in helping people to move on with life. In the body, the Gita is referred as the carrier of the soul. Death and reincarnation is inevitable as illustrated in the Gita. This will be helpful in minimizing the intensity of grief.

In interpersonal therapy, re-establishing interests and relationships are seen as crucial process in resolving grief (Bhatia,Madabushi, Kolli, Bhatia, & Madaan, 2013). "the supreme being carries off all things" is a key concept in Gita (Bhatia et al., 2013). Visiting this concept can facilitate the alleviation of guilt with regards to the deceased by directing responsibility towards God However, therapist has to ensure that exploration of beliefs of client was done before using extracts from the Gita.

Shlokas Useful in Addressing Grief

"Bereavement"

Thy tears are for those beyond tears; and are thy words of wisdom? The wise grieve not for those who live; and they grieve not for those who die for life and death shall pass away. (Mascaro, 1962, Chapter 2; Shloka 11)

"Imperishable nature of soul"

Weapons cannot hurt the Spirit and fire can never burn him. Untouched is he by drenching waters; untouched is he by parching winds. (Mascaro, 1962, Chapter 2; Shloka 23)

"Reincarnation"

For all things born in truth must die, and out of death in truth comes life. Face to face with what must be, cease thou from sorrow. (Mascaro, 1962, Chapter 2; Shloka 27)

This article is only the tip of the ice-burg in applications of Hinduism in Therapy.

CONCLUSION

Possible conflict may arise when counseling a client with Hindu values due to lack of congruence between values of a Hindu client as well as values of therapist primarily derived from western theories. As such if a therapist could enhance his or her cultural competence by understanding the worldviews of client, the therapeutic relationship between counselor and client could be further enhanced. However, it is very important for therapist to note that great diversity exists within the beliefs in Hinduism. Existence of the immortal soul, law of karma, reincarnation are some of the core concepts of Hinduism. The soul is believed to be immortal and as such death is seen as a natural event that would facilitate the process of atman attaining Moksha. Without proper enlightenment people will get trapped in the samsaric cycle (reincarnation). In addition to this, the concept of Shakti in Hinduism can be used to empower women in fighting against patriarchy. In Hinduism, women are acknowledged as the vessels of shakti with both creative and destructive power. Each forms of Shakthi are portrayed with different roles of a woman. Along this, it was also mentioned that expressing anger to god is a huge anger management method as it does not create bad karma for one unlike scolding or screaming to someone out of anger. Bhagavad Gita or better known as the Gita with approximately 700 verses from the Hindu scriptures is an important narrative in Hinduism. This chapter has also included some slokas which can be beneficial in therapy.

REFERENCES

Berkeley. (2017). *Karma Hinduism*. Berkeley Centre for religion, peace and worldly affairs. Retrieved from: https://berkleycenter.georgetown.edu/essays/karma-hinduism

Bhatia, S. C., Madabushi, J., Kolli, V., Bhatia, S. K., & Madaan, V. (2013). The Bhagavad Gita and Contemporary Psychotherapies. *Indian J Psychiatry 55: Indian Mental Concepts*. Retrieved from: www.indianjpsychiatry.org

Bhide, A. V. (2007). Anger and the Mahaabhaarata. *Indian Journal of Psychiatry*, *49*(2), 140. doi:10.4103/0019-5545.33265 PMID:20711400

Davis. (2001). *The Mahabharatha: A synopsis of the Great Epic of India*. Retrieved from: http://web.cs.ucdavis.edu/~vemuri/classes/freshman/Mahabharatasynopsis.htm

Hindu Dharma. (2017). *Anger (HinduDharma): Dharmas Common To All*. Retrieved from: http://www.kamakoti.org/hindudharma/part22/chap11.htm

Hinduism: beliefs about life after death. (2014). *Religious studies*. Retrieved from: http://www.bbc.co.uk/schools/gcsebitesize/rs/death/hindubeliefrev2.shtml

Jegathesan, A. J. (2016). Talk, Hindusim and Counselling. HELP University.

Johnson, J. (2017). Shakti: The Power of the Feminine. *Asia Society*. Retrieved from: iasociety.org/education/shakti-power-feminine

Kolluru, S. (2011). *Shakti: The Divine Element of the Feminine*. Retrieved from: http://www.stateofformation.org/2011/09/shakti-the-divine-element-of-the-feminine/

Lakhan, S. E. (2008). Hinduism: Life and Death. *Student BMJ Article.* Retrieved from: https://pdfs.semanticscholar.org/e64d/183c68d8f89f4817150742d458ea87b662df.pdf

Mascaro, J. (Ed.). (1962). *The Bhagavad Gita.* Penguin Books.

Ramakrishna. (n.d.). Hinduism: Death and Life Beyond Death. *Swami Adiswaraananda Ramakrishna Vivekananda Center.* Retrieved from: https://www.ramakrishna.org/activities/message/weekly_message43.htm

Reddy, M. S. (2012). Psychotherapy:Insights from Bhagavad Gita. *Indian Journal of Psychological Medicine, 34*(1). Retrieved from https://www.ncbi.nlm.nih.gov/pmc/articles/PMC3361835/ PMID:22661821

Sharp, R., & Hutchienson, J. F. (2008). Karma, reincarnation, and medicine: Hindu perspectives on biomedical research. *Springer Genomic Medicine, 2*(3-4). Retrieved from: https://www.ncbi.nlm.nih.gov/pmc/articles/PMC2694864/

Chapter 14
The Perception of Muslim Clients Towards Non-Muslim Counselors

Siti Salina Abdullah
University Malaysia Terengganu, Malaysia

Kamarul Md Shah
University Malaysia Terengganu, Malaysia

ABSTRACT

Having a counselor with a different religious background from the client might lead to conflicting perspectives. This chapter intends to explore the perceptive of a Muslim client in choosing a non-Muslim counselor. The concept of helping process, which is highly respectable in the teaching of Islam, is explicated. Muslims are encouraged to help each other, especially those who are in need. Preferably, a non-Muslim counselor should have some basic understanding of the Pillars of Islam prior to conducting a counseling session with a Muslim client. The knowledge will facilitate the counselor understanding process of the clients without bias. It is anticipated that the information presented herewith would benefit non-Muslim counselors and help them in understanding their Muslim clients better. This chapter also examines the cultural issues that may influence the effectiveness of a counseling session between Muslim clients and non-Muslim counselors.

INTRODUCTION

The challenges in human life today are highly complex. Counselor nowadays has become a place of reference to express a problem, seek advice, and a source of motivation. In addition, they also become a place of discussion about the various human scenario and diverse problems, which are getting increasingly critical and community-specific. Consequently, they need to equip themselves with vast knowledge and various skills not only to strengthen their existing counseling skills but also to deal with diverse clients of a different background. It is essential to streamline the counseling services offered to address the

DOI: 10.4018/978-1-5225-6073-9.ch014

growing societal complex problems. However, there are counseling methods that emphasized the Western way of thinking, which are incompatible with the culture, religion, and norms of the society in Malaysia.

A counselor with good counseling skills but lack knowledge in the field of religion, or vice versa, has limitation in offering counseling services. For instance, if a client is facing a critical religious issues, the counselor will not be able to help the client, effectively. This is because religious issues must be handled with due care, especially matter related to the legal aspect of the religion. Hence, the question; could a non-Muslim counselor provide an effective counseling service to a client, especially when it involves religion-related issues?

Counselling is a process that involves a counselor and a client in which the intention is to have a better outcome for the client. Both the client and the counselor are important to the counseling process. Having a counselor from a different religious background from the client might contribute to conflicting of perspectives between the counselor and the client. Multicultural counseling, as explained by Sue and Sue (2008), refers to the role and helping process that employed a method and a goal setting consistent with the client life experience and values. It also takes into account the client identity as an individual and a member of a society by using a strategy that is universal and specific to the client's culture when making an evaluation, diagnosis, and a treatment for the client. The cultural diversity between a counselor and the client makes the counseling process unique, which should be taken into account by the counselor. This is explained by Hays and Edford (2010) who asserted that the role of a client's cultural identity must be given due consideration during a counseling session because it has a strong influence on the client experience. A client who attends a counseling session with a counselor of a different religious belief is expected to undergo a unique experience. The limitation of understanding of the belief as well as the different values between a Muslim client and a non-Muslim counselor will somehow affect the counseling session effectiveness.

Counseling also occurs in the Islamic teaching. The concept of a helping process is highly commendable in the Islamic perspectives. It strongly indicates that Muslims are encouraged to help each other, especially towards those who are in need. The Quran and hadith also emphasize the need for a Muslim to be kind and helpful towards each other. A counselor needs to have some basic understanding of the Pillars of Islam to conduct counseling sessions with Muslim clients. The knowledge and understanding of this fundamental aspect of Islamic teaching help to ease the process of helping a client without prejudice. As a multicultural counselor, the combination of knowledge, awareness, and skills are the three main components required to conduct a counseling session, efficaciously. This paper explains counselling from the perspective of Islam, the duties of Muslim clients and issues regarding Muslim clients and non-Muslim counsellor. It is anticipated that the information offered in this paper would benefit non-Muslim counselor to have a better understanding towards their Muslim client. The non-Muslim counselor restricted understanding of the clients' belief as well as the different values between a Muslim client and a non-Muslim counselor will somehow affect the therapeutic relationship and the efficacy of the counseling process. This chapter also examines the cultural issues that may influence the effectiveness of the counseling session between a Muslim client and a non-Muslim counselor.

Counseling From the Perspective of Islam

Counseling is a process of a helping relationship between a counselor, who is trained and specialized in the field of counseling, and a client who needs an assistance and guidance. The helping nature of a counseling process between a counselor and a client is a noble feat, which is commendable in the Islam religion. This deed is clearly stated in Surah Al Ma'idah [5:2], which means, "Rather, help one another in acts of righteousness and piety, and do not help one another in sin and transgression." This verse indicates that the nature of counseling, which is to help a client resolve the test he or she is currently facing, is highly praiseworthy by the Islamic teaching.

The counselor role in encouraging a client who is experiencing an impasse is greatly regarded in Islam. This is evidenced by the numerous hadiths narrated with regard to helping others. The first hadith mentioning this notion was narrated by Abu Hurairah r.a., who said, Prophet Muhammad (PBUH) decrees that "If anyone relieves a Muslim believer from one of the hardships of this worldly life, Allah will relieve him of one hardship of the Day of Resurrection. If anyone makes it easy for the one who is indebted to him (while finding it difficult to repay), Allah will make it easy for him in this worldly life and in the Hereafter, and if anyone conceals the fault of a Muslim, Allah will conceal his fault in this world and the Hereafter. Allah helps His slaves as long as he helps his brother." Another hadith narrated by Tabarani and Daraqutni stated, "The best of people are those that bring the most benefit to the rest of mankind." This means that the earnest assistance provided by a counselor to a client will be rewarded in this life and his adversity in the Hereafter will be eased. Thus, a career as a counselor who benefits the client through the counseling sessions is regarded a noble and respected profession in Islam.

A counselor plays a role in helping a client in distress or facing difficulties. The Quran speaks of the challenges faced by humans. The tests take various forms including physical (property and poverty), emotional (fear and concern) and personal as well as family trials. Tests are considered a mechanism to strengthen the trust and belief of a client as a believer of Islam. The following are some verses from the Quran, which explain the trials that befall humans.

We shall certainly test you by afflicting you with fear, hunger, loss of properties and lives and fruits. Give glad tidings, then, to those who remain patient. Al Baqarah [2:155]

Do you supposed that you will enter Paradise untouched by the suffering endured by the people of faith who passed away before you? They were afflicted by misery and hardship and were so convulsed that the Messenger and the believers with him cried out: "When will Allah's help arrives?" They were assured: "Behold. Allah's help is close by." Al Baqarah [2:214]

(Believers!) You will certainly be put to test in respect of your properties and lives, and you will certainly hear many hurtful things from those who are granted the Book before you and those who have associated others with Allah in His divinity. If you remain patient and God-fearing this indeed is a matter of great resolution. Ali Imran [3:186]

Know well that your belongings and your children are but a trial and that with Allah there is a mighty reward. Al Anfal [8:28]

These Quranic verses clearly stated that God always tests humans with various trials. No matter what trials befell a person, they are resolvable. The verse of Surah Al Baqarah [2:286] said, *"Allah does not lay a responsibility on anyone beyond his capacity. In his favour shall be whatever good each one does, and against him whatever evil he does."* This verse specifies clearly that God does not test a man beyond his capacity. In other words, whatever issue faced by a client can be resolved with the help of a counselor.

Understanding Muslim Clients

The Muslims believed that God is to be worshipped. As a Muslim or a believer in Islamic teaching, there are two sources of reference underlying their life as a Muslim—the holy Quran and the Prophet Muhammad's (PBUH) Sunnah. These two sources play an important role in providing guidance to the Muslims in their daily living. The Quran is the main guide for the Muslim due to its comprehensive content that explain all the elements required in a man's life (Rosmizi, Fazrul, Munira, & Roslizawati, 2012; Sue & Sue, 2008), which include social matters, family life, economics and business, sexuality, and other fundamentals of life (Sue & Sue, 2016). In fact, the Quran stated laws and rules that the Muslim need to obey. The second source of reference is the Sunnah or hadith that serves as a guide to the way of life, such as speech, adherence, character, personal disposition, and the nature of events based on the Prophet Muhammad (PUBH) conduct. In terms of cultural and religious values, the Muslims engage in the ritual prayer five times a day. They are also committed to fast during daylight for the whole holy month of Ramadan. In addition, those who could afford, they would devote a certain amount of their wealth for *zakat* and almsgiving and perform the pilgrimage at the holy city of Mecca (Nobles & Sciarra, 2000).

In addition to the two main sources of reference, a Muslim is required to adhere to the teaching of Islam in the aspects of faith, Islamic law, and morals (Rosmizi, Fazrul, Munira, & Roslizawati, 2012). A Muslim gains knowledge and understanding of the divine and prophethood through the teaching of faith or *akidah* as outlined in the Pillars of Faith. Through the Islamic law and morals outlined in the Pillars of Islam, every Muslim learn about the relationship of life with God, man, and nature. With the general understanding of Islam, every Muslim client practiced the understanding and teaching in their daily lives. The Muslim clients practice the knowledge and teaching of Islam in their daily lives according to their religious belief.

Some knowledge of the Islamic teaching could help a non-Muslim counselor to understand a client from the client's cultural perspective. Knowledge is one of the important components required in order to increase the competency of a multicultural counselor apart from awareness and skills (Sue & Sue, 1996, 2008, 2016). Othman Mohamed (2017) also agreed on the need for the counselor to have a profound knowledge of a client's culture. A counselor that acts as a facilitator will strive to understand a client from a personal aspect and the client's cultural background (Mohamed, 2017). The need to understand a client's cultural aspect is highlighted in the Multicultural Counseling Theory as proposed by Sue and Sue (1996) through the following six suggestions:

1. Multicultural Counseling Theory was introduced to identify the cultural elements more clearly and objectively within the existing counseling theories. In the context of a Muslim client, counseling theories were applied to understand the client issues without neglecting the Muslim client's cultural aspect.
2. The identity of a counselor and a client is formed as a result of a certain level of experience and context. This means any intervention need to consider the client as a Muslim in entirety by looking at the root cause of the issue; not only focusing on the client but also the client's surrounding, such as the family, society, and his/her culture as a Muslim.
3. The development of the cultural identity as the core that shaped the attitude of the counselor and the client towards himself/herself and others, with the client or outside the client community group.

The attitude will affect one's feeling and behavior as well as one's worldview towards others. This means the level of development of the Muslim client cultural identity must be clearly understood so that the conceptualization of the issues and goal setting of the counseling can be made accordingly.

4. A counselors' competency increased when he/she take takes into account the experience and the Muslim client's cultural values when setting the goals of the session. This means any goal setting should consider the fundamental doctrine set out in the Islamic teaching. Hence, the need for the knowledge and experience about Islam is essential when conducting a session with a client to improve the counselor competency.
5. The importance of using the society's role, effectively, to help a client of a multicultural background. This means, in addition to the general organization such as the Welfare Department (JKM) and the National Population and Family Organization (LPPKN), organizations that are specific to Muslim clients such as the Department of Religious Affair and the State Islamic Religious Control can be utilized to assist the client further.
6. The counselor awareness towards the importance of the cultural aspect of a Muslim client in a counseling session. This means the counselor understanding of a Muslim client's issues should include his/her relationship with the family, society, and organizations related to the client as a Muslim.

Cultural Assumptions and Misunderstandings

The counseling practiced in Malaysia is mostly based on counseling practiced in the West. Theorist such as Sigmund Freud, Carl Rogers, and others in the field are well-known to the counseling practitioners in Malaysia because they are used as the main references in the study of counseling at various level of education. The theories describe aspects such as human events, goals, techniques and the counseling process, the roles of counselor–client, and their application in the counseling sessions. The descriptions are quite convincing that those theories were chosen to guide the local counseling practice.

However, the current development of counseling knowledge, especially in Malaysia, indicate the emergence of a view that the counseling theory from the West lack in the spiritual aspect. Undeniably, counseling of the West disregard the spiritual aspect in its analysis. Several researchers such as Badri (1994) and Langgulung (1990) found that spiritual aspect was not emphasized by the western psychologists. It indicates the inappropriateness of the western counseling to be practiced in Malaysia due to several reasons related to the local culture and Islamic teaching. Islam believes that if humankind does not adhere to the revelation of the Quran and the Sunnah, they will not find the true resolution and gain the Creator pleasure, which is the ultimate life goal of a Muslim.

Nevertheless, this does not mean that western counseling cannot be practiced in Malaysia, however, it has to be adapted according to the practice and teaching of Islam. Philosopher Imam Al-Ghazali said, "there is a relationship between faith and religion with the spiritual enrichment." As a result, Islamic researchers are constantly trying to adjust the practice of western counseling to make it relevant to the culture of Muslim society. The main reason for this is because the principles of Islamic teaching is pertinent to every aspect of human life. Raba and Othman (1998) opine that Islamic counseling is applicable to all target groups, including children, adolescent, and adult. Two important points that are part of the major differences between the western counseling approach and Islamic counseling approach are:

1. Religion and life are inseparable because religion rules a major part of the human lives. This means humans will not do things against the religious teaching on the principle of fearing God's punishment.
2. Values have many roles in counseling because they underlie the selection of counseling theories and techniques as well as determine the treatment process and decision-making. In other words, the counselor's values also play an important role in the counseling process undertaken towards the development of a therapeutic and conducive relationship.

The difference in view between the western and Islamic approaches as indicated by numerous findings has brought many benefits by means of improving the effectiveness of the counseling sessions. Any difference of view should become a reason to assess and examine the principle of counseling as the medium of helping service. A point of similarity should be sought and an appropriate adjustment should be made as both will contribute to the development of counseling knowledge. Misconception should be minimized and an understanding should be optimized so that the religious and cultural elements become part of the aspect that helps the development and success of the counseling sessions.

Hamdan (2007) states that Islam is a religion that covers all aspects of life, such as spiritual, social, economic, political, and family. Islam is considered a way of life that does not separate religion from other aspects of life. Furthermore, Islam provides a variety of functions, such as the provision of comfort, meaning, identity, spirituality, and society (Abu-Raiya & Pargament, 2010). Pew Research Centre (2007) conducted studies on American Muslims and found that 72% of the respondents affirmed that religion played an important role in their lives. In addition, although Islam is like other religions, there are unique factors to be understood and need to be given thoughtful consideration (Abu-Raiya & Pargament, 2011). Therefore, it is important to understand the effect of religion on the treatment of counseling and how it affects the counseling process.

There is a growing need for a definite information on how to treat Muslim clients and how to engage them in a treatment process. The implications of this for the current psychologists are that there is no available source of reference when working with Muslim clients. Amer (2009) states that psychologists often gave up looking for published research that could explain the appropriate services and eventually turned to the mainstream media or colleagues to seek for advice and resources that were usually inaccurate due to false and biased information. This may suggest that the therapists did not use the best practice for the Muslim clients. Abu-Raiya and Pargament (2010) propose that there is a need for empirical studies that examine the effectiveness of some of the techniques used as suggested by psychotherapists working with Muslim populations. Hence, creating an important gap in examining the effectiveness of the techniques in the previous studies. In other words, there is a need to provide therapy with empirical-based information to ensure the best treatment is given to the Muslim clients.

Prior to seeking a professional help, a Muslim may be more likely to seek help from religious leaders (Kobeisy, 2004; Springer et al., 2009). Springer et al. (2009) indicate the Muslims believe that in trying to solve personal and family problems, they have to turn to Islam (page 232). Padela et al. (2012) studied 13 focus groups of Muslims that revealed the majority of respondents reported they consulted the Imam instead of mental health professionals. In general, Muslims view their religion and religious leaders as entities that would help them in dealing with their problems.

Additionally, the cultural norm and religious belief emphasize families' responsibilities in teaching children on the proper behavior in the society; thus, problematic children reflect negatively on their parents and families (Daneshpour, 1998). This view suggests that the family will be blamed for any psychological problems arose and their inability to properly deal with the problem led them to seek out-of-the-kind assistance. This may be an important point for a non-Muslim counselor to consider when helping Muslim clients. Seeking out help may indicate that the person's faith is weak and a manifestation of a missing support system (Kobeisy, 2006).

Expectation of Muslim Client Toward Non-Muslim Counselors

The counseling process should take into account the cultural aspect of the counselor and client, thus, both the counselor and client should consider the meaning of culture. When an individual becomes a client, it means he/she is presenting his/her identity in the context of his/her culture to the counselor. The culture embodies the client identity, which comprises ethnicity, language, genus, economic status, family, learning style, and spirituality (Othman, 2005). A competent counselor always takes into account the cultural factor of the client and such counselor is said to have a multicultural competency. *Theory Multicultural Counseling and Therapy* by Sue, Ivey, and Pedersen (1996) and *Model Multicultural Counseling Competencies* by Sue, Arredondo, and McDavis (1992) suggest three characteristics or domains of competency, namely awareness, knowledge, and skill. Likewise, there are three dimensions of competency, which are:

1. Counselors' awareness of his/her own assumption, values, and cultural bias.
2. Understand the client's worldview from the perspective of the client's culture.
3. Develop appropriate intervention strategies and techniques for the client.

Counseling services in Malaysia are provided by counselors to clients of multicultural background. By the same token, clients met counselors of various cultural background including in the aspect of religion. A question arose; how does a Muslim client feels having a counseling session with a non-Muslim counselor? Ahmad Raba and Abdul Halim (1998) explicate that non-Muslim counselors have to master the knowledge of Islam as best they could before they can be a good counselor, particularly to the Muslim clients. This includes the understanding of the causes and the fundamental of helping in Islam. This requirement is deemed a major concern for non-Muslim counselors. Counseling from the perspective of Islam can be used to assist clients regardless of race and religion. The implementation of Islamic counseling has to be done systematically, similar to the western counseling. The Islamic counseling is based on the Al-Quran and Sunnah, which are being practiced by the Muslims. This aspect needs to be understood and taken into consideration in the counseling practice by non-Muslim counselors. If non-Muslim counselors can embrace this practice, it will give a good impression to the Muslim clients, hence, they will be more willing to undergo counseling sessions with non-Muslim counselors.

There is a growing need to get specific information on how to get Muslim client involved in the treatment process. The reason for this is because in the United State for instance, despite the increasing number of Muslim citizen, they are less likely getting psychological treatment (Kobeisy, 2004). Inayat (2007) notes several reasons for this occurrence, which include a feeling of distrust towards the counseling service provider, fear of the treatment process, fear of racial and discrimination, language barrier, communication differences, and cultural and religious issues. Khan (2006) conducted a survey on 459 Muslims in the Ohio region regarding client attitude towards therapy. Only about 11.1% indicated that they have been using a professional counseling service within two years while 15.7% of the respondents agreed that they actually need the service. The Muslim society is facing numerous difficulties, such as anxiety, depression, psychosomatic difficulties, PTSD, alcoholism, family problems, adjustment disorder, difficulties with prejudice and discrimination. For these reasons, Muslims need the clinical services as much as other population. Therefore, it is important to understand the concerns and uniqueness of Muslim society.

The study of 121 Muslim clients in Washington DC and Chicago by Kelly, Aridi, and Bakhtiar (1996) found that a small majority (52.9%) preferred Muslim counselors while 43.8% chose either Muslim or non-Muslim counselors. They also found that if they need to go to non-Muslim Counselors, more than 50% of respondents said it was very important and 25% felt it was important for the counselors to have similar religious values with them. It is also important for the counselors to understand Islam; 56.2% believed it is very important and 29.8% thought it is quite important. Carolan et al. (2000) found the same outcome in his study in which while seeking out help, a Muslim counselor was the Muslim client first choice. Nevertheless, non-Muslim counselors are known in the Muslim community as a cultural-sensitive professional (Carolan et al., 2000) and would be an ideal option if a Muslim professional is unavailable. In addition, there are some clients who may prefer non-Muslim counselors who are sensitive towards their culture (Keshavarzi & Haque, 2013; Kobeisy, 2004). These findings suggest that what is important for the Muslim client is to seek help from a professional, however, there is a concern of trust towards non-Muslim counselors and the need for them to understand Islamic teaching.

These studies reveal that Muslim clients also need professional counseling services although they could fulfil these needs according to their culture and beliefs. This is because Muslim clients are experiencing the same difficulties as other clients. Similarly, they are willing to undergo counseling sessions with non-Muslim counselors who are, professionally, deemed dependable counselors. However, the multicultural skills of non-Muslim counselors play an important role and could impact the perception and trust of the Muslim clients. This means that the multicultural competency of non-Muslim counselors should be improved from time to time in line with the changes that occur in the society, especially Muslim community.

In a counseling session involving a Muslim client, the role of the therapist may be different. A therapist can play a role as an advisor or a teacher and the client as a student (Ahmed & Amer, 2012; Keshavarzi & Haque, 2013). This situation differs from the western culture approach in which the therapist may suggest to a client an option of to do something but the client does not necessarily have to act on the suggestion. According to Hedayat-Diba (2000), even though Muslim clients do not believe in the therapists, they generally give a lot of power to the therapists and adhere to what is recommended or set by the therapist, at least in the initial stage. If they indicate otherwise, it would be considered offensive, hence, the client passive attitude in the treatment process. Hedayat-Diba (2000) also states that because psychological symptoms are often tangibly expressed, they are often expected to heal without involving the spiritual aspect; just like a person going for his/her doctor's appointment. Such circumstance gives a lot of power and responsibility to the therapists. However, Keshavarzi and Haque (2013) assert the role of a practitioner in assisting and guiding a client through the process towards self-realization and willingness to contemplate. It is important for the therapists to determine a collective approach; balancing the power given to them and keeping in mind the client wellbeing.

One of the concepts and fears felt by Muslim clients is likely to reflect their perceptions of how the therapeutic process will take effect. Kobeisy (2004) propose that the lack of information about the preparedness and expectation of counseling and misinformation on counseling from others may prevent Muslims from seeking professional help. This circumstance is different from those who are living in the United States or who have been receiving their education from the US academic institutions (Kobeisy,

2004). In general, information about therapy is rather limited. Kobeisy recommends the type of information considered beneficial for the clients, including therapeutic function, education and training of the therapists, helpful therapeutic issues, and counseling expectations. In addition, it is also important to inform clients of the therapy procedure, such as what to expect during the sessions and the financial liabilities (Kobeisy, 2004). Hedayat-Diba (2000) also suggest educating clients on the importance of time boundaries, such as appointment, delays, and non-attendance sessions. Graham et al. (2008) propose to improve the information and information sharing by safeguarding confidentiality and to clarify the roles and goals of social service agencies. Overall, the provision of information when giving a treatment to a client is deemed an important step to change clients' negative attitude towards therapy.

However, there are other challenges to be considered during a therapy session such as the religion aspect. One possible reason for this related to the psychological training. More than 90% of the psychologists studied revealed that their education and training in religious issues are scarce or non-existence (Shafranske & Malony, 1990; Shafranske, 1996), in other words, less than 20% reported that they have some knowledge of religious psychology. Therefore, a possible hypothesis for the difficulty of combining religion with the treatment is that psychologists lack training in the field of religion. Another possible reason for the difficulty of incorporating religion into the treatment is the therapists own religious belief (or lack of it). Religion seems to play a minimal role in the lives of most psychologists in the United States. The study by Jones (1996) found that only 33% of the clinical psychologists described religious beliefs as the most important influence on their lives. In addition, in a national survey, only 29% of the therapists found that religious beliefs were important in the treatment process of most of their clients (Bergin & Jensen, 1990). This may be another hypothesis of why psychologists are reluctant to consider religious belief as part of the therapy and this gives an indirect message to the clients that religion has no place in the treatment process. Consequently, this circumstance confirms the Muslim clients' reservation with regard to trust and values that seem to be ignored in the therapy process.

CONCLUSION

The difficulties faced by the Muslim clients in getting treatment call for a solution to include this group in professional treatments to address their apprehensions. The present researchers offered various suggestions to help Muslim clients going through the counseling process. These suggestions are largely based on the clinical work experiences with Muslim clients. The main objective is to build a relationship. Muslim clients may be reluctant to attend the counseling sessions, therefore, building a relationship at the initial stage is critical (Keshavarzi & Haque, 2013). Generally, if a counselor does not get involved with the clients or their family, the possibility of the counseling session to continue will decrease (Kobeisy, 2004). Kobeisy (2004) identifies several important factors that will ensure the continuity of the counseling sessions, which include clients' first impression of the counselors, clients' feelings towards the counselors, and positive expectations towards the counseling relationships. Apparently, creating a positive relationship with Muslim clients is an important initial task of the counseling process. Counselors should also be aware of bias and discrimination that could happen to Muslim clients. In general, counseling sessions may also be a medium of discussion for issues relating to Islam that lead to discrimination and bias, hence, augmenting mutual trust between the counselor and the client.

REFERENCES

Abu Raiya, H., & Pargament, K. I. (2010). Religiously integrated psychotherapy with Muslim clients: From research to practice. *Professional Psychology, Research and Practice*, *41*(2), 181–188. doi:10.1037/a0017988

Abu Raiya, H., & Pargament, K. I. (2011). Empirically based psychology of Islam: Summary and critique of the literature. *Mental Health, Religion & Culture*, *14*(2), 93–115. doi:10.1080/13674670903426482

Ahmed, S., & Amer, M. M. (Eds.). (2012). *Counseling Muslims: Handbook of mental health issues and interventions*. New York, NY: Routledge.

Amer, M. (2009). Editor's introduction: The role of journal thematic issues in developing an agenda and filling the literature gaps for mental health research with Muslim participants. *The Journal of Muslim Mental Health*, *4*(1), 1–4. doi:10.1080/15564900902801163

Bergin, A. E., & Jensen, J. P. (1990). Religiosity of psychotherapists: A national survey. *Psychotherapy (Chicago, Ill.)*, *27*(1), 3–7. doi:10.1037/0033-3204.27.1.3

Carolan, M. T., Basherinia, G., Juhari, R., Himelright, J., & Mouton-Sanders, M. (2000). Contemporary Muslim families: Research and practice. *Contemporary Family Therapy*, *22*(1), 67–79. doi:10.1023/A:1007770532624

Daneshpour, M. (1998). Muslim families and family therapy. *Journal of Marital and Family Therapy*, *24*(3), 355–368. doi:10.1111/j.1752-0606.1998.tb01090.x PMID:9677541

Graham, J. R., Bradshaw, C., & Trew, J. L. (2008). Social worker's understanding of the immigrant Muslim client's perspective. *The Journal of Muslim Mental Health*, *3*(2), 125–144. doi:10.1080/15564900802487527

Hamdan, A. (2007). A case study of a Muslim client: Incorporating religious beliefs and practices. *Journal of Multicultural Counseling and Development*, *35*(2), 92–100. doi:10.1002/j.2161-1912.2007.tb00052.x

Hays, D. G., & Erford, B. T. (2010). *Developing Multicultural Counseling Competence: A System Approach*. Pearson.

Hedayat-Diba, Z. (2000). Psychotherapy with Muslims. In P. S. Richards & A. E. Bergin (Eds.), *Handbook of psychotherapy and religious diversity* (pp. 289–314). Washington, DC: American Psychological Association. doi:10.1037/10347-012

Inayat, Q. (2007). Islamophobia and the therapeutic dialogue: Some reflections. *Counselling Psychology Quarterly*, *20*(3), 287–293. doi:10.1080/09515070701567804

Jones, S. L. (1996). A constructive relationship for religion with the science and profession of psychology: Perhaps the boldest model yet. Academic Press.

Kelly, E. W. Jr, Aridi, A., & Bakhtiar, L. (1996). Muslims in the United States: An exploratory study of universal and mental health values. *Counseling and Values*, *40*(3), 206–218. doi:10.1002/j.2161-007X.1996.tb00853.x

Keshavarzi, H., & Haque, A. (2013). Outlining a psychotherapy model for enhancing Muslim mental health within an Islamic context. *The International Journal for the Psychology of Religion*, *23*(3), 230–249. doi:10.1080/10508619.2012.712000

Khan, Z. (2006). Attitudes toward counseling and alternative support among Muslims in Toledo, Ohio. *The Journal of Muslim Mental Health*, *1*(1), 21–42. doi:10.1080/15564900600654278

Kobeisy, A. N. (2004). Counseling American Muslims: Understanding the faith and helping the people. Westport, CT: Praeger.

Kobeisy, A. N. (2006). Faith-based practice: An introduction. *The Journal of Muslim Mental Health*, *1*(1), 57–63. doi:10.1080/15564900600697749

Langgulung. (1990). *Kaunseling dalam Masyarakat Islam. Kertas Kerja Seminar Kebangsaan Kaunseling dalam Masyarakat Islam.* Yayasan Dakwah Islamiah Malaysia, Kuala Lumpur, Malaysia.

Mohamed, O. (2017). *Psikologi Kognitif Ad Din: Kaunseling Kesihatan Mental*. Serdang: Penerbit UPM.

Mohd, R. A. R., Wan, M. F. A. W. R., Marina, M. A. M., & Ramly, R. M. (2012). *Agama-agama di Dunia*. Negeri Sembilan: Penerbit Universiti Sains Islam Malaysia.

Nobles, A. Y., & Sciarra, D. T. (2000). Cultural determinants in the treatment of Arab Americans: A primer for mainstream therapist. *The American Journal of Orthopsychiatry*, *70*(2), 182–191. doi:10.1037/h0087734 PMID:10826030

Padela, A. I., Killawi, A., Forman, J., DeMonner, S., & Heisler, M. (2012). American Muslim perceptions of healing: Key agents in healing and their roles. *Qualitative Health Research*, *22*(6), 846–858. doi:10.1177/1049732312438969 PMID:22393065

Pew Research Center. (2007). *Muslim Americans: Middle class and mostly mainstream.* Washington, DC: Pew Research Center. Retrieved from http://pewresearch.org/assets/pdf/muslim-americans.pdf

Raba, A., & Othman, A. H. (1998). *Toward Islamization of Guidance and Counselling*. Sabah: Persatuan Kaunseling Malaysia.

Shafranske, E. P. (Ed.). (1996). *Religion and the clinical practice of psychology.* Washington, DC: American Psychological Association. doi:10.1037/10199-000

Springer, P. R., Abbott, D. A., & Reisbig, A. M. J. (2009). Therapy with Muslim couples and families: Basic guidelines for effective practice. *The Family Journal: Counseling and Therapy for Couples and Family*, *17*(3), 229–235. doi:10.1177/1066480709337798

Sue, D., Arredondo, P., & McDavis, R. (1992). Multicultural counseling competencies and standards: A call to the profession. *Journal of Multicultural Counseling and Development*, *20*(2), 64–88. doi:10.1002/j.2161-1912.1992.tb00563.x

Sue, D. W., Ivey. A. E., & Pedersen, P. B. (Eds.). (1996). *A Theory of Multicultural Counseling and Therapy.* Pacific Grove, CA: Brooks/Cole.

Sue, D. W., & Sue, D. S. (2008). *Counseling the Culturally Diverse: Theory and Practice* (5th ed.). John Wiley & Sons.

Sue, D. W., & Sue, D. S. (2016). *Counseling the Culturally Diverse: Theory and Practice* (7th ed.). John Wiley & Sons.

Chapter 15
Religion in Therapy:
Theravada Buddhism

Chandana Namal Kumara
HELP University, Malaysia

ABSTRACT

The absence of a central holy scripture in Buddhism and myriad manifestations coalesced into indigenous cultural communities across South and South-East Asia, presenting a formidable challenge to define Buddhism and its practices. This complexity may also be manifested in clients of Theravada background, making them elusive candidates in the therapy room. Complexity notwithstanding, Buddhism offers fertile learning ground for any optimistic multicultural counselor. For the purpose of this chapter, several selected fundamentals of Theravada Buddhism are presented with an emphasis on their possible cultural meanings and on therapeutic utility. This chapter is written from the perspective of Theravada school of Buddhism as it is taught, practiced, and seen in South-East Asia. The author's knowledge and personal experience in Buddhism as a former Buddhist monk, experience of Buddhism as a lay practitioner now, and as a practicing counselor inevitably influence, inspire, and may even limit the parameters of this chapter.

INTRODUCTION

Fundamental concepts of Theravada Buddhism such as mindfulness, loving-kindness, compassion, impermanence, non-self, dependent origination have already been introduced to the clinical and philosophical lexicon by practitioners and thinkers based in the west and these clinical and academic applications of Theravada fundamentals seem to complement or to advance the clinical and philosophical efforts toward the reduction of suffering and lasting happiness among professionals and clients they work with. The clinical application of Buddhist fundamentals have been endorsed and encouraged by notable authority figures of Buddhism such as Dalali Lama and people who are interested in meditation are increasingly received for retreat and ordination in monasteries in Thailand, Myanmar and Sri Lanka. It would be fair to state that this growing trend in the west is similar in spirit to the trend that was reported at the beginning of the historical Buddha's career when the teachings were received without the religious labeling

DOI: 10.4018/978-1-5225-6073-9.ch015

on them, making the practice and application of the teachings more direct and immediate. Many in the west encountered Buddhism through clinical exposure (Fulton, 2013) or while in a deliberate quest for alleviation of existential suffering and therefore the teachings and application were direct and immediate experiences for them, a self-evident epistemological quality that distinguished the teachings of the Buddha from his contemporary teachings. Many in fact recognize the teachings of the Buddha as a form of psychotherapy rather than a religion (Lee et al., 2017; Fulton, 2013; Segall, 2003; Michalon, 2001) and in that recognition they come closer to the central goal of the teacher as the healer (Rahula, 1978) and teachings as a means to end the sufferings (Bodhi, 2009). However, the clinical application of Buddhist concepts in societies where Buddhism is associated with orthodox religion with all the features of an organized religion may not be as straightforward as in non-Buddhist cultures.

As Ando (2008) recognized it, Buddhism in Asian societies is regarded as a religion and individual is born into a Buddhist cultural network without having to discover the teachings through an existential quest for happiness or freedom. From childhood, the individual is inducted in to religious culture in which Buddhist teachings are practiced blending them with indigenous beliefs, rituals and practices, a phenomenon that presents both opportunities and challenges for the integration of Buddhist fundamentals into counseling and psychotherapy in traditionally Buddhist societies. For example, the emphasis on values such as gratitude and generosity is notable and rituals such as making offerings to the monks are utilized to cultivate them in Asian societies. However, the application of fundamentals such as mindfulness in traditional Buddhist societies seems to be lagging behind the non-traditional Buddhist societies partly because the fundamentals with direct and immediate experiential benefits are covered with layers of cultural idiosyncrasies, rituals and hierarchies; many in traditional Buddhist societies tend believe that the spirituals benefits of Buddhist practice are too high-hanging fruits for them to reach and that they have not yet reached the stage to tune into those states. Many in traditional Buddhist societies are also influenced by the theistic thinking patterns and tend to live life hoping for a better afterlife. These self-defeating cognitive barriers may well be on your way when you begin to work with a Theravada Buddhist client and this juncture can be considered as a journey toward the rediscovery of the healing properties of the teachings of the Buddha that were diluted in the process of cultural evolution of Buddhism as a religion.

In the presentation of selected fundamentals of Buddhism in this chapter, while acknowledging the contributions of Buddhist scholars in the east and the west to the philosophical interpretations of Buddhism, attempt is made to inform the helping professionals of possible meanings these fundamentals may hold for the lay Theravada Buddhists. In doing so, the therapeutic utility of the fundamentals is highlighted much more than the philosophical depth of those concepts. Some case examples of working with Theravada Buddhist clients in counseling are presented and possible future directions and challenges in harmonizing psychotherapy and Buddhism in Theravada Buddhist societies are reflected upon at the end.

Selected Fundamentals of Theravada Buddhism

The Triple Gems: Source of Mental and Social Support

Though often overlooked in the western scientific community perhaps due to the absence of full-scale *Sangha* in respective societies, the triple gems may hold significant value for a Buddhist of Theravada background. These three gems and taking refuge in them by the way should not be confused with worshiping real precious stones like ruby or sapphire; triple gems symbolically refer to the *Buddha,* the

Dhamma and the *Sangha* and taking refuge in them means self-declared trust in these three elements by an aspirant Buddhist as reliable guiding principles for his or her spiritual cultivation. At one level taking refuge in triple gems may mean acknowledging that the Buddha is fully enlightened (*sammaā sambuddho*), that the *Dhamma* –his teachings – is well explained informing the aspirant Buddhist all what he or she needs to know about the practice (*suwakkhāto*), and that the *Sangha* – the community of practitioners – are on the right path of spiritual cultivation (*supatipanno*). This is the most common meaning of triple gems prevalent among Buddhists. At another level, particularly as one's practice becomes matured, the *Buddha* may also mean being fully aware of one's present moment reality and the *Dhamma* may mean not just the scriptures but the circumstances of life one encounters in reality such as loses, changing seasons, aging and natural disasters and the *Sangha* may include not only monks but also lay practitioners. While the *Buddha* and the *Dhamma* may act as a source of strength and security at a personal level, the *Sangha* may act as a source of social support particularly in times of crises. It would be useful for helping professionals to get to know the client's level of involvement in the *Sangha* – community – to assess the presence or the absence of social-spiritual support systems in his or her life.

Five Precepts: Self-Imposed Moral Code

Five precepts for Buddhists are what commandments are for followers of Abrahamic religion with one significant exception; five precepts are to be taken voluntarily as opposed to commandments that are imposed by higher spiritual authority. The precepts in Buddhism are considered to be the foundation of spiritual life (Lee et al., 2017; De Silva, 2014, 2005; Premasiri, 2001). Largely adopted from the contemporary religious forms in 5th century B.C. India, five precepts were presented as a universal code of ethics. Five precepts include voluntarily abstaining from killing, stealing, sexual misconduct, lying and verbal misconduct and abusing alcohol or intoxicating drugs. Clearly, these precepts can be interpreted more broadly than just killing or stealing. For example, first precept of abstaining from killing entails abstaining from any form of intentional physical harm to self and others. Self-harming behaviors and domestic violence can be technically interpreted as violation of first precept. Stealing may mean more than burglary; for example white-collar crimes, being late to work and leaving work early could also amount to stealing. Small lies or white lies can be observed closely for they might avail you with an opportunity to be honest or take a risk; for example, parents could benefit their children immensely by speaking the truth about the world than conveniently lying to them.

The successful maintenance of these precepts by a practitioner, however, depends on one's level of intrinsic motivation to observe them voluntarily without expecting any external rewards. Although the standard for five precepts is kept high, there are no moral reprisals for failing to uphold a precept once someone had observed them. In other words, one does not incur sinful loses if one transgresses on his or her commitments to five precepts. The moral consequences of such a transgression are to be borne by the individual and he or she is given the opportunity to repair the precepts and strive for more intrinsic form of practice. The individual practitioner is neither held responsible by religious or divine authority nor is he or she answerable to such an authority. One's conscience is the only authority one has to be answerable to.

Although the observance of five precepts by definition is voluntary and free from any sort of coercion from external authority, in reality it may not sound so forgiving for a lay person. It is not uncommon that many Theravada Buddhists perceive precepts in much the same way believers perceive commandments. For example, a lay Buddhist who consumes alcohol on a regular basis would be embarrassed to acknowledge that he breaks the fifth precept and even feels guilty about it leading to low self-evaluation on the spiritual domain and eventually to giving up on the spiritual efforts altogether. The forth and the fifth precept seem to put Buddhists through a test that they often failed to pass mainly due to the cultural misinterpretations of precepts as unbreakable sacred oaths and as compulsory moral commitments without which one cannot progress to the next level of spiritual pyramid. This is a cultural myth that needs to be addressed in counseling for several reasons.

First of all, life is lived by many under less than ideal conditions in which telling lies or having a drink is unavoidable, if not necessary for the survival of socioemotional life. In these less than ideal situations precepts can be a great source of distress if they were to be internalized as irreparable sacred oaths. But when precepts are taken as ideals one should strive to live by any transgressions become forgivable and less guilt-inducing. Second of all, it is understandable that the Buddhist teachings have been organized by generations of religious scholars just like any other subjects with stages starting from the preliminary levels leading all the way up to advance levels. But at a practical level, this stage model of spiritual organization runs straight in to troubles because the nature of the Buddhist teachings and their benefits are to be experienced on a here-and-now basis, not there-and-then after one has reached certain stages. When teachings are approached in this direct manner, it is possible for the person to build the spiritual life based on the strengths the person already has. For example, the fact that the person manages to keep first three precepts can be acknowledged as a source of strength to forgive the transgressions of the fourth and the fifth while tapping into other inner resources such as generosity and gratitude to draw strength. When precepts are approached in this broader sense of spiritual development, precepts become truly self-imposed guidelines because the person tends to perceive them as protective and self-regulatory framework rather than restrictive and retributive set of rules. Incidentally, precepts are acknowledged in positive psychology as a source of self-control and self-regulation (Falb and Pargament, 2014).

Four Noble Truths

Four truths provide a comprehensive framework for the investigation of the origin of unsatisfactory nature of human experience. Unlike any other religions, Buddhism focuses on banal yet universal human experience of unsatisfactoriness; once you start paying attention to your moment to moment experience it is not difficult to notice how this unsatisfactoriness creeps into our conscious experience irrespective of religion, gender, ethnicity or socioeconomic status of the person. Four noble truths identify in a therapeutic style human predicament, its origin, its cessation and the solution that leads to cessation of the predicament (Fulton, 2013; McWilliams, 2010; Gnanarama, 2000; Santina, 1984). For a curios therapist, four noble truths could work as a map in therapy similar to awareness, acknowledgement, acceptance and action, a framework that was postulated by Virginia Satir and her colleagues (Satir et al.,1991).

The first truth elaborates varieties of human suffering that include birth and death and everything unsatisfactory between those two notable life events. The second truth explains the cause of suffering paradoxically pointing, not to human desire, but to human's attachments to desires as the main killer; so desires is not suffering but the attachment to desire is suffering. For example, sexual desire in Buddhism is not condemned as an evil form of energy but recognized as a life force we are born with as part of nature. However, the moment one identifies with one's sexual energy and makes preferences and issues around it, sexual energy becomes a deep source of suffering. These desires are three fold: desire for sensual pleasure (*kāma tanhā*), desire for things to be specific way (*bhava tanhā*) and desire for things not to be specific way (*vibahva tanhā*). Attachment to sensual pleasures as a source of suffering is not difficult to understand given the nature of limited capacity of our sensory systems to accommodate sensory pleasures that await them. For example, each body has a 'set point' for fat intake and body naturally refuses to eat once it reached the set point; eyes and ears get fatigued if they are pushed to their limits. Any forceful feeding of these sensory systems would lead to abuse or even addiction, a common form of modern day suffering. The other two forms of desires are somewhat subtly intertwined. Once you start paying attention to them, it's not difficult to see that most of our unsatisfactory experiences revolve around our wanting for things to be specific way or not wanting for things to be specific way. These two experiences are triggered by our rejection of the way things are and demand for something other, better, faster than the way things are. In a way these two experiences are two side of the same coin. For example, someone who experiences strong suicidal ideation may contemplate ways to terminate life – an attachment for things *not* to be specific way – while believing in an imaginary peace after terminating life – an attachment for things to be specific way.

The third truth is concerned with the cessation of suffering by opening a window of opportunity to observe potential moments of experience where there is an absence of suffering. Philosophically speaking, this absence or the emptiness is attuned to by mindfully unwinding all the causes of sensory experiences. For example, think of someone who is suffering from a body image issue. There must be a potential beginning point for this person's suffering and this triggering point may well be a simple gaze this person picked up on the mirror or just by looking at someone else and comparing oneself with the other. Recognizing this triggering point and slowly dissecting that moment are critically important exercises in understanding the origin of human suffering. And at an experiential level, this is what is expected in meditation, to observe sensory experiences slowly by recognizing the way they affect the mind. Once one becomes skillful at recognizing these triggering moments, one is able to notice the cessation or the absence of unsatisfactoriness. This state of cessation is referred to as *nibbāna* (also referred to as *nirvana*), an imperturbable state that all Buddhists aspire to attain [*see* Premasiri (2001); Rahula (1978) for a philosophical treatment of this concept]. Below is a brief description of *nibbāna.*

Nibbāna is the enigmatic term attributed to the ultimate goal of Buddhism. *Nibbāna* is often (mis) understood as some kind of a final resting place (like heaven in theistic religions) that Buddhists aspire to arrive after death. Some misconceptions are inevitably created when Buddhism is viewed through religio-cultural lenses. For example, it is fair to state that theistic religions propose a union with the higher power as a reward for leading a faithful life only after the death of physical body and that union is considered the highest goal. Incidentally, discourse around death and funeral is full of words such as "going home", "going back to father", "sending him/her home". *Nibbāna* in Buddhism, however, represents a totally different paradigm, one that emphasizes an ultimate goal here and now. Teachers of Theravada Buddhism spend significant amount of time dispelling this myth and emphasize *nibbāna* or liberation as an existential experience to be witnessed here and now, not hereafter. As the semantics of *nibbāna* indicate, it refers to a state of the mind in which the burning fire of unsatisfactoriness is extinguished. The third noble truth that was explained earlier refers to this experience of cessation and should not be confused with some sort of spiritual bliss because blissful experiences, like any other sensory experiences, are transient sensorial illusions and such temporary states are not uncommon during meditative experiences. *Nibbāna* therefore should be recognized here and now as a state where there is no further desire, doubt or urge for anything unsatisfying.

The fourth truth proposes a holistic program to consolidate the experience of absence of suffering. This program is a life-long practice characterized by a shift in attitudes, ideals, behaviors, life-styles, livelihoods and life-goals. The fourth truth is usually expounded in the literature as Noble eight-fold path.

The path is not to be mistaken for a path that leads to a particular destination but an end in itself, a reality to be experienced here and now. This path is comprised of eight components that can be incorporated into daily life as a form of life style (*see* Gnanarama.2000; Santina,1984; Rahula,1978). These eight components include Right attitudes (*sammā ditthi*), Right concepts (*sammā sankappa*), Right speech (*sammā vāchā*), Right action (*sammā kammanta*), Right livelihood (*sammā ājiva*), Right efforts (*sammā vāyāma*), Right mindfulness (*sammā sati*), Right equilibrium (*sammā samādhi*).

First of all, the term "right" is not to be understood as opposed to "wrong", which might lead to a debate divided between right and wrong as moral binary oppositions. The term *sammā* in essence refers to a quality of wholesomeness that goes beyond the narrow definition of "right". For example, right livelihood for some people could mean making a living by fishing. The fact that the first precept in Buddhism is abstaining from killing does not limit fishermen from benefiting from the teachings of Buddhism. Few years ago I had the opportunity to visit a fishing village some distance from Penang Island in peninsular Malaysia. Most of the village men went out to the sea at night for fishing and came ashore in the morning. They usually offer sea food to the monks in the village temple and spend most of their afternoons meditating in the temple. Although I did not interview them to understand what they were contemplating on during their meditation, they appeared genuinely interested in mediation practice and peaceful in their postures during meditation. This is why Theravada Buddhism does not emphasize any form of exclusive practices such as vegetarianism, a practice that would potentially alienate certain group of people from practicing Buddhism who are living in a geographical region where vegetation is hardly possible. The bottom line is to be aware of one's circumstances and be reflective about them using the eight-fold path as a guideline. This approach makes the path a universally accessible method of bringing about mental equilibrium [*see* Fuller (2005) for a more philosophical discussion on this topic].

Dependent Co-origination: The Buddhist Genesis

Known as *paticca samuppāda* among Buddhists and often referred to as dependent co-origination or causality among scholars, this central concept of Buddhism presents a microscopic analysis of how basic sensory experiences are woven into complex life experiences with multiplying consequences. Understanding of dependent co-origin of phenomena is seen as a key prerequisite to break down the repetitive cycle of unsatisfactory life experiences (Kalupahana, 1986). While acknowledging the profound philosophical discussion on this subject by the Buddhist scholars, presentation of *paticca samuppāda* here is a practitioner-friendly interpretation of the concept aimed at providing a tool to work with Theravada Buddhist client.

In this presentation of *paticca samuppāda*, the twelve-fold formula (figure 1) is viewd as an analysis of human experience that can be utilized to dissect and understand patterns of client's suffering. The formula is presented in a cyclical model: from lack of awareness (*avijjā*) arises patterns and habits (*samkhārā*), from patterns and habits arises a particular consciousness (*viññāna*), that consciousness leads to a particular personhood (*nāma-rupa*), from the personhood arises patterns of sensing the world through sensory organs (*salāyatana*), depending on those patterns of sensing the world the environment is contacted in a particular way (*phassa*), depending on the way the environment is contacted feelings (*vedanā*) are triggered. Depending on the feelings a particular reaction (*tanhā*) is initiated. Depending on the reaction a particular attachment (*upādāna*) is formed. From the attachment arises a particular way of being (*bhava*) and this way of being is a transient experience subject to decaying (*jarā*), lack of awareness of which would lead to despair. Despite its technical nature this formula sheds light particu-

Figure 1. Wheel of existence

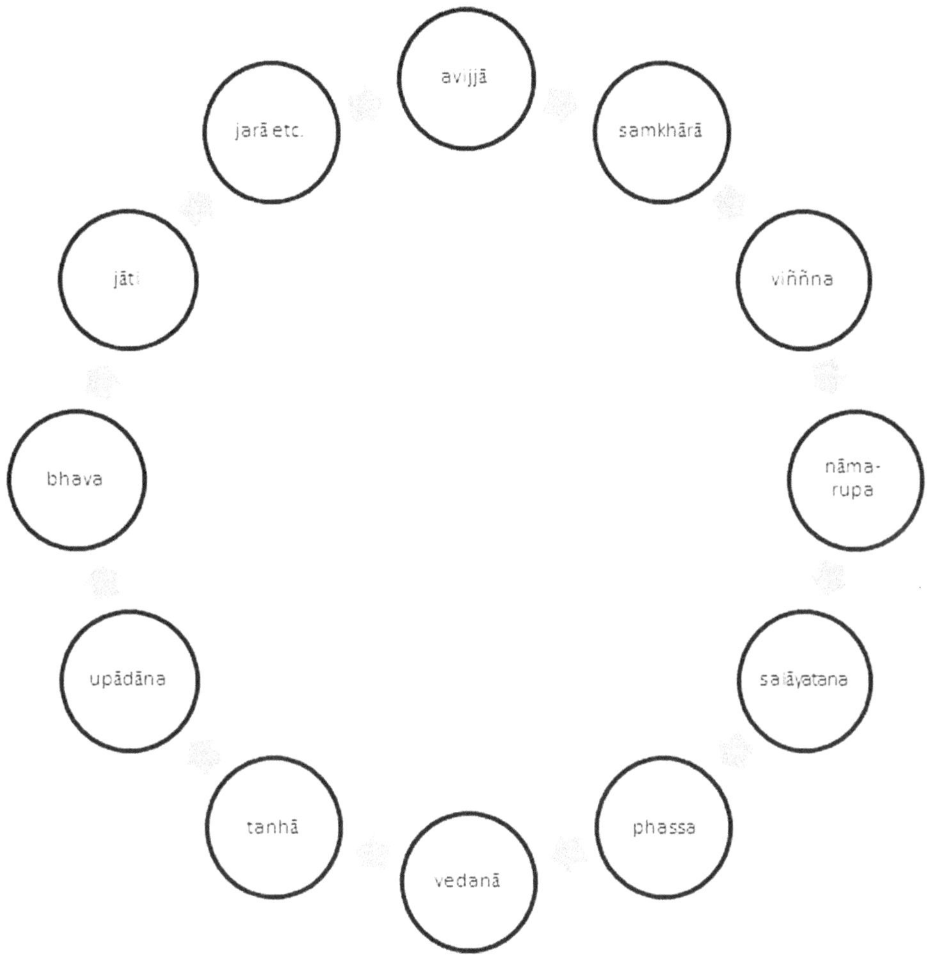

larly on dysfunctional ways of being, of feeling and of acting. For example, one would use blaming as a coping method without any awareness of what he or she is doing and it would lead to a formation of blaming pattern and habit. This blaming habit would give rise to a consciousness (a way of being aware at that moment – not a permanent repository of psychic content) which in turn leads to certain blaming personality formation – a representation of body and mind at that given moment. When the person is on blaming mode in a critical moment of life, the six sense organs – eyes, ears, nose, tongue, skin and mind – get conditioned in a way that perpetuates blaming personality. When the senses are conditioned in that way, the way person comes to contact with the environment is also affected by that conditioning. When the person is in contact with the environment through blame it might give rise to various ways of feeling ranging from relief, vindication, guilt to regrets. Based on any of these affective outcomes, the person may form an affiliation and attachment to whichever the feeling that is most rewarding. And this reward is so powerful that it reinforces the blaming method as a way of being, of feeling and of acting.

The whole point of this formula in Buddhism is to provide a potential exit plan from this pattern formation. This exit plan is to be implemented through meditation in which established patterns of thinking, feeling and acting are carefully dismantled by reflecting on their accumulative and conditioning nature.

Analogically, this process of dismantling can be called the way of breaking the cycle of repetitive unsatisfactory experience known as *samsāra* among Buddhists. As a practitioner, once you are familiar with this formula, it can be incorporated as a viable program for change. Because the formula is presented like a cycle you can initiate breaking of the cycle from any point. Incidentally contact here is somewhat similar to gestalt therapy concept of contact (Mann, 2010). Contact as an issue can be more visible in therapy than other underlying issues and clients would describe ways in which they are able or not able to be in contact with the environment. Therapists can use *paticca samuppāda* formula to closely analyze the situation by exploring how clients create a particular chain reaction that does not seem to be helpful for them to function normally. For example, when the person is able to see how he or she comes in contact with environment through blaming others, the person is able to reflect on moment-to-moment experience of blaming and unfolding toxic effects of that behavior [*See* Walpola et al. (2017) for a simulation model based on this concept].

Three Characteristics of Existence: A Buddhist Worldview

Three characteristics of existence, namely impermanence (*anicca*), unsatisfactoriness (*dukkha*) and non-self (*anatta*) provide a radically different view of the nature of human experience and these three concepts have been widely treated in the literature (McWilliams, 2010; De Silva, 2005; Karunadasa, 2001; Gnanarama, 2000; Kalupahana, 1987). Contrary to the popular perceptions of our reality as a lasting and satisfying experience that can be enjoyed by an individual, Buddhism invites us first, to look beyond the obvious and to examine our sensory and emotional experiences more closely to realize the transient nature of those experiences (*anicca*) and second, to realize the insatiable need we feel to desperately prolong those transient experiences, the inevitable failure of which results in lingering unsatisfactoriness (*dukkha*). And finally Buddhism points to the transient nature of the self by challenging the popular belief in personality as an individualist basis that can be identified with as self (*annatta*). Buddhism takes special interest in dismantling this well-established notion of self, an illusion, according to Buddhism, reinforced by cultural conditioning such as names, titles, education. Buddhism maintains that this fundamentally flawed idea fuels a culture of personality that is plagued with preoccupations about self-image, self-esteem, self-actualization and even self-realization leading to suffering (Karunadasa, 2001; Ganarama, 2000). If Heraclitus was heard saying "no one can jump into the same river twice", Buddha was heard saying "no same person can jump into the same river twice". This last point might be received with some resistance due to our own educated views about personality with many years of convincing research and expensive assessment tools to measure it. Buddhism, with its emphasis on transient and spontaneous nature of phenomena, dismisses the notion of self as an independent solid basis and encourages the intuitive capacity of human consciousness - a universal capacity with no sense of identity to it - to observe and reflect upon the creation of personality illusion on a moment-to-moment basis through our sensory experiences.

Loving-Kindness and Compassion

These two concepts have received increased attention in the areas of psychosocial interventions ranging from cultivation of prosocial behavior (Bankard, 2015), of altruism (Kristeller & Johnson, 2005), of empathy and wellbeing (Leppma & Young, 2016), to development of positive emotions and personal strengths (Fredrickson et al., 2008), to intergroup bias reduction (Kang et al., 2014), and reduction of negative emotions and increase of prosocial behavior (Kemeny et al., 2012). When practiced together with mindfulness (Salzberg, 2011) these concepts generate significant voltage of positive emotions that can be utilized to produce positive clinical outcomes as evidenced by the mounting empirical support.

Presented in Buddhism as two of the four divine abodes (*brahma vihāra*), loving-kindness and compassion raise the bar to an idealistic height for us to expand the horizon of love and care for oneself and for the others. Following descriptions of loving-kindness and compassion respectively by a renowned Buddhist teacher aptly sum up the depth of these concepts:

Love, without desire to possess, knowing well that in the ultimate sense there is no possession and no possessor: this is the highest love. Again the question is how to utilize them without promoting spiritual bypass in traditional societies? (Naynaponika, 1999, p-14)

It is compassion that removes the heavy bar, opens the door to freedom, makes the narrow heart as wide as the world. Compassion takes away from the heart the inert weight, the paralysing heaviness; it gives wings to those who cling to the lowlands of self. Through compassion the fact of suffering remains vividly present to our mind, even at times when we personally are free from it. It gives us the rich experience of suffering, thus strengthening us to meet it prepared, when it does befall us. (Nayanaponika, 1999, pp. 16-17).

Lay Buddhists may find these ideals to be somewhat intimidating, especially loving-kindness, as household notion of love is predicated upon possessiveness making it almost a prerequisite to love someone. Conversely, disclaiming the need to feel possessive may alarmingly indicate a lack of love or any sort of intimate interest in the other person. Again, lay Buddhists tend to openly declare that the bar is too high for them to live up to and that they would support any high-minded practitioners who can do the impossible so that they too can be inspired by such a superhuman endeavor to love without possession.

While acknowledging the idealistic descriptions of these concepts in the literature, it is useful to be informed by realistic experience of loving-kindness and compassion in order to go beyond the familiar self-defeating cognitive barrier. Possessive feelings toward loved ones become a source of suffering only when they are activated along the channels of wanting them to be specific way (*bhava tanhā*) or not wanting them to be specific way (*vibhava tanhā*). For example, when possessive demands are made for the loved ones to remain younger, prettier, sexier, smarter, richer or even faithful against the natural law of change, relationships between spouses, parents and children and friends fall apart. Integrating loving-kindness and compassion into life therefore does not require the person to renounce the need for possessiveness but to reflect upon the role played by the ego switching between *bhava* and *vibhava tanhā* on a here-and-now basis. During this exercise the person is able to realize the conditional nature of love and its limitations eventually leading to a greater acceptance of imperfections within the person and in others. There are two key points to ponder upon with regard to the cultivation of these virtues; firstly, the practice is to begin with an inward reflection focusing the person and to be expanded outwardly to other beings. Secondly, the cultivation is not about growing a brand-new benevolent virtue that the person never had before but about unlearning all the maleficent mental and behavioral habits thereby allowing the manifestation of a natural human tendency called unconditional love. It is noteworthy here that conventional approach to loving-kindness and compassion training may run the risk of reinforcing benevolent version of ego that is equally vulnerable to condemnation and comparison by the person because the nature of the reality does not permit the person to hold on to any ideals and feel at peace at the same time. This is a distressing situation for well-meaning Buddhists as they feel guilty about their inability to love and show compassion to someone from an out-group. But if they approach the out-group contempt for what it is at the first place and acknowledge it, the love and compassion will manifest without having to recite mantras for them to arise.

Karma, Death and Afterlife

It is fair to assert that the issue of kamma and rebirth does not occupy a central place [even death for that matter (Segall, 2003)] in Buddhism although the Buddha did make several references to the subject mainly to negate the contemporary deterministic views of kamma and rebirth in 5th centery B.C. India. Given the widespread loose usage of the term, it's inevitable to encounter lay Buddhist adherents who use karma loosely to understand and justify their circumstances [*see* Schlieter (2013) for a detailed analysis of metaphors of karma]. While it may be useful for the process of therapy to explore personal meanings of karma (taking a constructivist stance here) held by the client, positioning the concept of karma in its proper place can be very powerful in bringing about client's wellbeing especially in relation to helplessness versus responsibility dilemma. Contrary to the popular beliefs of karma as an action-reaction phenomenon (think of the instant karma videos on youtube), karma in Theravada Buddhism is defined as a basis for regulating mental, verbal and physical actions by being accountable for one's own actions and intentions. Karma therefore is defined as volition, a force driven by intention to act in a particular way either physically, verbally or mentally. The metaphors such as seeds (*bíja*), roots (*mūla*) used to refer to karma in early literature (Schlieter, 2013) indicate the vital role played by volition in producing karma. The emphasis here is on human tendency to act on auto-pilot without due diligence and leading therefore to proliferating consequences; raising one's voice during a conversation and slipping into an argument with lasting consequences is typical example of being on auto-pilot. However, when physical, verbal and mental actions are initiated with premeditated intentions, according to this formulation, they are meant to be regulated in a wholesome manner minimizing any harmful consequences to the doer as well as to the recipient. But this does not mean that well-thought-out actions do not generate consequences. Ironically, some of the most premeditated actions of our time happened to be criminal and fraudulent in nature. How does Buddhism explain the possibility of consequences of actions, wholesome or unwholesome?

Theravada formulation of karma challenges the popular belief of karma as a narrow action-reaction phenomenon and offers more realistic explanation as to when and how karma may produce consequences; there are several regulatory forces (niyāma) that are in action in the cosmos that produce certain circumstances (Kalupahana, 1986). For example, changing seasons bring about certain fortunes and misfortunes that are unrelated to any particular karma. Furthermore, one's ability or lack of ability to control impulses may produce favorable or unfavorable outcomes that may not be directly related to any karma. Think of, for example, Frank Abagnale Jr. whose life was depicted in the 2002 movie *Catch me if you can*. As a teenager he acted as a doctor, a pilot and a teacher and swindled millions of dollars from companies. However, after being apprehended by the authorities and serving short prison sentence he started working for the government and later became a security expert turning the very skills he used to deceive others to help others. Abagnale's story would have had a completely different end to it had he had born in a different culture where there is no such flexibility in criminal justice system. Bottom line here is to avoid any kind of reductionist view of karma and to execute actions mindfully by taking responsibility for their outcomes.

Rebirth (or reincarnation) also has not claimed a clear legitimate place in Theravada Buddhism although widely (mis)understood as a central "beliefs" in Buddhism. Instead of maintaining rebirth as a mystery behind the curtains of heaven or hell, Buddhism points to hear and now experience to witness the recurring transformative process of phenomenon in the form of birth and death. The practice of observing the inhaling and exhaling (or rising and falling of the breath) in mindfulness training at some level is meant to simulate the birth and death of phenomenon at here and now level. The widespread preoccupation with the physical death of human body and fears, myths and rituals around death, according to Buddhism, are cultural conditionings that need to be unlearned. The reason for the carefully placed emphasis on here and now and on mindfulness is to avoid philosophical, semantic and cultural entanglements around karma, rebirth, heaven and hell and to be available to the immediate sensory experience here and now; if the immediate sensory experience happens to be a confusion about karma, desire for heavenly rebirth or fear of hell that needs to be attended to for what it is, a sensory experience, without resorting to speculative philosophical discussions about those experiences [*see* Olendzki (2003) for a detailed account of constructing reality in the present moment].

Case Examples With Some Suggestions

It is common for Theravada Buddhists to be less informed or misinformed about these concepts and lack of centrally accepted way of being a Buddhist can make Theravada Buddhist client an elusive candidate. Having satisfactory knowledge of these concepts, therefore, can be a valuable asset for the therapist to organize the counseling process around these pillars and to explore views held by the client regarding these concepts to understand the discrepancy between the text book version and the personal meanings held by clients. Once a reference point has been established you can start working toward straightening up those views by exploring potential reasons for holding such meanings and secondary gains they may hold for the client.

Theravada Buddhists tend to use mantras such as "life is full of suffering", "everything is impermanent" or "letting go" to paint painful experiences with spiritual color so that trauma of the situation can be lessened or a painful dressing-up of an emotional wound can be avoided. These attempts certainly amount to spiritual bypassing, attempts by an individual to work on emotional issues only at spiritual level without working on cognitive, affective and behavioral levels (Clarke et al., 2012; Cashwell, 2010; Cashewell et al., 2007), while serving as temporary coping strategies.

As with any dysfunctional coping methods, they only serve a temporary purpose and clients' sufferings remain unchanged at a deeper level. Once the preconditions such as rapport and trust have been established these general remarks with a spiritual tone can lead to deeper conversations. The following case is an example of using the mantra "I must let go", a clear misuse of the four noble truths to subconsciously evade emotionally thorny path to acceptance. A woman who lost her husband due to a tragic accident two years prior to our meeting told me that she just couldn't let go of him; obviously she was frustrated with herself for holding on to him for two years; she condemned herself as a Buddhist for her failure to get it over with and move on. She had jumped straight to the last step of the four noble truths without reflecting deeply on the first three steps; she just wanted to let go of the painful memories of her husband without being fully aware of her feelings and acknowledging and accepting the tragic circumstances of his death. By exploring the reasons for her failure to let go of him after repeated attempts for two years, she was able to become aware of mixed feelings of guilt, frustration, fear and sadness and encounter them for the first time, allowing herself to be fully consumed by grief once and for all and leading to acknowledgement, acceptance and more functional actions toward meaning-making in the absence of her husband.

The following case highlights above all the role of the *Sangha* as a social support system. I worked with a middle-aged man who was struggling to get his life back on track after his wife left him together with their teenage children ending nearly two decades-long marriage. He was suicidal, anxious, depressed and hanging on to his stressful job by a thread at the time of our meeting. As a beginning counselor I considered this a challenging case and helping him through for a period of fifteen months would have been much toughter without the support I and he received from the community I called early the *Sangha*. As I was living at the time in a monastic community I was accessible to him literarily 24 seven and I was struggling to walk a fine line between professional standards I was getting used to through my master's in counseling program by having one session per week and monastic standards of limitless compassion by being available anytime, sometimes risking whatever that was achieved during the one hour session. As time went by his situation went from bad to worse as he had to go through a surgery on one of his eyes making it impossible for him to drive and attend to his basic needs. As he hanged around in the monastery after the counseling session, members of the community began to know his story and came forward to help him by taking turn to attend to him until he recovered fully. Once he recovered from the surgery he continued counseling while spending time on various volunteer activities in the community. After fifteen months of suffering he finally managed to move on with a renewed sense of meaning toward life. He was grateful for the role community – the *Sangha* – played during his predicament and was later seen giving back to the community as an avid volunteer member of the community.

The following case illustrates how high-minded ideals could become a source of distress if they are misunderstood at a practical level. A middle-aged woman sought help as she was struggling to overcome negative feelings she held toward her mother-in-law. At the time of our meeting she was embarrassed to acknowledge that she held a feeling of deep contempt toward her mother-in-law potentially due to some conflicts between them at the beginning of her fairly successful marriage some twenty years ago. Things have progressively improved between her and the mother-in-law and she was grateful for her role as a mother for bringing up a fine son who became her loving husband. The woman during counseling was able to articulate the issue with all the angles and told me that she had even received counseling sometime prior to our meeting. As an active member of Theravada Buddhist community, she felt guilty and was worried that her practice of Buddhism was going nowhere. She was even afraid that she would accumulate bad kamma and might behave the same way toward her future daughter-in-law when her own sons get married. It became clear as the sessions progressed that she was divided between the text book version of love and compassion and realities of her domestic life; she was beating herself up with "shoulds" and "musts" that generally come with any ideals including loving-kindness and compassion. The indoctrination of ideals of love and compassion as divine qualities was so strong that she took herself immediately to the guilty road without stopping to see the negative feelings for what they were, a breakthrough reflection that she was guided to do during the sessions. In these reflections, she was able to see the negative feelings as inevitable outcomes of those conditions that were present during the early period of her marriage and to realize that there was nothing surprising about negative feelings when the negative conditions were present. When the reality was seen for what it was, it led to some sort of depersonalization that diffused the guilty feelings. This was not a move to shift the blame to conditions and be anonymous in the situation but a liberating move to share the responsibility of the situation in a forgiving manner. Later she came to realization that she had been clouding her mind with obligatory feelings of love and automatic feeling of guilt leaving no room for the love or compassion to arise and her care for the aging mother-in-law had always been a half-hearted affair from her side. This realization also led to a growth in forgiving and relaxed attitude toward her allowing her to be imperfect and feel human after long time. Later in the sessions she revealed that she did not feel annoyed as she used to when her husband asked the other day if she could drive the mother to the clinic for a routine check-up.

A Theravada Problem

The psychotherapeutic relevance of Theravada Buddhism should be properly contextualized in traditionally Buddhist societies by addressing any misalignments of meanings that Theravada concepts and practices hold for laity. It is not uncommon to see Theravada Buddhists living a life divided between mundane and spiritual domains without being able to make a commitment to either one. It is noteworthy that this group is comprised of both men and women who tend to be well-educated, financially independent and single. Occasionally there are married couples that lead sexless marriages leading at some point to one of them leaving the marriage for monastic life. Also there are married couples who observe eight precepts, set of self-disciplinary rules intended for celibate renunciates and still continue to lead secular life. Theravada monastic ideals such as renunciation may attract a segment of the society that tends to be disenchanted by interpersonal, social, political and economic stressors in life and living a lay life according to monastic rules may create a moral ambivalence that could potentially jeopardize the prospects for both lay and spiritual life. This trend certainly shows signs of spiritual bypassing as a means of avoiding commitments required by lay life such as being in a relationship with someone, getting married, having children, having a career. While acknowledging the fact that lack of interest in worldly affairs is highly respected in Theravada societies and that people who renounce the worldly affairs and become monastics tend to go through a crisis period characterized by this confusion before resolving it successfully to become fully committed monastics, such tendencies must be carefully differentiated from any forms of dysfunctional thinking or maladaptive behavior.

CONCLUSION

In this chapter several fundamentals of Theravada Buddhism were presented while reflecting upon possible meanings they may hold for lay Buddhists. The triple gems and five precepts were particularly important concepts for lay Buddhists because these concepts provided the religious and cultural orientation for people in traditional Buddhist societies. Four noble truths encapsulated the essence of Buddhism as a way of understanding and alleviating human suffering. Three characteristics of existence and dependent co-origination provided a radical worldview and microscopic view of human experience enabling human capacity to dissect sensory experiences and consolidate the trust in the four noble truths. Some observations on karma and rebirth were presented to dispel myths around these beliefs by emphasizing the role of volition and responsibility in determining direction and the consequences of one's actions. Loving-kindness and compassion were highlighted as innate human capacity to love and care for oneself and others by unlearning the toxic habits of hatred and jealousy.

Both getting the Theravada Buddhists to come for therapy and getting them to see the therapeutic values of their religion are challenges located within the larger multicultural domain. While advancing the field of multicultural counseling, in order to help this segment of the population more effectively, new assessment protocols and tools that are sensitive issues and domains pertaining to Theravada Buddhism are needed.

REFERENCES

Ando, O. (2008). Psychotherapy and Buddhism: Spirituality underneath psychotherapies in East Asia. *International Medical Journal*, *15*(2), 115–118.

Bankard, J. (2015). Training emotions cultivates morality: How loving-kindness meditation hones compassion and increase prosocial behavior. *Journal of Religion and Health*, *54*(6), 2324–2343. doi:10.100710943-014-9999-8 PMID:25633082

Bodhi. (2009). Alagaddupama sutta: the simile of the snake. In *Middle length discourses of the Buddha* (pp. 224 - 236). Boston: Wisdom Publications.

Cashwell, C. S., Bently, P. B., & Yarborough, J. P. (2007). The only way out is through: The peril of spiritual bypass. *Counseling and Values*, *51*(2), 139–148. doi:10.1002/j.2161-007X.2007.tb00071.x

Cashwell, C. S., Glosof, H. L., & Hammond, C. (2010). Spiritual bypass: A preliminary investigation. *Counseling and Values*, *54*(2), 162–174. doi:10.1002/j.2161-007X.2010.tb00014.x

Clarke, P. B., Giodarno, A. L., Cashwell, C. S., & Lewis, T. F. (2013). The straight path to healing: Using motivational interviewing to address spiritual bypass. *Journal of Counseling and Development*, *91*(1), 87–94. doi:10.1002/j.1556-6676.2013.00075.x

De Silva, P. (2005). *Introduction to Buddhist psychology*. New York: Palgrave McMillan. doi:10.1057/9780230509450

De Silva, P. (2014). *An introduction to Buddhist psychology and counseling*. New York: Palgrave Mc-Millan. doi:10.1057/9781137287557

Falb and Pargament. (2014). Religion, spirituality and positive psychology: strengthening wellbeing. In J. T. Pedrotti & L. M. Edwards (Eds.), *Perspectives on the intersection of Multiculturalism and Positive psychology* (pp. 143–157). New York: Springer.

Fredrickson, B. L., Cohn, M. A., Coffey, K. A., Pek, J., & Finkel, S. M. (2008). Open hearts builds lives: Positive emotions, induced through loving-kindness mediation, build consequential personal resources. *Journal of Personality and Social Psychology*, *95*(5), 1045–1062. doi:10.1037/a0013262 PMID:18954193

Fuller, P. (2005). *The notion of ditthi in Buddhism*. London: Routledge Curzon.

Fulton, P. R. (2013). Contributions and challenges to clinical practice from Buddhist psychology. *Clinical Social Work Journal*, *42*(3), 208–217. doi:10.100710615-013-0469-7

Gnarama. (2000). *Essentials of Buddhism*. Singapore. Pathegama Gnarama.

Kalupahana, D. J. (1987). *Principles of Buddhist psychology*. Albany, NY: State University of New York Press.

Kalupahana. (1986). *Central philosophy of Buddhism*. Honolulu: The University Press of Hawaii.

Kang, Y., Gray, J. R., & Dovidio, J. F. (2014). The non-discriminating heart: Lovingkindness meditation training decreases implicit intergroup bias. *Journal of Experimental Psychology. General*, *143*(3), 1306–1313. doi:10.1037/a0034150 PMID:23957283

Karunadasa, Y. (2001). Buddhist doctrine of Anatta. In D. J. Kalupahana (Ed.), *Buddhist thought and ritual* (pp. 9–19). Delhi: Motilal Banarsidass.

Kemeny, M. E., Foltz, C., Cavanagh, J. F., Cullen, M., Giese-Davis, J., Jennings, P., ... Ekman, P. (2012). Contemplative/emotion training reduces negative emotional behavior and promotes prosocial responses. *Emotion (Washington, D.C.)*, *12*(2), 338–350. doi:10.1037/a0026118 PMID:22148989

Kristeller, J. L., & Johnson, T. (2005). Cultivating loving-kindness: A two stage model of the effect of meditation on empathy, compassion and altruism. *Zygon*, *40*(2), 391–407. doi:10.1111/j.1467-9744.2005.00671.x

Lee, K. C., Oh, A., Zhao, Q., Wu, F. Y., Chen, S., Diaz, T., & Ong, C. K. (2017). Buddhist counseling: Implications for mental health professionals. *Spirituality in Clinical Practice*, *4*(2), 113–128. doi:10.1037cp0000124

Leppma, M., & Young, M. E. (2016). Loving-kindness meditation and empathy: A wellness group intervention for counseling students. *Journal of Counseling and Development*, *94*(3), 297–305. doi:10.1002/jcad.12086

Mann, D. (2010). *Gestalt Therapy*. London: Routledge.

McWilliams, S. A. (2010). Inherent self, invented self, empty self: Constructivism, Buddhism and psychotherapy. *Counseling and Values*, *55*(1), 79–100. doi:10.1002/j.2161-007X.2010.tb00023.x

Michalon, M. (2001). "Selflessness" in the service of ego: Contribution, limitations and dangers of Buddhist psychology for western psychotherapy. *American Journal of Psychotherapy*, *55*(2), 202–2018. doi:10.1176/appi.psychotherapy.2001.55.2.202 PMID:11467257

Nyanaponika. (1999). *Four Sublime states*. Penang: Inward Path.

Olendzki, A. (2003). Buddhist Psychology. In S. R. Segalle (Ed.), Encountering Buddhism (pp. 9 – 30). Albany, NY: State University of New York Press.

Premasiri, P. D. (2001). Social relevance of the Buddhist nibbana ideal. In D. J. Kalupahana (Ed.), *Buddhist thought and ritual* (pp. 45–56). Delhi: Motilal Banarsidass.

Rahula, W. (1978). *What the Buddha taught*. London: Gordon Fraser.

Salzberg, S. (2011). Mindfulness and Loving – Kindness. *Contemporary Buddhism*, *12*(1), 177–182. doi:10.1080/14639947.2011.564837

Santina, P. D. (1984). *Fundamentals of Buddhism*. Singapore: Buddha Dharma Education Association Inc.

Satir, V., Banmen, J., Geber, J., & Gomori, M. (1991). *The Satir Model*. Palo Alto, CA: Science and Behavior Books, Inc.

Schlieter, J. (2013). Checking the heavenly 'bank account of karma': Cognitive metaphors for karma in Western perception and early Theravāda Buddhism. *Religion*, *43*(4), 463–486. doi:10.1080/0048721X.2013.765630

Segall. (2003). Psychotherapy practice and Buddhist practice. In S. R. Segalle (Ed.), *Encountering Buddhism* (pp. 165 – 178). Albany, NY: State University of New York Press.

Walpola, P. L., Walpola, D. Y., Walpola, I. C., & Toneatto, T. (2017). Mapping the Mind: A Model Based on Theravada Buddhist Texts and Practices. *Contemporary Buddhism*, *18*(1), 140–164. doi:10.1080/14639947.2017.1307575

Chapter 16
Faces of Grief:
Cross-Cultural Bereavement and Support in Malaysia

Anasuya Jegathevi Jegathesan
HELP University, Malaysia

ABSTRACT

Death, bereavement, and grief are natural processes that are experienced by every individual who is born into this world. The level of trauma experienced from such loss can be mitigated by internal factors and the external environment faced by the individual. Spiritual belief systems and culture play a critical role in the experience of bereavement. This qualitative study applies the phenomenological approach to explore the lived experience of bereavement of 15 Malaysians from five different religious groups, namely Buddhism, Christianity, Hinduism, Islam, and Taoism. Rituals and belief systems impact an individual's experience with bereavement. The likelihood of individuals to seek emotional and psychological support depends greatly on individual belief systems, family support, support facilities set up by religious groups, and the perceived availability of professional services.

INTRODUCTION

While 'Death' is a universal experience, the process and philosophical construct of death varies between cultures and religions. As Victor Frankl in his book 'Man's Search for Meaning' (pg. 51, 1984) said "When we are no longer able to change a situation… we are challenged to change ourselves." Death of a loved one or a family member is an ultimate example of a situation where we are unable to change. The event of death in a family is a universal experience that leads to changes in family roles and in an individual's life. Cultural norms and traditions have been developed by all groups to support and come together in the times of grief, examples of such norms are Wakes where friends and family come together to share memories of their loved ones, *Cheng Beng* festival by the Chinese to honor the graves of their ancestors, daily prayers from 10 to 35 days by the Hindus where family is supposed to take turns bringing food to ease the financial burdens of the family in mourning. Internal and external factors which

DOI: 10.4018/978-1-5225-6073-9.ch016

are possibly influenced by upbringing and culture have a mitigating effect on the trauma experienced upon the death of a loved one. Rituals to face grief and death is different in every culture and society worldwide, but according to Weeks (2004) the common factor of all these rituals is that they "enable us to remain connected with the past, the future and with each other. They also serve to provide us with comfort and security." (pg. 115)

Malaysia, with its rich multi-cultural and multi-religious heritage, allows for unique insights into the lived experience of individuals who may have differing religious backgrounds. However, it does share a common nationality, and a broadly common Asian upbringing.

The qualitative methodology is an appropriate means of studying the matter of multicultural approaches to grief because it aligns with the philosophical underpinnings of the approach as proposed by Cresswell (2013). The qualitative methodology is ontological, allowing for the study of the multi-dimensional reality of the nature, its properties and interrelated relationships of human experience. It is also epistemological, axiological and rhetorical. This allows for the study of knowledge and the justification of meanings, how experiences are value and made sense of in the daily experiences of the individuals. The approach allows the researcher to study grief from both an individual and societal standpoint.

A phenomenological qualitative research design was employed for purposes of conducting this study to provide insight into the essence of the lived experience of those whom are undergoing a particular phenomenon. The phenomenological approach allows for the identification of differences and commonalities in individuals' experiences of complex social phenomena (Barnard, McCosker & Garber, 1999). At the same time, generalizing these ontological narrations of subjective understanding to encompass broader social and cultural discourses. The approach provides insights into the objective as well as the subjective experiences as reported by individuals (*Ibid.*). Hence, ensuring that the discourse on the personal experience of bereavement provided by respondents was descriptive as well as reflective in nature. It also provided for rich and thick data that is relatively free of the researchers' personal framework (Edmonds & Hooker, 1992).

The subjective experiences of individuals in the phenomenological approach according to German philosopher Husserl looks at the subjective experiences of the moments that matter, moments that give meaning to an individual's experience. As quoted in Bailey (2013) "To live, Husserl says, is to experience (*leben ist erleben*)" (p. 39). Grief as experience by an individual is very much a personal experience and through the phenomenological approach the moments that creates meaning for individuals are captured and applied.

Therefore, in the context of this study, the phenomenological approach has allowed for an in-depth examination of how Malaysians responded to the universal phenomenon of grief and bereavement within their unique cultural and religious context.

METHODOLOGY

This qualitative study applies the phenomenological approach to explore the lived experience of bereavement of fifteen Malaysians from five different religious groups; namely, Buddhism, Christianity, Hinduism, Islam and Taoism. All respondents had completed the first year anniversary of the death of their loved ones and were English speakers. Semi-structured interviews were used to collect data from individuals.

The intentional-expressive approach of interviewing was applied to enter the life world of individuals and obtain narratives, concepts and in-depth experiences of individuals (Merriam, 2009; Salkind, 2009; Sin, 2010). To ensure the veracity of the research and to avoid unwarranted conclusions that may arise from personal bias, epoch and bracketing was employed in the course of data analysis. (Bryrne, 2001, as cited by Pitney & Parker, 2009; Merriam, 2009). Multiple means of data modification was employed. To ensure validity and reliability of the data finding two methods of triangulation was employed in the collection of data. Data was collected via multiple methods; namely, through semi-structured face-to-face interviews, researcher field notes, and review of existing literature on culture-specific grief and bereavement. This is for the dual purposes of broadening the scope of its focus as well as narrowing it down to one or several issues in the review scholarship that would benefit from further investigation (Richards, 2005). Further, three peer researchers were engaged to independently analyze the data and their individual findings were compared to ensure consistency of the analysis (Merriam, 2009).

Purposive sampling was used to ensure that all respondents had experienced the first anniversary of the death of their loved ones. The maximal sample variation was applied in selecting more than two respondents in each group in order to develop a comprehensive picture of the experience of bereavement as narrated by the respondents. The respondents were made up of three Hindus R1-R3, four Buddhists R4-R7, four Christians, two of whom were Protestant and Catholics R8-R11, two Muslims R12-13 and two Taoist R14-R15. All of the respondents had experienced deaths of close family members.

Data collected through fifteen face-to-face interviews were approximately 45 to 90 minutes in length. All interviews were audio recorded and transcribed. Transcripts were sent to the participants and were reviewed by peers for accuracy verification. The research was in compliance with the ethics standards of HELP University.

LITERATURE REVIEW

An inevitable consequence of life, is death. Yet, across nations, religions and cultures, the topic of death is not considered a topic of polite conversation. The experience of the death of a loved one may be met by tears, disorganization, and by a sense of helplessness and hopelessness. Bereavement is defined as the state of deprivation that arises from the death of a loved one, and from the continued feeling of loss that endures well past the actual death of the individual (Attig, 2004).

The permanence of death results in a unique loss in an individual's life, the loss of someone that can never be returned. This state of deprivation has a deep impact on individuals. The loss experience cuts across the mental, emotional, psychological, spiritual and even physiological state of the individual. (Love, 2007; Worden, 2009) Bereavement potentially disrupts the certainty one has in the ebb and flow of life, it can shake the foundation of one's core beliefs, priorities, values, worldview, spiritual and religious beliefs (Love, 2007; Gillies & Neimeyer, 2006). The grieving process is increasingly recognized as a method of preserving ties and connections with our loved one. These connections, memories and ties that have were formed with our loved ones in the past inform and mold out views of the present and help us shape our futures (Purkiss, 2006).

From the pyramids to the catacombs, death and the subsequent process of mourning is influenced by (and at the same time) greatly influences religious and philosophical beliefs, as well as the expression of culture. While the experience of bereavement may be universal, the expression and process of grief is culturally bound, with each culture providing a distinct approach to the loss and the transitions that follow after the death of a loved one (Anderson, 2010).

Strobe and Schut (1999) put forward a modal of grief to have a more universal application beyond gender and cultural specificity modals. Instead looking at the universal issues of stress and coping generated by the grieving process. The Dual Process model of coping with bereavement looks at how individuals go through two processes; loss orientation process and the restoration orientation process. These two processes are separate. Healthy grievers focus on the daily living challenges and then focus on the issues of managing their grief. The oscillation between these two processes promotes recovery and health coping.

Research has been done on the relationship between grief, spirituality and coping, where Bruke and Neimeyer (2014) found that religion provides mourners with an opportunity to seek meaning; to get some level of inner control and receive comfort and love from the Divine. Beyond the personal comfort, religion provides a shared platform to provide support and gives structure that can facilitate the process of managing the loss of a loved on. Religion is seen as providing a positive coping experience as it creates a sense of spiritual alliance and support system with those of the same faith and group.

Malaysia, as a multi-ethnic society has a rich diversity of culture and religions. The rationale of this research is to understand the bereavement experience of individuals, who while sharing a nationality (Malaysian) are from different and unique cultural and religious backgrounds. While the research adds to the literature of Asian grief and bereavement studies, it is also a potentially solid guide to counselors and therapists in dealing with bereaved clients in a culturally sensitive and professional manner.

DISCUSSION OF LIVED EXPERIENCES OF RESPONDENTS

Respondents reported that many factors played into the experiences of grief and loss. There are universal experiences that are nuanced by the personalized cultural experiences.

Emotions elicited by grief are complex and overwhelming. As a universal experience, all respondents felt the loss but how that loss was expressed varied between respondents. All respondents reported experiencing sadness and pain in a highly personalized manner. R8 reported, "Grief means I feel acute pain, a sharp pain...", and R5 reported, "I was really in a great depression… most of the time I will cry alone." While expressing and describing grief was actionable for most, some of the respondents were unable to articulate their grief experience. R7 for instance said "Ok, em, ok, it feels sad that this person is not around (M...), guess you'll miss um...his guidance and advice (Ok...), but other than that I can't think of a.. Can't think of anything say...very traumatic ah...". The individual could express the cognitive loss but was unable to express the emotions that went with it. In the respondent's voice and manner the sadness was apparent but they were unable to express the depth of their emotions because their family saw crying as a 'luxury' and that they needed to be logical about the situation.

An important emotional impact of death is that it generates within human beings a sense of helplessness and being overwhelmed by the situation. "I was very confused at the time, I particularly like blank-out" R4. "I couldn't cope with it" R2. "I wasn't very well prepared, I broke down" R8. In remembering the death of their loved one during the interviews, some respondents still displayed an emotional reaction to the loss by tearing up, stuttering and other minor physical cues. However, the lack of external displays of grief does not indicate a person in unaffected, the opposite may be true. R3 who faced the sudden loss of a sibling stated "it's like being in a situation, being and seeing from the outside what is actually happening. It's like I didn't feel part of the…I felt like I was watching a movie. I didn't feel that I was part of the... one of the actors in that scene. I felt like I was standing out of the whole thing and I was watching what was happening, because I couldn't believe what was happening before me….. I may not be able to, would have been able to... would not have been able to handle myself at that time. So, I don't know, maybe it's a system working within myself that took me out of that." Respondent R3 was hurt by the situation so much that till today she is able to recall the moment and feel a similar sense of pain. But at the event to others she seemed in control and slightly aloof. This may be very much part of Asian cultures where those in charge need to appear strong and in control, therapists approaching this situation need to trend lightly to ensure clients have the space to manage their internal state.

Psychologically, this can be seen as a sign of the individuals' defense mechanisms reacting to the painful situation and a sense of disassociation is generated. This feeling of numbness or aloofness allows the individual to function, albeit somewhat mechanically in this situation, temporarily locking down the otherwise deliberating emotions.

In terms of anticipated death, emotional expressions of loss that was reported was no different from when there was no prior warning of the death. R14 who was caring for her terminally ill mother was still surprised at the moment of death "you were prepared, but did not expect it to really come that fast la, it was so sudden, so sudden, ya, and your immediate reaction to it was stunned, shock and you know, you just can't cry, right?' Respondent R2 who was in hospital with her father experienced a similar sense of overwhelm, "… my dad is gone.. there was a lot of blankness is like, the cold you know this thing that he is supposed to get up.. never got up. I cannot think." Despite being the main care-giver, despite being hospitalized and aware on a cognitive level of the impending death of the loved one, the actual moment of death is still a uniquely overwhelming experience. The anticipation of the death seems to have little impact on the actual emotional experience of the moment of death. Reasons for this is layered and varied ranging from the loss of a role of care-giver in the family, feelings of guilt related to robustness of caregiving, physical loss of the individual and loss of a sense of identity and purpose.

Among respondents, reactions to the death was reported to be mitigated by the sense of responsibility that they bore to making arrangements and looking after the last rights. Respondent R14 for instance had to maintain calm while her younger sister could kick the wall and shout at people around her. Respondent R2 related that she had to keep it together for her mother's sake. At the time of the funeral she could not give in to the grief as her mother needed her to be strong. Even in grief respondents were empathetic and aware of the needs of those around them, tampering their responses to support those they perceived as more needy around them.

Aside from emotional control, the roles one plays in the family also influences expressions of grief. When a key family figure is gone, the role has to be taken over by surviving members. R11 as an eldest son felt keenly the new responsibilities on the death of his father, "Er I was I was sad, the thing that immediately I..I feel that I am the er....responsibility, to...to handle, all my younger... My brothers, and uh and and the children, and and..to settle the.. er.. all the..job after he died." The need to fulfil obligations and care for those around, to an extent blocked an individual's ability to openly express their loss. So while all felt loss and sorry, the emotions are not expressed the same way across the board. Cultural and societal roles mitigate the freedom respondents had to express their grief.

The range of emotions experienced by those in the first few hours of grief covers almost the entire darker spectrum of emotions; from pain to numbness, even hidden relief. It is therefore best to not make assumptions of what the grieving should be doing or how they should be acting. The impact can be expressed or internalized but the impact of the loss of a loved one is there.

In the face of such personalized uncertainty, the rituals, prayers and cultural activities surrounding funerals provides a sense of structure and guidance. Which is sorely needed in a time of such acute upheaval.

Respondents reported that prayer was a common coping mechanism used to mitigate the pain of bereavement. Common elements in the prayers to cope with bereavement included a prayer for guidance, a sense of companionship or strength to face the painful situation that they are in. Respondent R1 stated that she prayed that for "...the wound to heal, you have to have some kind of a guidance or some support or something to that extent for me to heal from within." R10 prayed for a sense of 'relinquishment' asking God to support her in moving forward. She was able to hold it together and not have a breakdown at home because "but God really was with me, with me la. God was with me." Respondent R15 stated that the chanting and the many days of prayer brought the family together. The chanting gave her a sense of "being connected to the ground, connected to ourselves, connected to the, the Buddha" thus supporting her in the process.

While prayer is a common element in the bereavement process, the nature and focus of prayer between the religious groups seems to differ. For instance, the Christian respondents reported that in prayer, they connected with Jesus to save the soul of their loved ones: "I hoped Jesus will come and save his soul" R9. The Hindus, who believe in the rebirth of the soul in their prayers, focused on being connected with the soul of their loved one as the soul continues its journey after death: "I speak to them through my prayers"R2. The Muslim respondent R12 believes that the prayers help the soul of the departed to find peace and gave a sense of control in the situation. He stated "..for those who really, really believe that, yes this is what you should do, you know, when people who pass on, and that you're gonna help their soul, and stuff like that, this is what you should do. So, in that sense, you know, because you can't really help anybody when they've, they've, you know (passed away) passed away right. And if you think that you know this might help by saying a few prayers here and there and then you feel like you're doing your part la." From the rituals this respondent received a sense of purpose and direction.

The Buddhist focused on the sense of community, continuance and comfort provided by their prayers and chanting, R6 'We are coming together, offering prayers." The Taoist had rituals to ensure the wealth and happiness of their loved on after death. The difference in the nature of their prayers is most likely due to the different views of death and afterlife held by each religious group. The benefit of the prayers as experienced by the respondents therefore ranged from a sense of community, personal support, to empowerment from assisting the souls of their loved ones, to a continued sense of connection with their loved one.

Whatever an individual's personal opinion of religion and rituals for death, respondent R7 said it very nicely"… the departed has departed, and you know it's just the living needs some way of coming to terms with their grief and we've got all these funeral rituals... if it makes my mom and family feel better, then they are okay."

Among the Buddhist respondents, there was a willingness to address the topic of death before the loved ones passed on. Planning for the passing and subsequent funeral was reported by all respondents. According to R6, "I already discuss with him before that, when he was alive we sort of discuss what I want, what he wants for his funeral." With the numerous taboos, sensitivities and cultural norms in the Asian context, this is neither a normal nor an easy conversation. None of the respondents from the other groups reported similar conversations among family member. On a personal level, most of the respondents reported that they have not had discussions of death issues with their family.

Discussions of death did however occurs on a more philosophical and spiritual level among the Muslim and Christian community, where death reactions from a religious perspective was discussed. The Muslim respondents in particular reported having deeper discussions on death and the relationship between death and religious belief. This philosophical view of death allowed for a more cognitive processing. It is the respondent's belief that the philosophy supported him in moving forward from his personal loss.

Funeral rites return a sense of purpose and power to the individuals on two distinct levels. Firstly, there is a solid belief that the rituals have a positive impact on their loved one's after life. A Hindu respondent went as far as having a second funeral ceremony conducted in India. The individual felt that upon having the second ceremony that was more traditionally complete and detailed, he had truly advanced the liberation of his loved one's soul. Respondent R10, a Catholic shared that, "It was frustrating that we could not do anything, but we prayed for her soul that she will have a better time in heaven."

The second and more pragmatic purpose provided by funerals is that the funeral itself forces the grieving into motion. It provides a clear purpose that allows grieving space, to avoid emotional overload because they are dealing with physical and societal needs. As reported by R5 who stated, "I was holding on, you know, short of holding on to it lah. Because I have to make sure everything is done perfectly well." The need to conduct the funeral, to an extent, allows the space to process and filter emotions so that individuals can function without being overwhelmed immediately after a traumatic loss.

While the rituals helped respondents focus on what needed to be done, some respondents felt that they rituals put extra pressure on them and interfered with their grieving process. "When my mother-in-law passed away I had no time to cry." R1. People were coming to her home all day, there were things to do. The respondents were unable to make time for themselves to grieve. There is a clear need to strike a proper balance and ensure that grievers have space for themselves to do what is necessary for the funeral and the family around them.

One of the most common problems noted by the grievers was adapting to the change of role that the death of the loved ones created. Death impact individuals and families in every aspect of their lives--emotionally, mentally, physiologically, financially and spiritually. In the collectivistic cultures of the East, death creates a tremendous shift in an individual's role in their family. Respondents were at loss when they are faced with new responsibilities, on top of the grief-reduction in household income, changes in maturity and emotional responses that were required of them. This was especially apparent in the loss of a parent or the loss of a major care giver in the family. Children felt the need to be "tougher" than their surviving parent and to support them in their time of need. Others felt as though, "I was just thrust into this role that I couldn't.. I couldn't turn back you know" R2.

Across cultures at the time of need, friends and family were a source of support and comfort. Human presence, kind empathic words and touch are important in times of need. While all participants were supported by family and friends, it is important to note that Christian participants received direct support from their church. Christian respondents recognized their church pastors, religious counselors and support groups as being an active part of their grieving process. The Buddhist and Hindu participants, while receiving a great deal of support from family, friends and the rituals of their religious practice, neither identified their place of prayer, nor their prayer group, as an active source of support.

Eight respondents however reported that while family and friends were supportive, their support was ineffective at the time. Use of platitudes such as "I know how you feel" and "they are in a better place" was not helpful in minimizing the experience of grief. One respondent felt that there is an artificial social guideline to how long and how much a person should grieve. The misconception that one should recover fast led to inappropriate and hurtful comments being made during the funeral.

Respondents reported that friends and family who attended funerals seemed to be confused on how to console those in grief. Some of the more unhelpful statements by family and friends are as follows. "When someone around you dies, the people around you keep telling you don't cry. Don't cry for your parents, don't cry for your mom, don't cry for your brother" R10. If one cannot cry in mourning, when else can they cry? It is perhaps good to realize that when in funerals the words 'Don't cry" translates into "I am uncomfortable with your tears, so please stop crying." The supports are asking grievers to stop crying not for their sake but for their own.

Statements such as "be strong" to those already taking charge and leading the funerals placed extra pressure. Contrary to the healing of the respondents. They felt that telling someone to stay strong was not supportive and locked them in a role they were unprepared for. Respondent R11 reported "I have no idea how to let go of being strong" and felt that they had still not properly grieved.

Grievers reported that they were inundated by platitudes such as "Are you okay". Although the respondents were not okay, what else they could say except 'I'm fine thank you.' Griever also reported feeling unsupported when people offered help without really meaning it. ".. they tell me what they feel is respectable to say for example, please let me know if you need anything. I believe that is a scripted speech." R15. Vague statements of support and generalized offers of help did little to actually support the respondents, who would be rote give negative responses to offers to help.

Grievers also felt pressured and alienated by having to repeat what happened over and over again. When friends and family visited, they often out of natural curiosity asked what happened. Repeating the story was painful to the respondents. It created a feeling as if their own emotional state were being disregarded by the supporters. Gossip, passing negative remarks and judgements made during funerals within ear-shot distance of the griever is obviously the exact opposite of support. These are negative habits but given that even funerals are social gatherings, it is an unfortunate outcome of being unable to filter the guests, where some carry their bad behaviors with them.

Most helpful behaviors experienced by grievers was when people were there for the bereaved. Respondents felt what was most beneficial was having a friend or a family member by their side, providing comfort. "People wanted to spend time with me," R1, "People actually took the time to get to know me and listen to my thoughts" R8, "Just being there is important, just think I am there." R14. The presence of genuinely caring individuals or a warm hug provided the most positive support. When griever felt that they were not being judged or criticized, was when they were most consoled. "She said look you don't have to stay strong, you don't have to do anything. If you want to cry – cry… if you want to scream-scream. Do anything you want and there is no how to do this thing." R13. The unconditional acceptance of the griever's needs and behavior conveyed the most active support on those in grief. Finally what was most helpful post the death of a loved one was consistent support. Not just turning up during the funeral, but being there and being available over a period of time to support the grieving was important.

The final aspect of the culture of grief looked at were the meta-physical manifestations of loved ones in dreams and various symbolic forms. These symbols were obviously very influenced by the religious belief and spiritual philosophy of the individual. Dreams of loved ones seemed to be common occurrence, and the dreams shared corresponded with the cultural and religious context of the dreamer. For a Muslim respondent, the visitations of the departed in dreams was not a good sign as it meant that they had blocks in their journey. Other religious groups seemed to see it as a positive occurrence. They saw their loved ones in familiar settings, such as the swing in the back garden, in their bedrooms, at places of prayer, and during special festivals. These kinds of dreams gave respondents a sense of a continued bond with the deceased and were in themselves a source of comfort. However, unresolved issues with the deceased were a source of disturbance. Two respondents dreamed of their loved ones in need, crying and lost. The dreams seem to correspond with the relationship of the living to those who had deceased. Perhaps as means by which unresolved issues can be processed and even overcome.

INTERTWINING GRIEF AND RECOVERY

The process of grief emerging from this research is that of an intertwining modal, where the socio-cultural environment and the grieving process is very much intertwined. The death rites and rituals of cultural groups are perhaps not so much for the benefit of the deceased but for the benefit of those that they leave behind. Certain rites of cultural group facilitate both the grieving and the process of moving forward in the bereaved journeys through life.

The sharing of Damma in Buddhism allows individuals to feel that they are actively supporting the soul of the departed as it is carried on its journey. The prayers of the living mitigate and ease the burdens of pain and sin carried by their dearly departed. Prayers of all the groups while aimed at the departed, have the more practical impact of giving those in grief a feeling of purpose. It has, can and does have an impact on the positive fortunes of those who have departed. This is a huge buffer to of the feelings of hopelessness and helplessness, providing guidance, purpose and a sense of direction in an otherwise unmanageable situation.

The processes are intertwined with the act of grieving and the activities of reconciliation with a new lifestyle without the loved ones, occurring together in mentally healthy individuals. Some acts may require the focus to be more on an emotional grief journey, but both states of a person move forward.

Moving forward and emotional processing of grief are not the only two intertwining threads in an individual's journey through grief. Other threads of shame, loss, fear, guilt and so forth are intertwined in the individuals' grief experience. Methods of managing these darker emotional threads can be sourced from spiritual practices, wellness plans and therapeutic interventions. It is in the experience of the author as a counsellor practitioner whom has worked with grief that the negative emotions can be elevated to an extent, if individuals are able to accept their grieving as a sign of the respect and love that they have of their loved ones. Regardless of time and space, the reality that the ones we love are gone remains. The pain and loss is unique and will last as long as we live. If individuals are able to see their grief not as a continued sign of trauma, but rather as he legacy of love and reverence that they carry for their loved one, the moments of STUG (Sudden Temporary upsurge of Grief) can be seen as moments of bitter sweet nostalgia and moments of reverence. Also reflecting the importance and the enduring impact of the one who has passed on, rather than traumatic reminder of death.

Culturally and traditionally, there are events that honor the passing of our loved ones. From Cheng Beng among the Chinese, to yearly death anniversary prayers of the Indians, it is to achieve the purpose of giving reverence to the memory of those who have departed. These traditions make individuals pause in their busy hustle and bustle of life to give moments of deep importance, respect and reverence to the memory of individuals who impacted us. These traditions allows for the intertwining of grief, family unification and reconciliation to occur in an organic and family focused manner.

When these threads become entangled, the grieving process may be choked to a halt. The halting of the grieving process, potentially interferes with an individual's ability to move forward and function in their everyday life. Thus the situation develops into complicated grief. Complicated grief here is in reference to grieving that interferes with daily functioning.

Individual philosophy on death and bereavement, which may be very much influenced by religious beliefs, is a critical factor that allows for the processing of bereavement in a healthy manner.

DISCUSSION: IMPLICATIONS FOR COUNSELORS

In working with one of the most traumatic times that an individual may experience, the first call to any counsellor, social worker or supporter is respect. Respect for the individual's grieving process, their personal beliefs, the unique emotional state they are in and respect for the culture that is governing the last rites. Counsellors may not believe in the faith, philosophy and religion of the clients. But therapists, in order to work with grief and loss must be able to respect the rights of the clients to believe and worship as they see fit.

The second criteria is to recognize and understand the client's current state of mind. Any intervention therapy is only effective if the client is functioning both emotionally and mentally. Clients who have just experienced loss are in a state of crisis. They are emotionally overwhelmed and their normal coping strategies are unable to meet the unique challenge of grief, leading to a state of cognitive and emotional disequilibrium. This is a classic sign of disequilibrium that is associated with crisis management. The death of a loved one is a state of personal crisis and individuals to an extent must be treated as if there are in crisis. In the first few days after a loss, therapy focuses on Crisis Management rather than counselling per say. The role of the counsellor is to ensure immediate safety of the client rather than trying to start the healing process. The healing process only begins after the state of crisis is over and this can be a few weeks or even a few months after the funeral.

The third criteria needed by therapists in multi-cultural grief work is to be open, curious and courageous. An open and curious therapists is willing to learn about other religions and cultures. While it is impossible and not recommended that one try to learn everything about other religions, it is crucial that the therapists have some knowledge of the basic principles of the various major religions in their area or country. The researcher will always recall a pointed lesson that occurred in a group therapy session, the facilitator said to a member, "How do you think God would feel about that action." The participant responded "I'm a Buddhist, I don't believe in God." A very awkward moment followed that statement, as the facilitator stammered and changed the subject. If a therapist is going to embark on any form of spiritual therapy, that basic understanding of major concepts is critical for long term success. Courage is needed because we are talking about religion. We are breeching a topic in therapy that has caused wars through the centuries. But when it is relevant to the client's healing we need to be courageous enough to address the issue in a supportive and respectful manner.

From the experiences of respondents shared across the different religious groups, it is apparent that while grief and bereavement is a universal experience, the religious, social and cultural context of those going through grief makes it a highly unique experience (Cowles, 1996). This uniqueness calls for the need for sensitivity and understanding of cultural and religious norms when managing grief. The universality of grief response can be seen by how all spiritually inclined respondents used prayer as a key coping mechanism. The differences between groups arose in terms of what was the content of the prayer and the meaning the prayer carried for the individual that was highly influenced by their religious philosophies. In therapy it is probably prudent to check with spiritually inclined clients on how they can incorporate prayer into their healing. Assuming that prayer is universal and that individuals approach prayer in the same way with similar intentions (especially if the therapist is from the same religious group) can lead to the activity missing the mark and the client feeling that the therapist has imposed their beliefs on them.

In terms of coping current literature indicates that the Dual Process Model suggests that in managing grief, individuals either coped with the loss caused by the death of a loved one, or with restoration-orientated coping that refers to the reorganization of life. It's only after they masters new skills required in meeting daily challenges post bereavement (Stroebe & Schut, 2001 as cited in Neimeyer, 2001). Current literature suggests that grievers alternate between loss and restoration orientation, with both orientations a necessary part of grief work. The findings of this research suggests that in the collectivistic cultures of the East, especially in from Buddhist and Hindu perspectives, the rights and rituals focus on loss and restoration simultaneously. The Buddhist transfer of merit and the offerings of the Hindu's to feed the needy as part of their funerals, address both orientations. It addresses loss as the ritual is done for the deceased and the restoration orientation as it adds meaning to the rituals besides fulfilling obligation to culture and society. The significance of the rites and rituals surrounding death, therefore, play numerous roles in ensuring the continued welfare of the living.

In dealing with the grieving process incorporating activities unique to that culture and religion may have a more intense impact than simply relying on generic activities such as journaling or simple service activities. Feeding the needy in the name of those who have passed on is highly significant to Hindu's and Buddhists. Reciting the Al-Fatihah is important to the Muslims. Reading the Holy Books, chanting, activities in memorial can all be incorporated into a comprehensive grief management plan with clients, that is highly personalized and meaningful to them.

In Western literature, the continuing bond that an individual maintains with the deceased is viewed at times as an unresolved source of grief (Bowlby, 1980) or a part of the global meaning making mechanism of certain cultural groups (Benore & Park, 2004). Findings of this study were more aligned to studies on grief done in Japan (Klass, 2001) which found that the continuing bonds, impacted moral, social and spiritual growth. Both Hindu and Buddhist respondents found continuing bonds with the deceased a normal part of life and karma. Their task in mourning is not to move on, instead it is to "find an enduring connection with the deceased in the midst of embarking on a new life" (Worden, 2010, p.50). This means that it is important that therapists understand what the continuing bond means to the culture and religion the client. This is a nuanced difference that can in the opinion of the researcher be critical to the healing of the client.

How the therapists develops the continuing bond between the client and their dearly departed is important. Especially in terms of catching the client's internal view of the death and the afterlife as well as the theoretical or therapeutic approach. Individuals may see themselves in ways such as carrying on the legacy of the departed, as the one who remembers, as the one who has picked up the burdens, source of spiritual solace, as a guardian and so on. Spending time exploring and understanding the clients view will allow for a robust development of the continuing bond that is match to the client's needs.

Mental health workers need to appreciate that this may mean what can be considered delusional or imaginary by other cultures, may be wholly culturally appropriate to the grieving individual. With the exception of the Muslim respondents who saw dreams of the departed as a sign that not all is well on their journey, most of the religious respondents took comfort in dreams and even saw having visions of the departed as a positive occurrence. Dreams, visions, signs and ghosts may be normal and appropriate to the clients world view and not in any way a sign of developing mental aberrations. Therapists need to process that at times 'supernatural' occurrences with a sense of confidence and detachment are only pathological if they interfere with the daily functioning and the mental health of the client. If these events do not interfere with a client's functioning, therapist need to monitor the situation, be respectful to the client's needs (silence is golden), listen empathically and focus on the emotional content of the client's story rather than trying to align cognitive and physical beliefs.

The likelihood of individuals to seek emotional and psychological support depends greatly on individual belief systems, family support, support facilities set up by religious groups and the perceived availability of professional services. Among grieving Malaysians, there is still a high resistance and lack of awareness of counseling services for the grieving. Those who grieve will attend prayer meetings, general sharing session and talks offered by their religious groups, but two participants, both who were already involved in helping services reported that they approached a counselor for support.

In order to reduce the stress created by funerals, it is important for mental health workers to have a conversation of the best practices during a funeral. First off avoid platitudes, be genuine and if you do not know what to say just say "My deepest condolences" and provide a warm hug. No other statements is needed when individuals can lend active presence. At times, we can just stand beside the mourner for a period of time allowing the person to know they are not alone without needing them to say more. If individuals sincerely want to provide help it is the advice of the researcher that we ask specific questions. Instead of asking the general "Do you need anything" ask "When was the last time you ate / had a drink / slept?" People are more likely to give correct information to well-thought questions. From that specific answer, you will know what needs to be done to best support the individual in grief.

There is a definite need for counseling to be provided to grieving. Such service, to be effective, must cover the grief process, the cultural and religious idiosyncrasies of their clients, as well as, address the changes in the roles of those going through grief. Dreams and manifestations of the deceased need to be understood within correct cultural contexts in order to avoid misinterpretations of the phenomenon.

The role of spirituality and religion in mitigating and processing grief cannot be denied. It was perhaps best expressed by respondent R3 who said, "I know he is there. If you think death is removing, completely wiping out somebody's existence, soul, then you should grieve." Cultural and religious grounding allows the perceived bond with the loved ones to persist after death. They provide support and structure in an overwhelming situation and are an active part of individual coping mechanisms. Thus it is the responsibility of those who venture into grief work. To recognize and appreciate the influence of culture and religion in the healing process, to gain relevant knowledge and develop the skills that will allow for active support of clients.

REFERENCES

Anderson, H. (2010). Common grief, complex grieving. *Pastoral Psychology*, *59*(2), 127–136. doi:10.100711089-009-0243-5

Atig, T. (2004). Meanings of death seen through the lens of grieving. *Death Studies*, *28*(4), 341–360. doi:10.1080/07481180490432333 PMID:15129689

Bailey. (2013). *Philosophy of Mind: The Key Thinkers*. British Library.

Barnard, A., McCosker, H., & Gerber, R. (1999). Phenomenography: A qualitative research approach for exploring understanding in health care. *Qualitative Health Research*, *9*(2), 212–226. doi:10.1177/104973299129121794 PMID:10558364

Becker, C. S. (1986). Interviewing in human science research. *Methods (San Diego, Calif.)*, *1*, 101–124.

Benore, E. L., & Park, C. L. (2004). Death-Specific religious belieds and bereavement: Belief in the afterlife and continued attachment. *The International Journal for the Psychology of Religion*, *14*(1), 1–22. doi:10.120715327582ijpr1401_1

Bowlby, J. (1980). Attachment and loss: Vol. 3. *Loss*. New York: Basic Books.

Colaizzi, P. F. (1978). Psychological research as the phenomenologist views it. In R. S. Valle & M. King (Eds.), Existential-phenomenological alternatives for psychology (pp. 48-71). New York: OUP.

Cowles, K. V. (1996). Cultural perspectives of grief: An expanded concept analysis. *Journal of Advanced Nursing*, *23*(2), 287–294. doi:10.1111/j.1365-2648.1996.tb02669.x PMID:8708241

Creswell, J. W. (2013). *Research Design Qualitative, Quantitative, And Mixed Method Approaches*. SAGE Publications CA.

Edmonds, S., & Hooker, K. (1992). Perceived changes in life meaning following bereavement. *Omega*, *25*(4), 307–318. doi:10.2190/TE7Q-5G45-BETY-X1TT

Frankle, V. E. (1992). *Man's Search for Meaning; An Introduction to Logotherapy* (4th ed.). Boston: Beacon Press.

Gillies, J., & Neimeyer, R. A. (2006). Loss, grief and the search for significance: Toward a model of meaning reconstruction in bereavement. *Journal of Constructivist Psychology*, *19*(1), 31–65. doi:10.1080/10720530500311182

Klass, D. (2001). Continuing the bonds in the resolution of grief in Japan and North America. *The American Behavioral Scientist*, *44*(5), 742–763. doi:10.1177/00027640121956476

Kvale, S. (1983). The qualitative research interview: A phenomenological and a hermeneutical mode of understanding. *Journal of Phenomenological Psychology*, *14*(1-2), 171–196. doi:10.1163/156916283X00090

Love, A. W. (2007). Progress in understanding grief, complicated grief and carig for the bereaved. *Contemporary Nurse*, *27*(1), 73–83. doi:10.5172/conu.2007.27.1.73 PMID:18386957

Merriam, S. B. (2009). *Qualitative Research –A Guide to Design and Implementation*. Jossey-Bass.

Neimeyer, R., Prigreson, H. G., & Davies, B. (2002). Mourning and meaning. *The American Behavioral Scientist*, *46*(2), 235–254. doi:10.1177/000276402236676

Park, C. L. (2005). Religion as a meaning-making framework in coping with life. *The Journal of Social Issues*, *61*(4), 707–729. doi:10.1111/j.1540-4560.2005.00428.x

Pitney, W., & Parker, J. (2009). *Qualitative research in Physical activity and the health profession*. Human Kinetic.

Richards, L. (2005). *Handling qualitative data: A practical guide*. London: Sage Publications.

Salkind, N. J. (2009). *Exploring Research*. Pearson Education, Inc.

Sin, S. (2010). Considerations of quality in phenomenographic research. *International Journal of Qualitative Methods*, *9*(4), 305–319. doi:10.1177/160940691000900401

Worden, J. W. (2009). *Grief Counselling and grief therapy: A handbook for mental health practitioners* (4th ed.). New York: Springer Publishing.

Compilation of References

20/20: A Vision for the Future of Counseling. (2010, March). Consensus definition of counseling. Retrieved from http://www.counseling.org/knowledge-center/20-20-a-vision-for-the-future-of-counseling/consensus-definition-of-counseling.

Abu Raiya, H., & Pargament, K. I. (2010). Religiously integrated psychotherapy with Muslim clients: From research to practice. *Professional Psychology, Research and Practice*, *41*(2), 181–188. doi:10.1037/a0017988

Abu Raiya, H., & Pargament, K. I. (2011). Empirically based psychology of Islam: Summary and critique of the literature. *Mental Health, Religion & Culture*, *14*(2), 93–115. doi:10.1080/13674670903426482

Ahmad, M. M. (2002). Who cares? The personal and professional problems of NGO fieldworkers in Bangladesh. *Development in Practice*, *12*(2), 177–191. doi:10.1080/09614520220127694

Ahmad, N., Cheong, S. M., Ibrahim, N., & Rosman, A. (2014). Suicidal ideation among Malaysian adolescents. *Asia-Pacific Journal of Public Health*, *26*(5), 63–69. doi:10.1177/1010539514540746 PMID:25005932

Ahmad, N., MuhdYusoff, F., Ratnasingam, S., Mohamed, F., Nasir, N. H., MohdSallehuddin, S., ... Aris, T. (2015). Trends and factors associated with mental health problems among children and adolescents in Malaysia. *International Journal of Culture and Mental Health*, *8*(2), 125–136. doi:10.1080/17542863.2014.907326 PMID:26000035

Ahmed, S., & Amer, M. M. (Eds.). (2012). *Counseling Muslims: Handbook of mental health issues and interventions*. New York, NY: Routledge.

Akinsulure-Smith, A. M., Dachos, N., & Jones, W. L. (2013). Nah We Yone's De Fambul Camp: Facilitating Resilience in Displaced African Children. *Journal of Immigrant & Refugee Studies*, *11*(3), 221–240. doi:10.1080/15562948.2013.801721

Alias, R., Alias, N. A., Ibrahim, A. B., Attan, H., & Kadir, A. L. (2013). What do the disabled students need? A study on the needs of the special educational needs (SEN) learners in Malaysian public universities. *The European Journal of Social & Behavioural Sciences*, 603-623.

Ali, M., Briskman, L., & Fiske, L. (2016). Asylum Seekers and Refugees in Indonesia: Problems and Potentials. *Cosmopolitan Civil Societies Journal*, *8*(2). doi:10.5130/ccs.v8i2.4883

Alivandi Vafa & Ismail. (2009). Reaching Out to Single Parent Children through Filial Therapy. *Online Submission*, *6*(2), 1–12. Retrieved from https://manowar.tamucc.edu/login?url=http://search.ebscohost.com/login.aspx?direct=true&db=eric&AN=ED504968&site=eds-live&scope=site&scope=cite

Alphonsus, A. (2012, June 18). Chinese youths top suicide list. *Free Malaysia Today.* Retrieved from http://www.freemalaysiatoday.com/category/nation/2012/06/18/chinese-youths-top-suicide-list/

American Counselling Association. (2014). ACA Code of Ethics. Retrieved from http://www.counseling.org/docs/ethics/2014-aca-code-of-ethics.pdf

American Psychological Association. (2002). Ethical principles of psychologists and code of conduct. *American Psychologist*, 57, 1060–1073. Retrieved from http://apa.org/ethics/code/index.aspx?item=3

American Psychological Dictionary. (2017). Washington, DC: American Psychological Association.

Amer, M. (2009). Editor's introduction: The role of journal thematic issues in developing an agenda and filling the literature gaps for mental health research with Muslim participants. *The Journal of Muslim Mental Health*, *4*(1), 1–4. doi:10.1080/15564900902801163

Anderson, H. (2010). Common grief, complex grieving. *Pastoral Psychology*, *59*(2), 127–136. doi:10.100711089-009-0243-5

Ando, O. (2008). Psychotherapy and Buddhism: Spirituality underneath psychotherapies in East Asia. *International Medical Journal*, *15*(2), 115–118.

Andres-Hyman, R. C., Ortiz, J., Anez, L. M., Paris, M., & Davidson, L. (2006). Culture and clinical practice: Recommendations for working with Puerto Ricans and other Latinas(os) in the United States. *Professional Psychology, Research and Practice*, *37*(6), 694–701. doi:10.1037/0735-7028.37.6.694

Ang, I. (2014). Beyond Chinese groupism: Chinese Australians between assimilation, multiculturalism and diaspora. *Ethnic and Racial Studies*, *37*(7), 1184–1196. doi:10.1080/01419870.2014.859287

Arifin, M., Roshaidai, S., Cheyne, H., & Maxwell, M. (2015, June). Postnatal depression across cultures: A qualitative study in Malaysia. *Paper presented at NMAHP Research Unit Mini Conference 2015*, Glasgow, Scotland.

Armstrong, K. (2009). *The Case for God: What Religion Really Means*. London: The Bodley Head.

Arredondo, P., & Glauner, T. (1992). *Personal dimensions of identity model*. Boston, MA: Empowerment Workshops, Inc.

Arshad, A. H. (2005). *The Protection of Refugee Children in Malaysia: Wishful Thinking or Reality.* Retrieved from http://www.malaysianbar.org.my/human_rights/the_ protection_of_refugee_children_in_malaysia_wishful_thinking_or_reality_.html

ASEAN. (2016). *HIV in the ASEAN region: Second regional report on HIV & AIDS 2011 -2015.* Retrieved from http://asean.org/storage/2016/11/08ASEAN-Regional-Report-on-HIV-AIDS-1dec.pdf

Atig, T. (2004). Meanings of death seen through the lens of grieving. *Death Studies*, *28*(4), 341–360. doi:10.1080/07481180490432333 PMID:15129689

AVERT. (2017). *HIV and AIDS in Asia & The Pacific regional overview.* Retrieved from https://www.avert.org/professionals/hiv-around-world/asia-pacific/overview

Bailey. (2013). *Philosophy of Mind: The Key Thinkers*. British Library.

Bala, J., & Kramer, S. (2010). Intercultural Dimensions in the Treatment of Traumatized Refugee Families. *Traumatology*, *16*(4), 153–159. doi:10.1177/1534765610369262

Ballve. (2015). Messaging apps are overtaking social networks to become the dominant platforms on phones. *Business Insider*. Retrieved from http://www.businessinsider.com/messaging-apps-have-completely-overtaken-social-networks-to-become-the-dominant-platforms-on-phones-2015-4/?IR=T&r=MY

Bankard, J. (2015). Training emotions cultivates morality: How loving-kindness meditation hones compassion and increase prosocial behavior. *Journal of Religion and Health*, *54*(6), 2324–2343. doi:10.100710943-014-9999-8 PMID:25633082

Bansal, S. (2012, December 2). Volunteers on the frontline of services delivery. *The Guardian*. Retrieved from https://www.theguardian.com/global-development-professionals-network/2012/dec/05/volunteers-frontline-services-delivery

Banyan. (2013, April 28). Malaysia's close-fought election: The Penang effect. *The Economist*. Retrieved from https://www.economist.com/blogs/banyan/2013/04/malaysias-close-fought-election

Barnard, A., McCosker, H., & Gerber, R. (1999). Phenomenography: A qualitative research approach for exploring understanding in health care. *Qualitative Health Research*, *9*(2), 212–226. doi:10.1177/104973299129121794 PMID:10558364

Barnes, J. (2014). *Christianity vs. modern psychology: Centered ministry or problem centered counseling?* Retrieved October 19, 2017, from http://www.the-gospel.org/stdy_psych/christ-centered.php

Barret, B., & Logan, C. (2002). Counselling Gay Men and Lesbians: A Practice Primer. Brooks/Cole, Cengage Learning.

Baumeister, R. F., Campbell, J. D., Krueger, J. I., & Vohs, K. D. (2003). Does high self-esteem cause better performance, interpersonal success, happiness, or healthier lifestyles? *Psychological Science in the Public Interest*, *4*(1), 1–44. doi:10.1111/1529-1006.01431 PMID:26151640

Bavin-hoffman, R., Jennings, G., & Landreth, G. (1996). Filial Therapy: Parental Perceptions of the Process. *International Journal of Play Therapy*, *5*(5), 45–58. doi:10.1037/h0089109

BBC. (2009b, August 14). *Religions - Christianity: The basics of Christian beliefs*. Retrieved October 19, 2017, from http://www.bbc.co.uk/religion/religions/christianity/beliefs/basics_1.shtml

BBC. (2011b, June 30). *Religions - Christianity: Christianity at a glance*. Retrieved October 19, 2017, from http://www.bbc.co.uk/religion/religions/christianity/ataglance/glance.shtml

BBC. (2015). *Asia Migrants: Malaysia Orders Search and Rescue for Boats*. Retrieved from http://www.bbc.com/news/world-asia-32822508

Becker, C. S. (1986). Interviewing in human science research. *Methods (San Diego, Calif.)*, *1*, 101–124.

Beck, J. R. (1997). Value tensions between evangelical Christians and Christian counseling. *Counseling and Values*, *41*(2), 107–116. doi:10.1002/j.2161-007X.1997.tb00393.x

Bellaire, C., & Young, J. S. (2005). Inclusion of religious behaviors and attitudes in counseling expectations of conservative Christians. *Counseling and Values*, *49*(2), 82–94. doi:10.1002/j.2161-007X.2005.tb00255.x

Belle, C. V. (1998, May). *Consultative Report: The Future Directions of Rural Counselling in South Australia*. Prepared for the Hon. Rob Kerin, Minister for Primary Industries, Natural Resources and Regional Development, South Australia, Adelaide, Australia.

Belle, C. V. (2005). *Evaluation Report: Funding for AIDS in Rural South Australia*. Adelaide: South Australian Farmers' Federation.

Belle, C. V. (1992). *Towards Truth: An Australian Spiritual Journey*. Kuala Lumpur: Pacific Press.

Belle, C. V. (2012). *Keynote Address: Religious Minorities in Australia: Past and Present*. Adelaide: Tertiary Ministries Conference of Australia.

Bemak, F., & Chung, R. C. Y. (2017). Refugee Trauma: Culturally Responsive Counseling Interventions. *Journal of Counseling and Development*, *95*(3), 299–308. doi:10.1002/jcad.12144

Benore, E. L., & Park, C. L. (2004). Death-Specific religious belieds and bereavement: Belief in the afterlife and continued attachment. *The International Journal for the Psychology of Religion*, *14*(1), 1–22. doi:10.120715327582ijpr1401_1

Bergin, A. E., & Jensen, J. P. (1990). Religiosity of psychotherapists: A national survey. *Psychotherapy (Chicago, Ill.)*, *27*(1), 3–7. doi:10.1037/0033-3204.27.1.3

Bergin, A. E., Payne, R. I., & Richards, P. S. (1996). Values in psychotherapy. In E. Shafranske (Ed.), *Religion and the clinical practice of psychology* (pp. 297–325). Washington, DC: American Psychological Association. doi:10.1037/10199-011

Berkeley. (2017). *Karma Hinduism*. Berkeley Centre for religion, peace and worldly affairs. Retrieved from: https://berkleycenter.georgetown.edu/essays/karma-hinduism

Bernama. (2016, September 12). Mental health of Malaysian students cause of worry: Health Ministry. *The New Straits Times*. Retrieved from https://www.nst.com.my/news/2016/09/172683/mental-health-malaysian-students-cause-worry-health-ministry

Berry, K., & Haddock, G. (2008). The implementation of the NICE guidelines for schizophrenia: Barriers to the implementation of psychological interventions and recommendations for the future. *Psychology and Psychotherapy: Theory, Research and Practice*, *81*(4), 419–436. doi:10.1348/147608308X329540 PMID:18652741

Bhatia, S. C., Madabushi, J., Kolli, V., Bhatia, S. K., & Madaan, V. (2013). The Bhagavad Gita and Contemporary Psychotherapies. *Indian J Psychiatry 55: Indian Mental Concepts*. Retrieved from: www.indianjpsychiatry.org

Bhide, A. V. (2007). Anger and the Mahaabhaarata. *Indian Journal of Psychiatry*, *49*(2), 140. doi:10.4103/0019-5545.33265 PMID:20711400

Billy Graham Evangelistic Association. (2004). *What is the Apostles' Creed?* Retrieved October 19, 2017, from https://billygraham.org/answer/what-is-the-apostles-creed/

Bodhi. (2009). Alagaddupama sutta: the simile of the snake. In *Middle length discourses of the Buddha* (pp. 224 - 236). Boston: Wisdom Publications.

Bond, M. H. (Ed.). (2006). *Handbook of Chinese Psychology*. New York: Oxford University Press.

Bond, M. H. (Ed.). (2010). *The Oxford handbook of Chinese psychology*. New York: Oxford University Press. doi:10.1093/oxfordhb/9780199541850.001.0001

Bonn, B., & Tam, C. L. (2015). Imagining a good life in Malaysia and China: Cultural beliefs among Mainland Chinese, Malaysian Chinese, and Malay University students. *Asian Journal of Social Psychology*, *19*(2), 145–153. doi:10.1111/ajsp.12120

Borwick, S., Schweitzer, R. D., Brough, M., Vromans, L., & Shakespeare-Finch, J. (2013). Well-Being of Refugees from Burma: A Salutogenic Perspective. *International Migration (Geneva, Switzerland)*, *51*(5), 91–105. doi:10.1111/imig.12051

Bowker, J. (2015). *Why Religions Matter*. Cambridge, UK: Cambridge University Press. doi:10.1017/CBO9781316048023

Bowlby, J. (1979). *Seperation and anxiety*. London, UK: Routledge Classics.

Bowlby, J. (1980). Attachment and loss: Vol. 3. *Loss*. New York: Basic Books.

Brassard, C., Sherraden, M. S., & Lough, B. J. (2010). Emerging Perspectives on International Volunteerism in Asia. *The International FORUM on Development Service. IVCO.*

Buscher, D., & Heller, L. (2010). Desperate Lives: Urban Refugee Women in Malaysia And Egypt. *Forced Migration Review*, *34*, 20–21. Retrieved from http://ezproxy.help.edu.my:2052/eds/pdfviewer/pdfviewer?vid=22&sid=a0d7a383-ea6a-4ec6-bd99-0ad8ad602574%40sessionmgr4008&hid=4205

CARE. (2014). *Marginalised Urban Women in Southeast Asia.* Retrieved from https://www.care.org.au/wp-content/uploads/2014/12/MUW-in-SE-Asia-Report.pdf

Carolan, M. T., Basherinia, G., Juhari, R., Himelright, J., & Mouton-Sanders, M. (2000). Contemporary Muslim families: Research and practice. *Contemporary Family Therapy*, *22*(1), 67–79. doi:10.1023/A:1007770532624

Carstens, S. A. (2005). *Histories, cultures, identities: Studies in Malaysian Chinese worlds.* Singapore: Singapore University Press.

Cashwell, C. S., Bently, P. B., & Yarborough, J. P. (2007). The only way out is through: The peril of spiritual bypass. *Counseling and Values*, *51*(2), 139–148. doi:10.1002/j.2161-007X.2007.tb00071.x

Cashwell, C. S., Glosof, H. L., & Hammond, C. (2010). Spiritual bypass: A preliminary investigation. *Counseling and Values*, *54*(2), 162–174. doi:10.1002/j.2161-007X.2010.tb00014.x

Chan, D. W. (1990). The meaning of depression: The Chinese word associations. *Psychologia*, *33*, 191–196.

Chang, M. L., Tam, A., & Mohd Suki, N. (2017). Moderating effect of races towards consumers' feeling of TCM usage. In Handbook of Research on Leveraging Consumer Psychology for Effective Customer Engagement. doi:10.4018/978-1-5225-0746-8.ch020

Chang, K. H., & Horrocks, S. (2006). Lived experiences of family caregivers of mentally ill relatives. *Journal of Advanced Nursing*, *53*(4), 435–443. doi:10.1111/j.1365-2648.2006.03732.x PMID:16448486

Chapman, R. T. (2006). Internalized racism of the clinician and the treatment dynamic. *Journal of Emotional Abuse*, *6*(2-3), 219–228. doi:10.1300/J135v06n02_13

Chau, I. Y., & Landreth, G. L. (1997). Filial therapy with Chinese parents: Effects on parental empathic interactions, parental acceptance of child and parental stress. *International Journal of Play Therapy*, *6*(2), 75–92. doi:10.1037/h0089409

Chelliah,. K. (2012). *Hinduism: A Brief Study of It's* (sic) *Origins, Traditions and Practice.* Bukit Berunding: Kandiah Chelliah.

Chen, L.-S., & Liew, S.-A. (2015, February). Factors influencing career decision making difficulties among graduating students from Malaysian private higher educational institutions. In *Proceedings of the 8th Asia Pacific Business Research Conference*, Kuala Lumpur, Malaysia.

Chen, P. C. Y. (1981). Traditional and modern medicine in Malaysia. *Social Science & Medicine. Part A: Medical Psychology & Medical Sociology*, *7*, 127–136. doi:10.1016/0271-7123(81)90032-8

Chen, S. W. H., & Davenport, D. S. (2005). Cognitive-Behavioral therapy with Chinese American clients: Cautions and modifications. *Psychotherapy (Chicago, Ill.)*, *42*(1), 101–110.

Ching, M. S., & Ng, K. M. (2010). Counseling in Malaysia: History, current status, and future trends. *Journal of Counseling and Development*, *88*(1), 18–22. doi:10.1002/j.1556-6678.2010.tb00144.x

Chin, J. M. (1981). *The Sarawak Chinese*. NY: Oxford University Press.

Choi, F. H. (2013). *The Faithful and the Distressed: How Likely are Christians to Seek Psychotherapy Treatment for Psychological Distress?* (Doctoral dissertation).

Christian Federation of Malaysia. (n.d.). *Christian Federation of Malaysia*. Retrieved from http://cfmsia.org/

Christian Research Institute. (2009). *Psychology and the church (part one)*. Retrieved October 19, 2017, from: http://www.equip.org/article/psychology-and-the-church-part-one/

Chuah, S. M. (2017). *Reporting Behaviours of Children-Centric NGO Workers on Child Abuse in Southeast Asia* (Unpublished dissertation). HELP University, Kuala Lumpur, Malaysia.

Chung, R. C. Y., Bemak, F., & Grabosky, T. K. (2011). Multicultural-Social Justice Leadership Strategies: Counseling and Advocacy with Immigrants. *Journal for Social Action in Counseling and Psychology*, *3*(1). Retrieved from http://www.psysr.org/jsacp/chung-v3n1-11_86-102.pdf

Civil movement to call for self-government, nationhood for Malaysia's Sarawak. (2013, April 15). *Nationalia Aureli Argemí*. Retrieved from https://www.nationalia.info/new/9822/civil-movement-to-call-for-self-government-nationhood-for-malaysias-sarawak

Clark, C. M. H. (1962). *A History of Australia: From the Earliest Times to the Age of Macquarie*. London: Cambridge University Press.

Clarke, P. B., Giodarno, A. L., Cashwell, C. S., & Lewis, T. F. (2013). The straight path to healing: Using motivational interviewing to address spiritual bypass. *Journal of Counseling and Development*, *91*(1), 87–94. doi:10.1002/j.1556-6676.2013.00075.x

Clement, S., Schauman, O., Graham, T., Maggioni, F., Evans-Lacko, S., Bezborodovs, N., ... Thornicroft, G. (2015). What is the impact of mental health-related stigma on help-seeking? A systematic review of quantitative and qualitative studies. *Psychological Medicine*, *45*(1), 11–27. doi:10.1017/S0033291714000129 PMID:24569086

Cochran, S. D. (n.d.). Lifetime Prevalence of Suicide Symptoms and Affective Disorders Among Men Reporting Same-Sex Sexual Partners: Results From NHANES III. *American Journal of Public Health*, *90*(4), 573–578. PMID:10754972

Cocker, F., & Joss, N. (2016). Compassion fatigue among healthcare, emergency and community service workers: A systematic review. *International Journal of Environmental Research and Public Health*, *13*(6), 618. doi:10.3390/ijerph13060618 PMID:27338436

Colaizzi, P. F. (1978). Psychological research as the phenomenologist views it. In R. S. Valle & M. King (Eds.), Existential-phenomenological alternatives for psychology (pp. 48-71). New York: OUP.

Cole. (1993). *Christians and psychology: Some common questions answered*. Retrieved October 19, 2017, from: https://bible.org/article/christians-and-psychology-some-common-questions-answered

ComScore. (2012). *The Power of Like 2*. Retrieved from http://www.comscore.com/Insights/Presentations_and_Whitepapers/2012/The_Power_of_Like_2_How_Social_Marketing_Works

Conte, C. (2009). *Advanced techniques for counseling and psychotherapy* (pp. 7–8). New York: Sprinter Publishing Company.

Corey, G. (2013). *Theory and Practice of Counseling and Psychotherapy*. Brooks/Cole.

Cornett, N., & Bratton, S. C. (2014). Examining the impact of child parent relationship therapy (CPRT) on family functioning. *Journal of Marital and Family Therapy*, *40*(3), 302–318. doi:10.1111/jmft.12014 PMID:24749890

Cornett, N., & Bratton, S. C. (2015). A Golden Intervention : 50 Years of Research on Filial Therapy. *International Journal of Play Therapy*, *24*(3), 119–133. doi:10.1037/a0039088

Corrigan, P. W., & Wassel, A. (2008). Understanding and influencing the stigma of mental illness. *Journal of Psychosocial Nursing and Mental Health Services*, *46*(1), 42–48. doi:10.3928/02793695-20080101-04 PMID:18251351

Covey, S. M. R. (2006). *The Speed of Trust: The one thing that changes everything*. London: Simon & Schuster UK Ltd.

Cowan, G. (2007). *Understanding and conducting research in education: A user-friendly approach* (2nd ed.). Dubuque, IA: Kendall/Hunt Publishing Company.

Cowles, K. V. (1996). Cultural perspectives of grief: An expanded concept analysis. *Journal of Advanced Nursing*, *23*(2), 287–294. doi:10.1111/j.1365-2648.1996.tb02669.x PMID:8708241

Cragun, C. L., & Friedlander, M. L. (2012). Experiences of Christian clients in secular psychotherapy: A mixed-methods investigation. *Journal of Counseling Psychology*, *59*(3), 379–391. doi:10.1037/a0028283 PMID:22563669

Creswell, J. W. (2013). *Research Design Qualitative, Quantitative, And Mixed Method Approaches*. SAGE Publications CA.

Crisp, J. (2017). *An Inside Account of UNHCR's Urban Refugee Policy*. Retrieved from https://www.newsdeeply.com/refugees/community/2017/04/14/an-inside-account-of-unhcrs-urban-refugee-policy

Cross, W. E. Jr. (1971). The Negro-to-Black conversion experience. *Black World*, *20*(9), 13–27.

Cummings, E. J. (2009). Trends in mental health googling. *The Psychiatrist*, *33*(11), 437–437.

Daneshpour, M. (1998). Muslim families and family therapy. *Journal of Marital and Family Therapy*, *24*(3), 355–368. doi:10.1111/j.1752-0606.1998.tb01090.x PMID:9677541

David, L. E., & Gelsomino, J. (1994). An assessment of practitioner cross-racial treatment experiences. *Social Work*, *39*, 116–123. PMID:8310317

Davis. (2001). *The Mahabharatha: A synopsis of the Great Epic of India*. Retrieved from: http://web.cs.ucdavis.edu/~vemuri/classes/freshman/Mahabharatasynopsis.htm

De Silva, P. (2005). *Introduction to Buddhist psychology*. New York: Palgrave McMillan. doi:10.1057/9780230509450

De Silva, P. (2014). *An introduction to Buddhist psychology and counseling*. New York: Palgrave McMillan. doi:10.1057/9781137287557

Department of Statistics Malaysia Official Portal. (2011, July 29). Retrieved October 19, 2017, from https://www.dosm.gov.my/v1/index.php?r=column/cthemeByCat&cat=117&bul_id=MDMxdHZjWTk1SjFzTzNkRXYzcVZjdz09&menu_id=L0pheU43NWJwRWVSZklWdzQ4TlhUUT09

Department of Statistics, Malaysia. (2001). Population and Housing Census 2000. In *Distribution and Basic Demographic Characteristics Report*. Retrieved from http://www.statistics.gov.my/English/pageDemo.htm

Department of Statistics, Malaysia. (2011). *Population Distribution and Basic Demographic Characteristic Report 2010.* Retrieved from https://www.dosm.gov.my/v1/index.php?r=column/cthemeByCat&cat=117&bul_id=MDMxdHZjWTk1SjFzTzNkRXYzcVZjdz09&menu_id=L0pheU43NWJwRWVSZklWdzQ4TlhUUT09

Department of Statistics, Malaysia. (2016). *Current Population Estimates, Malaysia, 2014 – 2016. Retrieved from* https://web.archive.org/web/20160812014710/ https://www.statistics.gov.my/index.php?r=column%2FcthemeByCat&cat=155&bul_id=OWlxdEVoYlJCS0hUZzJyRUcvZEYxZz09&menu_id=L0pheU43NWJwRWVSZklWdzQ4TlhUUT09

Disability News and Information Service. (2010). *The needs of disabled persons in Malaysia are still seen largely as a welfare function, Maniam Sinnasamy.* Retrieved from http://www.dnis.org/interview.php?issue_id=6&volume_id=7&interview_id=150

Donnellan, M. B., Trzesniewski, K. H., & Robins, R. W. (2011). Self-esteem: Enduring issues and controversies. In T. Chamorro-Premuzic, S. von Stumm, & A. Furnham (Eds.), *The Wiley-Blackwell handbook of individual differences* (pp. 718–746). Chichester, UK: Wiley-Blackwell.

Donnellan, M. B., Trzesniewski, K. H., Robins, R. W., Moffitt, T. E., & Caspi, A. (2005). Low self-esteem is related to aggression, antisocial behavior, and delinquency. *Psychological Science, 16*(4), 328–335. doi:10.1111/j.0956-7976.2005.01535.x PMID:15828981

Dotevall, C., Winberg, E., & Rosengren, K. (2017). Nursing Students' Experience with Refugees with Mental Health Problems in Jordan: A Qualitative Control Analysis. *Nurse Education Today, 61*, 155–161. doi:10.1016/j.nedt.2017.11.025 PMID:29207287

Drury, J., Cocking, C., & Reicher, S. (2009). Everyone for themselves? A comparative study of crowd solidarity among emergency survivors. *British Journal of Social Psychology, 48*(3), 487–506. doi:10.1348/014466608X357893 PMID:18789185

Dueck, A., Ting, S.-K., & Cutiongco, R. (2007). Constantine, Babel, and Yankee Doodling: Whose indigeneity? Whose psychology? *Pastoral Psychology, 56*(1), 55–72. doi:10.100711089-007-0082-1

Earnest, J., Mansi, R., Bayati, S., Earnest, J. A., & Thompson, S. C. (2015). Resettlement Experiences and Resilience in Refugee Youth in Perth, Western Australia. *BMC Research Notes, 8*(1), 1–10. doi:10.118613104-015-1208-7 PMID:26054946

Eastman, R. (Ed.). (1993). *The Ways of Religion: An Introduction to the Major Traditions* (2nd ed.). New York: Oxford University Press.

Editors, C. T. (2018). *What Made Mental Illness a 'Sin'? Paganism.* Retrieved from https://www.christianitytoday.com/ct/2018/february-web-only/mental-illness-sin.html

Edman, J. L., & Koon, T. Y. (2000). Mental illness beliefs in Malaysia: Ethnic and intergeneration comparisons. *The International Journal of Social Psychiatry, 46*(2), 101–109. doi:10.1177/002076400004600203 PMID:10950358

Edmonds, S., & Hooker, K. (1992). Perceived changes in life meaning following bereavement. *Omega, 25*(4), 307–318. doi:10.2190/TE7Q-5G45-BETY-X1TT

EduAdvisor. (2017). *Find and compare psychology degree courses in Malaysia.* Retrieved from https://eduadvisor.my/psychology-degree-institutions/

Edwards, N. A., Ladner, J., & White, J. (2007). Perceived effectiveness of filial therapy for a Jamaican mother: A qualitative case study. *International Journal of Play Therapy, 16*(1), 36–53. doi:10.1037/1555-6824.16.1.36

Ehntholt, K. K., & Yule, W. (2006). Practitioner Review: Assessment and Treatment of Refugee Children and Adolescents Who Have Experienced War-Related Trauma. *Journal of Child Psychology and Psychiatry, and Allied Disciplines*, *47*(12), 1197–1210. doi:10.1111/j.1469-7610.2006.01638.x PMID:17176375

El-Shaarawi, N. (2015). Living An Uncertain Future. Temporality, Uncertainty, and Well Being Among Iraqi Refugees in Egypt. *Social Analysis*, *59*(1), 38–56. doi:10.3167a.2015.590103

Ely, G. E., Koury, S., Bennett, K., Hartinger, C., Green, S., & Nochajski, T. (2017). "I Feel Like I am Finding Peace": Exploring the Use of a Combined Art Therapy and Seeking Safety Progam with Refugee Support Groups. *Advances in Social Work*, *18*(1), 103. doi:10.18060/21130

Encyclopædia Britannica. (2017, February 15). *Reformation*. Retrieved October 19, 2017, from https://www.britannica.com/event/Reformation

Esau, T. G. (1998). The evangelical Christian in psychotherapy. *American Journal of Psychotherapy*, *52*(1), 28–36. doi:10.1176/appi.psychotherapy.1998.52.1.28 PMID:9553638

Etkin, A., Egner, T., & Kalisch, R. (2011). Emotional processing in anterior cingulate and medial prefrontal cortex. *Trends in Cognitive Sciences*, *15*(2), 85–93. doi:10.1016/j.tics.2010.11.004 PMID:21167765

Falb and Pargament. (2014). Religion, spirituality and positive psychology: strengthening wellbeing. In J. T. Pedrotti & L. M. Edwards (Eds.), *Perspectives on the intersection of Multiculturalism and Positive psychology* (pp. 143–157). New York: Springer.

Farsimadan, F., Draghi-Lorenz, R., & Ellis, J. (2007). Process and outcome of therapy in ethnically similar and dissimilar therapeutic dyads. *Psychotherapy Research*, *17*(5), 567–575. doi:10.1080/10503300601139996

Farzana, K. F. (2016). Voices of Burmese Rohingya Refugees: Everyday Politics of Survival in Refugee Camps in Bangladesh. *Pertanika Journal of Social Science & Humanities*, *24*(1), 131–150. Retrieved from http://ezproxy.help.edu.my:2057/eds/pdfviewer/pdfviewer?vid=2&sid=690dc86c-c8bd-4fae-8c90-9e0e677b12ec%40sessionmgr102

Fazel, M., Wheeler, J., & Danesh, J. (2005). Prevalence of Serious Mental Disorderin 7000 Refugees Resettled in Western Countries: A Systemic Review. *Lancet*, *365*(9467), 1309–1314. doi:10.1016/S0140-6736(05)61027-6 PMID:15823380

Fisher-Smith, A. M. (1999). *From value neutrality to value inescapability: A qualitative inquiry into values management in psychotherapy*. Unpublished doctoral dissertation, Brigham Young University, Provo, UT.

Flood, G. (2012). *The Importance of Religion: Meaning and Action in Our Strange World*. Chichester, UK: Wiley Blackwell.

FMT Reporters. (2017, December 8). MP censures Najib for 'insensitive' remark about Penang floods. *Free Malaysia Today*. Retrieved from http://www.freemalaysiatoday.com/ category/nation/2017/12/08/mp-censures-najib-for-insensitive-remark-about-penang-floods/

FMT Reporters. (2017, November 17). Report: Chinese community has the biggest income gap. *Free Malaysia Today*. Retrieved from http://www.freemalaysiatoday.com/category/ nation/2017/11/17/report-chinese-community-has-the-biggest-income-gap/

Francis, J., & Yan, M. C. (2016). Bridging the Gaps: Access to Formal Support Services Among Young African Immigrants and Refugees in Metro Vancouver. *Canadian Ethnic Studies*, *48*(1), 77 – 100. Retrieved from: http://ezproxy.help.edu.my:2057/eds/pdfviewer/pdfviewer?vid=5&sid=690dc86c-c8bd-4fae-8c90-9e0e677b12ec%40sessionmgr102

Frankle, V. E. (1992). *Man's Search for Meaning; An Introduction to Logotherapy* (4th ed.). Boston: Beacon Press.

Fredrickson, B. L., Cohn, M. A., Coffey, K. A., Pek, J., & Finkel, S. M. (2008). Open hearts builds lives: Positive emotions, induced through loving-kindness mediation, build consequential personal resources. *Journal of Personality and Social Psychology*, *95*(5), 1045–1062. doi:10.1037/a0013262 PMID:18954193

Freedman, A. L. (2000). *Political participation and ethnic minorities: Chinese overseas in Malaysia, Indonesia, and the United States*. New York: Routledge.

Fu, C. Q. (2007). *A different Chinese. Petaling Jaya, Malaysia*. Malaysia: Strategic Information and Research Development Centre.

Fuller, P. (2005). *The notion of ditthi in Buddhism*. London: Routledge Curzon.

Fulton, P. R. (2013). Contributions and challenges to clinical practice from Buddhist psychology. *Clinical Social Work Journal*, *42*(3), 208–217. doi:10.100710615-013-0469-7

Gadamer, H. G. (2004). *Truth and method* (2nd ed.). (J. Weinsheimer & D. G. Marshall, Trans.). New York: Continuum.

Gass, C. S. (1984). Orthodox Christian values related to psychotherapy and mental health. *Journal of Psychology and Theology*, *12*(3), 230–237. doi:10.1177/009164718401200308

GE13. Movement wants full autonomy for Sarawak. (2013, April 14). *The Star Online*. Retrieved from https://www.thestar.com.my/news/community/2013/04/14/ge13-movement-wants-full-autonomy-for-sarawak/

Gelso, C. J., & Mohr, J. J. (2001). The working alliance and the transference/countertransference relationship: Their manifestation with racial/ethnic and sexual orientation minority clients 106 and therapists. *Applied & Preventive Psychology*, *10*(1), 51–68. doi:10.1016/S0962-1849(05)80032-0

Gergen, K. J., Gulerce, A., Lock, A., & Misra, G. (1996). Psychological science in cultural context. *The American Psychologist*, *51*(5), 496–503. doi:10.1037/0003-066X.51.5.496

Ghazali, K. (2012, November 2). National identity and minority languages. *UN Chronicle*. Retrieved from https://web.archive.org/web/20121102173228/http://www.un.org/wcm/content/site/chronicle/home/archive/issues2010/un_academic_impact/national_identity_and_minority_languages?ctnscroll_articleContainerList=1_0&ctnlistpagination_articleContainerList=true

Ghazali, S. R., & Azhar, A. (2015). Depressive symptoms, gender, and ethnicity: An exploratory study among cross ethnic adolescents in Sarawak, Malaysia. *Malaysian Journal of Youth Studies*, *13*, 141–152.

Giacco, D., Laxhman, N., & Priebe, S. (2017). Prevalence of and Risk Factors for Mental Disorders in Refugees. *Seminars in Cell & Developmental Biology*. doi:10.1016/j.semcdb.2017.11.030 PMID:29174456

Gialelis, J. (2016). *Massage improves quality of life for the cerebral palsy patients*. Retrieved from https://www.massagemag.com/massage-improves-quality-of-life-for-the-cerebral-palsy-patient-40731/

Gillies, J., & Neimeyer, R. A. (2006). Loss, grief and the search for significance: Toward a model of meaning reconstruction in bereavement. *Journal of Constructivist Psychology*, *19*(1), 31–65. doi:10.1080/10720530500311182

Glasser, W. (2011). *Take charge of your life: How to get what you need with Choice Theory psychology*. Bloomington, IN: iUniverse.

Glasser, W. (1998). *Choice theory: a new psychology of personal freedom*. New York: Harper Perennial.

Glasser, W. (2000). *Every student can succeed*. Chula Vista: Black Forest Press.

Glasser, W. (2005). *How the brain works chart*. Tempe: The William Glasser Institute.

Gnarama. (2000). *Essentials of Buddhism*. Singapore. Pathegama Gnarama.

Gomez, E. T. (1999). *Chinese Business in Malaysia: Accumulation, Ascendance, Accommodation*. Psychology Press.

Gonslaves, C. J. (1992). Psychological Stages of the Refugee Process: A Model for Therapeutic Interventions. *Professional Psychology, Research and Practice*, *23*(5), 382–389. doi:10.1037/0735-7028.23.5.382

Goodkind, J. R., Hess, J. M., Isakson, B., LaNoue, M., Githinji, A., Roche, N., ... Parker, D. P. (2014). Reducing Refugee Mental Health Disparities: A Community Based Intervention to Address Postmigration Stressors with African Adults. *Psychological Services*, *11*(3), 333–346. doi:10.1037/a0035081 PMID:24364594

gotquestions.org. (2017, January 4). *What is praying in tongues? Is praying in tongues a prayer language between a believer and God?* Retrieved October 20, 2017, from https://www.gotquestions.org/praying-in-tongues.html

Graham, J. R., Bradshaw, C., & Trew, J. L. (2008). Social worker's understanding of the immigrant Muslim client's perspective. *The Journal of Muslim Mental Health*, *3*(2), 125–144. doi:10.1080/15564900802487527

Greenaway, K. H., Wright, R. G., Willingham, J., Reynolds, K. J., & Haslam, S. A. (2015). Shared identity is key to effective communication. *Personality and Social Psychology Bulletin*, *41*(2), 171–182. doi:10.1177/0146167214559709 PMID:25416042

Griner, D., & Smith, T. B. (2006). Culturally adapted mental health interventions: A meta-analytic review. *Psychotherapy (Chicago, Ill.)*, *43*(4), 531–548. doi:10.1037/0033-3204.43.4.531 PMID:22122142

Guan, T. E., & Rahimi, C. A. (2015). Prevalence of self-hurt behaviour among Chinese adolescents in Malaysia. *International Journal of Humanities. Arts and Social Sciences*, *1*(2), 108–113.

Guo, Y. (2005a). Emotional Problems in Mainland China. *Journal of Child and Adolescent Psychiatric Nursing*, *18*(4), 171–180. doi:10.1111/j.1744-6171.2005.00028.x PMID:16236099

Hall, E. T. (1966). *The Hidden Dimension*. New York: Anchor Press/Doubleday.

Hamdan, A. (2007). A case study of a Muslim client: Incorporating religious beliefs and practices. *Journal of Multicultural Counseling and Development*, *35*(2), 92–100. doi:10.1002/j.2161-1912.2007.tb00052.x

Han, B. (2015, November 10). Malaysia's Chinese diaspora: The other side of the story. *The Diplomat*. Retrieved from https://thediplomat.com/2015/11/malaysias-chinese-diaspora-the-other-side-of-the-story/

Haque, A. (2005). Mental health concepts and program development in Malaysia. *Journal of Mental Health (Abingdon, England)*, *14*(2), 183–195. doi:10.1080/09638230500059997

Haque, A., & Masuan, K. A. (2002). Religious psychology in Malaysia. *The International Journal for the Psychology of Religion*, *12*(4), 277–289. doi:10.1207/S15327582IJPR1204_05

Hashim, J., Chongsuvivatwong, V., Phua, K. H., Pocock, N., Teng, Y. M., Chhem, R. K., . . . Lopez, A. (2012). *Health and healthcare systems in Southeast Asia*. Retrieved from https://unu.edu/publications/articles/health-and-healthcare-systems-in-southeast-asia.html

Haslam, S. A. (2001). *Psychology in organizations: The social identity approach*. London: Sage.

Haslam, S. A., Oakes, P. J., Reynolds, K. J., & Turner, J. C. (1999). Social identity salience and the emergence of stereotype consensus. *Personality and Social Psychology Bulletin*, *25*(7), 809–818. doi:10.1177/0146167299025007004

Haslam, S. A., & Reicher, S. D. (2012). When prisoners take over the prison a social psychology of resistance. *Personality and Social Psychology Review*, *16*(2), 154–179. doi:10.1177/1088868311419864 PMID:21885855

Hays, D. G., & Erford, B. T. (2010). *Developing Multicultural Counseling Competence: A System Approach*. Pearson.

Hedayat-Diba, Z. (2000). Psychotherapy with Muslims. In P. S. Richards & A. E. Bergin (Eds.), *Handbook of psychotherapy and religious diversity* (pp. 289–314). Washington, DC: American Psychological Association. doi:10.1037/10347-012

Heide, F. J. J. T., Mooren, T. M., & Kleber, R. J. (2015). Complex PTSD and Phased Treatment in Refugees: A Debate Piece. *Eurpoean Journal of Psychotraumatology*, *7*(1). Retrieved From http://www.tandfonline.com/doi/full/10.3402/ejpt.v7.28687%40zept20.2016.7.issue-s1

Heilman, S. C., & Witztum, E. (1997). Value-sensitive therapy: Learning from ultra-orthodox patients. *American Journal of Psychotherapy*, *51*(4), 522–541. doi:10.1176/appi.psychotherapy.1997.51.4.522 PMID:9470959

Heng, P. K. (2006). Patterns of Chinese settlement. In L. Pan (Ed.), *The encyclopedia of the Chinese overseas* (2nd ed.). Singapore: Editions Didier Millet.

Hijazi, A. M., Lumley, M. A., Ziadni, M. S., Haddad, L., Rapport, L. J., & Arnetz, B. B. (2014). Brief NarrativeExposure Therapy for Posttraumatic Stress in Iraqi Refugees: A Preliminary Randomized Clinical Trial. *Journal of Traumatic Stress*, *27*(3), 314–322. doi:10.1002/jts.21922 PMID:24866253

Hindu Dharma. (2017). *Anger (HinduDharma): Dharmas Common To All*. Retrieved from: http://www.kamakoti.org/hindudharma/part22/chap11.htm

Hinduism: beliefs about life after death. (2014). *Religious studies*. Retrieved from: http://www.bbc.co.uk/schools/gcsebitesize/rs/death/hindubeliefrev2.shtml

Hing, L. K., & Tan, C.-B. (Eds.). (2000). *The Chinese in Malaysia*. New York: Oxford University Press.

Hinton, D. E., Chhean, D., Pich, V., Safren, S. A., Hofmann, S. G., & Pollack, M. H. (2005). A Randomized Controlled Trial of Cognitive-Behavior Therapy for Cambodian Refugees with Treatment Resistant PTSD and Panic Attacks: Across-Over Design. *Journal of Traumatic Stress*, *18*(6), 617–629. doi:10.1002/jts.20070 PMID:16382423

Hinton, D. E., Rivera, E., Barlow, D. H., & Otto, M. W. (2012). Adapting CBT for Traumatized Refugees and Ethnic Minority Patients: Examples from Culturally Adapted CBT (CA- CBT). *Transcultural Psychiatry*, *49*(2), 340–365. doi:10.1177/1363461512441595 PMID:22508639

Hofstede, G. (2003). *Culture's consequences: comparing values, behaviors, institutions, and organizations across nations* (2nd ed.). CA: Sage Publication.

Hogg, M. A., & Hains, S. C. (1996). Intergroup Relations and Group Solidarity. *Journal of Personality and Social Psychology*, *70*(2), 295–309. doi:10.1037/0022-3514.70.2.295

Hogg, M. A., & Hardie, E. A. (1991). Social Attraction, Personal Attraction, and Self-Categorization-, A Field Study. *Personality and Social Psychology Bulletin*, *17*(2), 175–180. doi:10.1177/014616729101700209

Holcomb, J. (n.d.). *The Five Solas - Points from the Past that Should Matter to You*. Retrieved October 19, 2017, from http://www.christianity.com/church/church-history/the-five-solas-of-the-protestant-reformation.html

Horyniak, D., Melo, J. S., Farrell, R. M., Ojeda, V. D., & Strathdee, S. A. (2015). Epidemiology of Substance Use among Forced Migrants: A Global Systematic Review. *PLoS One*, *11*(7), 1–34. doi:10.1371/journal.pone.015913 PMID:27411086

How life is tough for transgender in conservative Malaysia, who face violence, religious and official bias, and abusive media. (2017, November 15). *South China Morning Post*. Retrieved from http://www.scmp.com/lifestyle/article/2119847/how-life-tough-transgenders-conservative-malaysia-who-face-violence

Human Rights Watch. (2017). *HRW: Deteriorating outlook for human rights in Southeast Asia*. Retrieved from https://www.voanews.com/a/human-rights-watch-southeast-asia/3674978.html

Hussein, H., & Yaacob, N. M. (2012). Development of accessible design in Malaysia. *Procedia: Social and Behavioral Sciences*, *68*, 121–133. doi:10.1016/j.sbspro.2012.12.212

Hwang, K. K. (2006). Constructive realism and Confucian relationalism: An epistemological strategy for the development of indigenous psychology. In U. Kim, K. Yang, & K. Hwang (Eds.), *Indigenous and cultural psychology: Understanding people in context*. New York: Springer. doi:10.1007/0-387-28662-4_4

Inayat, Q. (2007). Islamophobia and the therapeutic dialogue: Some reflections. *Counselling Psychology Quarterly*, *20*(3), 287–293. doi:10.1080/09515070701567804

Indramalar, S. (2017, November 21). Study shows that Malaysians don't understand disability. *The Star Online*. Retrieved from https://www.star2.com/people/2017/11/21/disability-prejudice-malaysia/

Inter-Agency Standing Committee. (2010). *Mental Health and Psychosocial Support in Humanitarian Emergencies: What Should Humanitarian Health Actors Know?* Retrieved from: www.who.int/mental_health/emergencies/what_humanitarian_health_actors_should_ know.pdf

IntraHealth. (2016). *The case for frontline health workers in addressing non-communicable diseases globally*. Retrieved from https://www.intrahealth.org/sites/ihweb/files/files/media/the-case-for-frontline-health-workers-in-addressing-non--communicable-diseases-globally/NCDBrief.pdf

Jackson, A. P., Hansen, J., & Cook-Ly, J. M. (2013). Value conflicts in psychotherapy. *Issues in Religion and Psychotherapy, 35*, 6–15. Retrieved from http://scholarsarchive.byu.edu/irp/vol35/iss1/3

James, K. (2010). Domestic Violence Within Refugee Families: Intersecting Patriarchal Culture and the Refugee Experience. *ANZJFT Australian and New Zealand Journal of Family Therapy*, *31*(3), 275–284. doi:10.1375/anft.31.3.275

Jegathesan, A. J. (2016). Talk, Hindusim and Counselling. HELP University.

Johnson, J. (2017). Shakti: The Power of the Feminine. *Asia Society*. Retrieved from: iasociety.org/education/shakti-power-feminine

Jones, E. (2017). *Life in Limbo: The Refugee Experience in Southeast Asia*. Retrieved from https://www.trtworld.com/opinion/life-in-limbo-the-refugee-

Jones, G. W. (2013). *The Population of Southeast Asia*. Retrieved from http://www.ari.nus.edu.sg/wps/wps13_196.pdf

Jones, S. L. (1996). A constructive relationship for religion with the science and profession of psychology: Perhaps the boldest model yet. Academic Press.

Judge, T. A., & Bono, J. E. (2001). Relationship of core self-evaluations traits—self-esteem, generalized self-efficacy, locus of control, and emotional stability—with job satisfaction and job performance: A meta-analysis. *The Journal of Applied Psychology*, *86*(1), 80–92. doi:10.1037/0021-9010.86.1.80 PMID:11302235

Jung, Y. (2010). *Successful Models on achieving the Millennium Development Goals in South East Asia* (Unpublished dissertation). London School of Economics and Political Science, London, UK.

Jusoh, A. J., Mahmud, Z., & Ishak, N. M. (2008). The patterns of reality therapy usage among Malaysian counselors. *International Journal of Reality Therapy*, *28*, 5–14.

Kalupahana. (1986). *Central philosophy of Buddhism*. Honolulu: The University Press of Hawaii.

Kalupahana, D. J. (1987). *Principles of Buddhist psychology*. Albany, NY: State University of New York Press.

Kanekar, A. S. (2011). HIV/AIDS Counseling Skills and Strategies: Can Testing and Counseling Curb the Epidemic? *International Journal of Preventive Medicine*, *2*(1), 10–14. PMID:21448398

Kang, Y., Gray, J. R., & Dovidio, J. F. (2014). The non-discriminating heart: Lovingkindness meditation training decreases implicit intergroup bias. *Journal of Experimental Psychology. General*, *143*(3), 1306–1313. doi:10.1037/a0034150 PMID:23957283

Kartal, D., & Kiropoulos, L. (2015). Effects of Acculturative Stress on PTSD, Depressive and Anxiety Symptoms Among Refugees Resettled in Australia and Austria. *European Journal of Psychotraumatology*, *7*, 1–11. doi:10.3402/ejpt.v7.28711 PMID:26886488

Karunadasa, Y. (2001). Buddhist doctrine of Anatta. In D. J. Kalupahana (Ed.), *Buddhist thought and ritual* (pp. 9–19). Delhi: Motilal Banarsidass.

Katila, R., Chen, E. L., & Piezunka, H. (2012). All the right moves: How entrepreneurial firms compete effectively. *Strategic Entrepreneurship Journal*, *6*(2), 116–132. doi:10.1002ej.1130

Kelly, E. W. Jr, Aridi, A., & Bakhtiar, L. (1996). Muslims in the United States: An exploratory study of universal and mental health values. *Counseling and Values*, *40*(3), 206–218. doi:10.1002/j.2161-007X.1996.tb00853.x

Kemeny, M. E., Foltz, C., Cavanagh, J. F., Cullen, M., Giese-Davis, J., Jennings, P., ... Ekman, P. (2012). Contemplative/emotion training reduces negative emotional behavior and promotes prosocial responses. *Emotion (Washington, D.C.)*, *12*(2), 338–350. doi:10.1037/a0026118 PMID:22148989

Keshavarzi, H., & Haque, A. (2013). Outlining a psychotherapy model for enhancing Muslim mental health within an Islamic context. *The International Journal for the Psychology of Religion*, *23*(3), 230–249. doi:10.1080/10508619.2012.712000

Khan, Z. (2006). Attitudes toward counseling and alternative support among Muslims in Toledo, Ohio. *The Journal of Muslim Mental Health*, *1*(1), 21–42. doi:10.1080/15564900600654278

Kim, R. I., & Hwang, M. (2006). A meta-analysis of reality therapy and choice theory group programs for self-esteem and locus of control in Korea. *International Journal of Choice Theory*, *1*, 25–30.

Klass, D. (2001). Continuing the bonds in the resolution of grief in Japan and North America. *The American Behavioral Scientist*, *44*(5), 742–763. doi:10.1177/00027640121956476

Kleinman, A. (1982). Neurasthenia and depression: A study of somatization and culture in China. *Culture, Medicine and Psychiatry*, *6*(2), 117–190. doi:10.1007/BF00051427 PMID:7116909

Knezevic, B., & Olson, S. (2014). Counseling People Displaced by War: Experiences of Refugees from the Former Yugoslavia. *The Professional Counselor*, *4*(4), 316–331. doi:10.15241/bkk.4.4.316

Knight, N. (2014, September 18). Why Do We Cry? The Science of Tears. *The Independent*. Retrieved from http://www.independent.co.uk/life-style/health-and-families/features/why-do-we-cry-the-science-of-tears-9741287.html

Kobeisy, A. N. (2004). Counseling American Muslims: Understanding the faith and helping the people. Westport, CT: Praeger.

Kobeisy, A. N. (2006). Faith-based practice: An introduction. *The Journal of Muslim Mental Health*, *1*(1), 57–63. doi:10.1080/15564900600697749

Kolluru, S. (2011). *Shakti: The Divine Element of the Feminine*. Retrieved from: http://www.stateofformation.org/2011/09/shakti-the-divine-element-of-the-feminine/

Krishnaswamy, S., Subramaniam, K., Jemain, A. A., Low, W. Y., Ramachandran, P., Indran, T., & Patel, V. (2012). Common mental disorders in Malaysia: Malaysian mental health survey, 2003–2005. *Asia-Pacific Psychiatry*, *4*(3), 201–209. doi:10.1111/j.1758-5872.2012.00180.x

Kristeller, J. L., & Johnson, T. (2005). Cultivating loving-kindness: A two stage model of the effect of meditation on empathy, compassion and altruism. *Zygon*, *40*(2), 391–407. doi:10.1111/j.1467-9744.2005.00671.x

Kushner, J. (2016, March 22). The Voluntourist's Dilemma. *The New York Times*. Retrieved from https://www.nytimes.com/2016/03/22/magazine/the-voluntourists-dilemma.html

Kvale, S. (1983). The qualitative research interview: A phenomenological and a hermeneutical mode of understanding. *Journal of Phenomenological Psychology*, *14*(1-2), 171–196. doi:10.1163/156916283X00090

Lakhan, S. E. (2008). Hinduism: Life and Death. *Student BMJ Article*. Retrieved from: https://pdfs.semanticscholar.org/e64d/183c68d8f89f4817150742d458ea87b662df.pdf

Landau, E. (2017, July 1). Malaysia needs 3,000 registered psychiatrists to meet WHO recommendation: Lee. *New Straits Times Online*. Retrieved from https://www.nst.com.my/news/nation/2017/07/253500/malaysia-needs-3000-registered-psychiatrists-meet-who-recommendation-lee

Landreth, G. L., & Lobaugh, A. F. (1998). Filial therapy with incarcerated fathers: Effects on parental acceptance of child, parental stress, and child adjustmend. *Journal of Counseling and Development*, *76*(2), 157–165. doi:10.1002/j.1556-6676.1998.tb02388.x

Langgulung. (1990). *Kaunseling dalam Masyarakat Islam. Kertas Kerja Seminar Kebangsaan Kaunseling dalam Masyarakat Islam.* Yayasan Dakwah Islamiah Malaysia, Kuala Lumpur, Malaysia.

Latiff, L. A., Tajik, E., Ibrahim, N., Abubakar, A. S., & Ali, S. S. B. A. (2016). Depression and its associated factors among secondary school students in Malaysia. *The Southeast Asian Journal of Tropical Medicine and Public Health*, *47*(1), 131–141. PMID:27086434

Lauritzen, C., & Sivertsen, H. (2012). Children and Families Seeking Asylum in Northern Norway: Living Conditions and Mental Health. *International Migration (Geneva, Switzerland)*, *50*(6), 195–210. doi:10.1111/j.1468-2435.2012.00774.x

Lee, K. C., Oh, A., Zhao, Q., Wu, F. Y., Chen, S., Diaz, T., & Ong, C. K. (2017). Buddhist counseling: Implications for mental health professionals. *Spirituality in Clinical Practice*, *4*(2), 113–128. doi:10.1037cp0000124

Lee, M. N., Abdullah, Y., & Mey, S. C. (2011). Employment of People with Disabilities in Malaysia: Drivers and Inhibitors. *International Journal of Special Education*, *26*(1), 112–124.

Lee, M.-K., & Landreth, G. L. (2003). Filial therapy with immigrant Korean parents in the United States. *International Journal of Play Therapy*, *12*(2), 67–85. doi:10.1037/h0088879

Lehnung, M., Shapiro, E., Schreiber, M., & Hofmann, A. (2017). Evaluating the EMDR Group Traumatic Episode Protocol with Refugees: A Field Study. *Journal of EMDR Practice and Research*, *11*(3), 129–139. doi:10.1891/1933-3196.11.3.129

Lembaga Kaunselor Malaysia. (2016). *Laporan Tahunan 2016 Lembaga Kaunselor*. Retrieved from https://www.lkm.gov.my/kpwkm/uploads/files/LAPORAN%20TAHUNAN%20 LEMBAGA%202016%20%20.pdf

Leppma, M., & Young, M. E. (2016). Loving-kindness meditation and empathy: A wellness group intervention for counseling students. *Journal of Counseling and Development*, *94*(3), 297–305. doi:10.1002/jcad.12086

Levine, M., Prosser, A., Evans, D., & Reicher, S. (2005). Identity and emergency intervention: How social group membership and inclusiveness of group boundaries shape helping behavior. *Personality and Social Psychology Bulletin*, *31*(4), 443–453. doi:10.1177/0146167204271651 PMID:15743980

Lim, V. W. L., & Staines, A. (2007). Pathways to Services for Children with Cerebral Palsy in Selangor and the Federal Territory, Kuala Lumpur. *The Medical Journal of Malaysia*, *62*(5), 398. PMID:18705475

Ling, H. S. (2008). Negotiating Malaysian Chinese ethnic and national identity across borders. Unpublished Master thesis. Retrieved from https://etd.ohiolink.edu/rws_etd/document/get/ohiou1226957088/inline

Lin, R. K., & Ting, R. S. K. (2014). Acculturation process of returned overseas Chinese refugees from Southeast Asia: A textual analysis on 10 returned oversea Chinese cases in Zhuba Overseas-Chinese farm, Xiamen. *Hua Ren Yan Jiu Guo Ji Xue Bao*, *6*, 1–26. (in Chinese)

Liu, E. S. K., Ching, C. W. L., & Wu, J. (2017). Who is a volunteer? A cultural and temporal exploration of volunteerism. *Journal of Human Behavior in the Social Environment*, *27*(6), 530–545. doi:10.1080/10911359.2017.1295715

Love, A. W. (2007). Progress in understanding grief, complicated grief and carig for the bereaved. *Contemporary Nurse*, *27*(1), 73–83. doi:10.5172/conu.2007.27.1.73 PMID:18386957

Low, S. K., Kok, J. K., & Lee, M. N. (2013). A holistic approach to school-based counselling and guidance services in Malaysia. *School Psychology International*, *34*(2), 190–201. doi:10.1177/0143034312453398

Loyd, B. D. (2005). The Effects of Reality Therapy/Choice Theory Principles on High School Students' Perception of Needs Satisfaction And Behavioral Change. *International Journal of Reality Therapy*, *25*, 5–9.

Mahanta, L. B., Choudhury, M., Borthakur, S., Bhagabati, R., & Gogoi, P. (2015). Can communication media improve the KAP status of frontline health workers? A cross-sectional study on MCH indicators from Assam, India. *South East Asia Journal of Public Health*, *5*(2), 57–64. doi:10.3329eajph.v5i2.28314

Mak, W. W. S., & Chen, S. X. (2010). Illness behaviour among the Chinese. In M. H. Bond (Ed.), *The Oxford handbook of Chinese psychology* (pp. 421–439). New York: Oxford University Press.

Malaysia, R. (n.d.). *Persons with disabilities act 2008.* Retrieved from https://relate.com.my/persons-with-disabilities-act-2008/

Malaysian Psychiatric Association. (2013). *Mental health: With compassion we can help them cope*. Retrieved from https://www.psychiatry-malaysia.org/article.php?aid=1757

Malaysiancare.org. (2018). *Service Directory for People with Disabilities.* Retrieved from https://www.malaysiancare.org/pwd_list?pg=8

Mann, C. M., & Fazil, Q. (2006). Mental Illness in Asylum Seekers and Refuges. *Primary Care Mental Health, 4*(1), 57 – 66. Retrieved from http://ezproxy.help.edu.my:2057/ eds/pdfviewer/pdfviewer?vid=2&sid=d6f96970-d20c-4eb3-9fbf-a522f8dd2 30e%40sessionmgr103

Mann, D. (2010). *Gestalt Therapy*. London: Routledge.

Manson, M. (2014). *Facebook zero: Considering life after the demise of organic reach*. Retrieved from https://social.ogilvy.com/facebook-zero-considering-life-after-the- demise-of-organic-reach/

Manson, M. (2014, March 6). *Analysis of 100 Facebook Pages conducted by Social@Ogilvy [Digital image]*. Retrieved November 18, 2017, from https://social.ogilvy.com/facebook-zero-considering-life-after-the-demise-of-organic-reach/

Marini, I., & Stebnicki, M. A. (2009). *The professional therapist's desk reference*. New York: Springer.

Marsh, H. W., & Craven, R. G. (2006). Reciprocal effects of self-concept and performance from a multidimensional perspective: Beyond seductive pleasure and unidimensional perspectives. *Perspectives on Psychological Science, 1*(2), 133–163. doi:10.1111/j.1745-6916.2006.00010.x PMID:26151468

Marzabadi, E. A., & Hashemi, S. M. (2014). The Effectiveness of Mindfulness Training in Improving the Quality of Life of the War Victims with Post Traumatic Stress Disorder (PTSD). *Iran Journal of Psychiatry, 9*(4), 228 – 236. Retrieved from http://ezproxy.help.edu.my:2057/eds/pdfviewer/pdfviewer?vid=28&sid=ef7edb83-181d-48df-8108-368ddbf3b20e%40sessionmgr104

Mascaro, J. (Ed.). (1962). *The Bhagavad Gita*. Penguin Books.

Mavros, K. (2015). *The importance of being an ally*. Retrieved from https://www.forbes.com/sites/strategyand/2015/06/16/the-importance-of-being-an-ally/#5caacc1d35c9

Mazlan, L. B., Bahari, F., & Ardillah, F. (2012). Stress and coping skills among university students: A preliminary research on ethnicity. *Southeast Asia Psychology Journal, 1*, 31–37.

McCloskey, L. A., & Southwick, K. (1996). Psychosocial Problems in Refugee Children Exposed to War. *Pediatrics, 97*(3), 394-398. Retrieved from http://ezproxy.help.edu.my:2057/eds/pdfviewer/pdfviewer?sid=7f55c8c8-f3d9-4f9-3a7 afb1f9e507e30b%40sessionmgr105&vid=21&hid=111

McDermott, G. (2016). *Mormons and Christians: So Close, Yet So Far Away*. Retrieved from https://www.christianity-today.com/ct/2016/june-web-only/mormons-and-christians-so-close-yet-so-far-away.html

McWilliams, S. A. (2010). Inherent self, invented self, empty self: Constructivism, Buddhism and psychotherapy. *Counseling and Values, 55*(1), 79–100. doi:10.1002/j.2161-007X.2010.tb00023.x

MDG Achievement Fund. (2017). *Millennium Development Goals*. Retrieved from http://www.mdgfund.org/node/922

Merriam, S. B. (2009). *Qualitative Research –A Guide to Design and Implementation*. Jossey-Bass.

Merriam, S. B. (2009). *Qualitative Research: A guide to design and interpretation*. San Francisco: Jos-sey-Bass.

Michalon, M. (2001). "Selflessness" in the service of ego: Contribution, limitations and dangers of Buddhist psychology for western psychotherapy. *American Journal of Psychotherapy, 55*(2), 202–2018. doi:10.1176/appi.psychotherapy.2001.55.2.202 PMID:11467257

Ministry of Health Malaysia. (2015). *National health and morbidity survey 2015 volume II: Non-communicable diseases, risk factors & other health problems*. Retrieved from http://www.iku.gov.my/images/IKU/Document/REPORT/nhmsreport2015vol2.pdf

Ministry of Women, Family, and Community Development. (2017). *KASIH package module*. Retrieved from http://www.lppkn.gov.my/index.php/en/family-development-services/168-pk0003.html

Minkov, M., & Bond, M. H. (2017). A Genetic component to national differences in happiness. *Journal of Happiness Studies*, *18*(2), 321–340. doi:10.100710902-015-9712-y

Mirdal, G. M., Ryding, E., & Sondej, M. E. (2012). Traumatized Refugees, Their Therapists, and Their Interpreters: Three Perspectives on Psychological Treatment. *Psychology and Psychotherapy. Research and Practice*, *85*, 436–455. doi:10.1111/j.2044- 8341.2011.02036.x PMID:23080532

Miremadi, S., Ganesan, S., & McKenna, M. (2011). Pilot Study of the Prevalence of Alcohol, Substance Use and Mental Disorders in a Cohort of Iraqi, Afghani and Iranian Refugees in Vancouver. *Asia-Pacific Psychiatry*, *3*(3), 137–144. doi:10.1111/j.1758-5872.2011.00136.x

Mohamed, O. (2017). *Psikologi Kognitif Ad Din: Kaunseling Kesihatan Mental*. Serdang: Penerbit UPM.

Mohamed, Z., & Rahman, A. (2011). Counseling practitioners in Malaysia: Socio-Demographic profile and theoretical approaches in counseling process. *International Journal of Business and Social Science*, *2*(22), 184–188.

Mohanty, C. T. (1988). Under Western eyes: Feminist scholarship and colonial discourses. *Feminist Review*, *30*(1), 65–88. doi:10.1057/fr.1988.42

Mohd, R. A. R., Wan, M. F. A. W. R., Marina, M. A. M., & Ramly, R. M. (2012). *Agama-agama di Dunia*. Negeri Sembilan: Penerbit Universiti Sains Islam Malaysia.

Moosa, A., & Koorankot, J. K. N. (2017). Solution Focused Art Therapy Among Refugee Children. *Indian Journal of Health and Wellbeing*, *8*(8), 811 – 816. Retrieved from http://ezproxy.help.edu.my:2057/eds/pdfviewer/pdfviewer?vid=0&sid=3f93fbb4-6a8f-49e2-ae1f-6f940b69925e%40sessionmgr120

Mpofu, E., & Conyers, L. M. (2004). A representational theory perspective of minority status and people with disabilities: Implications for rehabilitation education and practice. *Rehabilitation Counseling Bulletin*, *47*(3), 142–151. doi:10.1177/00343552040470030301

Mustafa, L. (2017, June 27). Doing more for disabilities. *News Straits Times*. Retrieved from https://www.nst.com.my/news/2017/03/155019/doing-more-disabilities

MyChild at CerebralpPalsy.org. (n.d.). *Massage Therapy*. Retrieved from http://www.cerebralpalsy.org/about-cerebral-palsy/treatment/therapy/massage-therapy

MyChild at CerebralpPalsy.org. (n.d.). *Social Therapy*. Retrieved from http://www.cerebralpalsy.org/about-cerebral-palsy/treatment/therapy/social-therapy

Nah, A. M. (2010). Refugees and Space in Urban Areas in Malaysia. *Forced Migration Review*, *1*(34), 29 – 31. Retrieved from: http://ezproxy.help.edu.my:2057/ eds/pdfviewer/pdfviewer?vid=6&sid=60d55cda-e435-419d-94ce-cc2b503ff642%40sessionmgr102&hid=120

National Association of Christian Counsellors. (n.d.). *National Association of Christian Counsellors*. Retrieved from https://www.nacc-malaysia.org/

National Center for Complementary and Integrative Health. (2016). *Relaxation Techniques for Health*. Retrieved from https://nccih.nih.gov/health/stress/relaxation.htm

Neimeyer, R., Prigreson, H. G., & Davies, B. (2002). Mourning and meaning. *The American Behavioral Scientist*, *46*(2), 235–254. doi:10.1177/000276402236676

Neuner, F., Schauer, M., Klaschik, C., Karanukara, U., & Elbert, T. (2004). A Comparison of Narrative Exposure Therapy, Supportive Counseling, and Psychoeducation for Treating Posttraumatic Stress Disorder in an African Refugee Settlement. *Journal of Consulting and Clinical Psychology*, *72*(4), 579–587. doi:10.1037/0022-006X.72.4.579 PMID:15301642

Ng, J. H. (2015). *Lived Experiences of Chinese Adolescents Who From Failing In Their Academic Studies Journey into Passing Grades*. unpublished master's thesis, HELP University.

Ng, L. O. (2008). Clinical psychology update: Challenges for practice and training [Unpublished manuscript].

Ng, S. (1999, August 15). Students react to hostel policy. *The Star*. Retrieved April 26, 2004, from http://thestar.com.my/news/storyx1000.asp?file=/1999/8/15/education/15lasaro&sec=

Ng, W. S. (2005). *Psychotherapists in Malaysia: A preliminary study of clinical psychologists.* [Unpublished doctoral Clinical Research Project completion of the Doctor of Psychology].

Ng, W. S. (2007, August). Cultural identity of psychotherapists in Malaysia. *Paper presented at the World Mental Health Congress*, Hong Kong Polytechnic University, Hong Kong.

Ng, C. H. (1997). The stigma of mental illness in Asian cultures. *The Australian and New Zealand Journal of Psychiatry*, *31*(3), 382–390. doi:10.3109/00048679709073848 PMID:9226084

Ng, C. T. C., & James, S. (2013). "Directive approach" for Chinese clients receiving psychotherapy: Is that really a priority. *Frontiers in Psychology*, *4*(49), 1–13. PMID:23408043

Ng, J. H., & Jegathesan, A. J. (in press). Malaysian Chinese youths: Learning CTRT is fun and impactful! *International Journal of Choice Theory and Reality Therapy.*

Ng, L. O. (2007). A brief study into the awareness of the field of clinical psychology among medical and health science professionals in Malaysia. *Malaysian Journal of Health Sciences*, *5*, 23–30.

Ng, L. O., Teoh, H.-J., & Haque, A. (2003). Clinical psychology in Malaysia: A brief overview. *ASEAN Journal of Psychiatry*, *6*, 11–16.

Ng, M. N., Bhugra, D., Mcmanus, F., & Fennell, M. (2011). Filial piety as a protective factor for depression in survivors of childhood abuse. *International Review of Psychiatry (Abingdon, England)*, *23*(1), 100–112. doi:10.3109/09540261.2010.544645 PMID:21338305

Nielsen. (2012, April). Global Trust in Advertising and Brand Messages. Retrieved from http://www.nielsen.com/content/dam/corporate/us/en/reports-downloads/2012-Reports/global-trust-inadvertising-2012.pdf

Nobles, A. Y., & Sciarra, D. T. (2000). Cultural determinants in the treatment of Arab Americans: A primer for mainstream therapist. *The American Journal of Orthopsychiatry*, *70*(2), 182–191. doi:10.1037/h0087734 PMID:10826030

Novelli, D., Drury, J., & Reicher, S. (2010). Come together: Two studies concerning the impact of group relations on personal space. *British Journal of Social Psychology*, *49*(2), 223–236. doi:10.1348/014466609X449377 PMID:19523278

Nunis, A. (2017). *The Lived Experience of Refugees (Illegal Immigrants): A Malaysia Context* (Unpublished Dissertation). HELP University, Kuala Lumpur, Malaysia.

Nyanaponika. (1999). *Four Sublime states.* Penang: Inward Path.

O'Connor, S., & Vandenberg, B. (2005). Psychosis or faith? Clinicians' assessment of religious beliefs. *Journal of Consulting and Clinical Psychology, 73*(4), 610–616. doi:10.1037/0022-006X.73.4.610 PMID:16173848

Olendzki, A. (2003). Buddhist Psychology. In S. R. Segalle (Ed.), Encountering Buddhism (pp. 9 – 30). Albany, NY: State University of New York Press.

Ong, K. H., & Tan, J. (2017). Penang Hokkien on life support. *Penang Monthly.* Retrieved from http://penangmonthly.com/article.aspx?pageid=7412&name=penang_hokkien_on_life_support

Ong, L. C., Afifah, I., Sofiah, A., & Lye, M. S. (1998). Parenting stress among mothers of Malaysian children with cerebral palsy: Predictors of child-and parent-related stress. *Annals of Tropical Paediatrics, 18*(4), 301–307. doi:10.1080/02724936.1998.11747964 PMID:9924586

Othman, A., & Abdullah, S. S. (2015). Counselling in Malaysia: Trends and Practice with the Malays. *International Journal of Business and Applied Social Science, 1*, 1–10.

Padela, A. I., Killawi, A., Forman, J., DeMonner, S., & Heisler, M. (2012). American Muslim perceptions of healing: Key agents in healing and their roles. *Qualitative Health Research, 22*(6), 846–858. doi:10.1177/1049732312438969 PMID:22393065

Pan, L. (Ed.). (2006). *The encyclopedia of the Chinese overseas* (2nd ed.). Singapore: Editions Didier Millet.

Park, C. L. (2005). Religion as a meaning-making framework in coping with life. *The Journal of Social Issues, 61*(4), 707–729. doi:10.1111/j.1540-4560.2005.00428.x

Patel, C. (2017, February 25). Time for ASEAN to take human rights seriously. *The Diplomat.* Retrieved from https://thediplomat.com/2017/02/time-for-asean-to-take-human-rights-seriously/

Persons with Disabilities Act. (2008). (Act 685). Retrieved from http://ilo.org/dyn/natlex/docs/ELECTRONIC/86297/97318/F1567227890/MYS86297.pdf

Pew Research Center. (2007). *Muslim Americans: Middle class and mostly mainstream.* Washington, DC: Pew Research Center. Retrieved from http://pewresearch.org/assets/pdf/muslim-americans.pdf

Phillips, J. (2011). *Asylum seekers and refugees: What are the facts? Background note, Parliamentary Library, Parliament of Australia, Canberra.* Retrieved from http:// www.aph.gov.au/library/pubs/BN/sp/Asylumfacts.htm

Piper, J. (2008, February 13). *What does it mean to have a relationship with God?* Retrieved October 19, 2017, from https://www.desiringgod.org/interviews/what-does-it-mean-to-have-a-relationship-with-god

Pitney, W., & Parker, J. (2009). *Qualitative research in Physical activity and the health profession.* Human Kinetic.

Pitsuwan, S., & Parameswaran, P. (2015). *Why Southeast Asia Refugee Crisis Matters.* Retrieved from https://thediplomat.com/2015/07/southeast-asia-refugees-in-crisis/

Pochelli, M. (2015). *This is what happens to your brain when you experience happiness.* Retrieved from http://reset.me/story/this-is-what-happens-to-your-brain-when-you-experience-happiness/

Posselt, M., Procter, N., Galletly, C., & de Crespigny, C. (2014). Aetiology of Coexisting Mental Health and Alcohol and Other Drug Disorders: Perspectives of Refugee Youth and Service Providers. *Australian Psychologist, 50*(2), 130–140. doi:10.1111/ap.12096

Post, B. C., & Wade, N. G. (2009). Religion and spirituality in psychotherapy: A practice-friendly review of research. *Journal of Clinical Psychology*, *65*(2), 131–146. doi:10.1002/jclp.20563 PMID:19132737

Premasiri, P. D. (2001). Social relevance of the Buddhist nibbana ideal. In D. J. Kalupahana (Ed.), *Buddhist thought and ritual* (pp. 45–56). Delhi: Motilal Banarsidass.

Priebe, S., Giacco, D., & El-Nagib, R. (2017). Public Health Aspects of Mental Health Among Migrants and Refugees: A Review of the Evidence of Mental Health Care for Refugees, Asylum Seekers and Irregular Migrants in the WHO European Region. *Health Evidence Network Synthesis Report, 47*. Retrieved from https://www.ncbi.nlm.nih.gov/books/NBK391045/

Raba, A., & Othman, A. H. (1998). *Toward Islamization of Guidance and Counselling*. Sabah: Persatuan Kaunseling Malaysia.

Rahula, W. (1978). *What the Buddha taught*. London: Gordon Fraser.

Ramakrishna. (n.d.). Hinduism: Death and Life Beyond Death. *Swami Adiswaraananda Ramakrishna Vivekananda Center.* Retrieved from: https://www.ramakrishna.org/activities/message/weekly_message43.htm

Raman, V., & Singhal, M. (2015). Play therapy with children: Its relevance and utility in the Indian context. *Journal of Indian Association for Child & Adolescent Mental Health*, *11*(2), 121–157.

Randle, M., & Dolnicar, S. (2012). Attracting volunteers in highly multicultural societies: A marketing challenge. *Journal of Nonprofit & Public Sector Marketing*, *24*(4), 351–369. doi:10.1080/10495142.2012.733668

Razali, S. M., Aminah, K., & Khan, U. A. (2002). Religious–cultural psychotherapy in the management of anxiety patients. *Transcultural Psychiatry*, *39*(1), 130–136. doi:10.1177/136346150203900106

Reddy, M. S. (2012). Psychotherapy:Insights from Bhagavad Gita. *Indian Journal of Psychological Medicine*, *34*(1). Retrieved from https://www.ncbi.nlm.nih.gov/pmc/articles/PMC3361835/ PMID:22661821

Religions - Christianity. The basics of Christian history. (2009a, June 08). Retrieved October 19, 2017, from http://www.bbc.co.uk/religion/religions/christianity/history/history_1.shtml

Religions-Christianity. Paul. (2011a, June 21). Retrieved October 19, 2017, from http://www.bbc.co.uk/religion/religions/christianity/history/paul_1.shtml

Renger, D., & Simon, B. (2011). Social recognition as an equal: The role of equality-based respect in group life. *European Journal of Social Psychology*, *41*(4), 501–507. doi:10.1002/ejsp.814

Richards, C. L., & Malouin, F. (2013). Cerebral palsy: Definition, assessment and rehabilitation. *Handbook of Clinical Neurology*, *111*, 183–195. doi:10.1016/B978-0-444-52891-9.00018-X PMID:23622163

Richards, L. (2005). *Handling qualitative data: A practical guide*. London: Sage Publications.

Rintod, L. (2013, May 30). Working towards reinstating Sarawak's sovereignty. *Free Malaysia Today*. Retrieved from http://www.freemalaysiatoday.com/category/nation/2013/05/30/ working-towards-reinstating-sarawaks-sovereignty/

Robinson, B. A. (2008). *Christianity: A brief history*. Retrieved October 19, 2017, from http://www.religioustolerance.org/chr_intr1.htm

Robjant, K., & Fazel, M. (2010). The Emerging Evidence for Narrative Exposure Therapy: A Review. *Clinical Psychology Review*, *30*(8), 1030–1039. doi:10.1016/j.cpr.2010.07.004 PMID:20832922

RoketKini.Com. (2013). *DAP mohon kerajaan sediakan pendidikan khusus kanak-kanak lumpuh otak atau Cerebral Palsy*. Retrieved from https://www.roketkini.com/2013/10/03/sediakan-pendidikan-cerebral-palsy/

Ross, M., Svajlenka, N. P., & Williams, J. (2014). *Part of the solution: Pre-Baccalaureate healthcare workers in a time of health system change*. Retrieved from https://www.brookings.edu/wp-content/uploads/2014/07/Healthcare-Workers-Report.pdf

Rousseau, C., Pottie, K., Thombs, B. D., Munoz, M., & Jurcik, T. (2011). *Post Traumatic* Stress Disorder: Evidence Review for Newly Arriving Immigrants and Refugees. *Canadian Medical Association Journal*, *11*(Appendix). Retrieved from http://www.cmaj.ca/content/suppl/2010/06/07/cmaj.090313.DC1/imm-ptsd-11-at.pdf

Roxborogh, J. (1989). *A Short Introduction to Malaysian Church History: A Guide to the Story of Christianity in Malaysia and How to Go About Discovering the History of Your Church* (2nd rev. Ed.). Seremban: Seminari Theoloji Malaysia.

Rural Youth of South Australia. (2001). *A Practical Counsellor's Handbook*. Gawler: Rural Alliance Network.

Sahri, M., Murad, K., Alias, A., & Sirajuddin, M. (2013). Empowering Youth Volunteerism: The Importance and Global Motivating Factors. *Journal Of Educational And Social Research*, *3*(7), 502. Retrieved from http://www.mcser.org/journal/index.php/jesr/article/view/995

Salkind, N. J. (2009). *Exploring Research*. Pearson Education, Inc.

Salzberg, S. (2011). Mindfulness and Loving – Kindness. *Contemporary Buddhism*, *12*(1), 177–182. doi:10.1080/14639947.2011.564837

Sangganjanavanich, V. F., Cook, K., & Rangel-Gomez, M. (2010). Filial therapy with monolingual Spanish-speaking mothers: A phenomenological study. *The Family Journal (Alexandria, Va.)*, *18*(2), 195–201. doi:10.1177/1066480710364320

Santina, P. D. (1984). *Fundamentals of Buddhism*. Singapore: Buddha Dharma Education Association Inc.

Sarfo-Manch, A. G. (2009). *Coping Methods and Meaning Making of Liberian Refugees in the Buduburam Refugee Camp of Ghana*. Retrieved from http://digitalcommons.uconn.edu/cgi/viewcontent.cgi?article=1113&context=srhonor_theses

Satir, V., Banmen, J., Geber, J., & Gomori, M. (1991). *The Satir Model*. Palo Alto, CA: Science and Behavior Books, Inc.

Schiff, J. W., & Lane, A. (2016). *Burnout and PTSD in workers in the homeless sector in Calgary*. Retrieved from http://calgaryhomeless.com/content/uploads/Calgary-Psychosocial-Stressors-Report.pdf

Schlieter, J. (2013). Checking the heavenly 'bank account of karma': Cognitive metaphors for karma in Western perception and early Theravāda Buddhism. *Religion*, *43*(4), 463–486. doi:10.1080/0048721X.2013.765630

Schouten, K.A., de Niet, G.J., Knipscheer, J.W., Kleber, R.J., & Hutschemaekers, G.J.M. (2014). The Effectiveness of Art Therapy in the Treatment of Traumatized Adults: A Systemic Review on Art Therapy and Trauma. *Trauma Violence and Abuse*, 1 - 9. doi:10.1177/1524838014555032

Schuh, J. H., & Upcraft, M. L. (2001). *Assessment practice in student affairs: An applications manual*. San Francisco, CA: Jossey-Bass.

Schuller, M. (2016). *Humanitarian Aftershocks in Haiti*. Rutgers University Press.

Schweitzer, R. D., Brough, M., Vromans, L., & Asic-Kobe, M. (2011). Mental Health of Newly Arrived Burmese Refugees in Australia: Contributions of Pre-Migration and Post Migration Experience. *The Australian and New Zealand Journal of Psychiatry*, *45*(4), 299–307. doi:10.3109/00048674.2010.543412 PMID:21303193

Schweitzer, R., van Wyk, S., & Muray, K. (2015). Therapeutic Practice with Refugee Clients: A Qualitative Study of Therapist Experience. *Counselling & Psychotherapy Research, 15*(2), 109–188. doi:10.1002/capr.12018

Segall. (2003). Psychotherapy practice and Buddhist practice. In S. R. Segalle (Ed.), *Encountering Buddhism* (pp. 165 – 178). Albany, NY: State University of New York Press.

Shafranske, E. P. (Ed.). (1996). *Religion and the clinical practice of psychology*. Washington, DC: American Psychological Association. doi:10.1037/10199-000

Shakespeare-Finch, J., Schweitzer, R. D., King, J., & Brough, M. (2014). Distress, Coping and Posttraumatic Growth in Refugees from Burma. *Journal of Immigrant & Refugee Studies, 12*(3), 311–330. doi:10.1080/15562948.2013.844876

Sharp, R., & Hutchienson, J. F. (2008). Karma, reincarnation, and medicine: Hindu perspectives on biomedical research. *Springer Genomic Medicine, 2*(3-4). Retrieved from: https://www.ncbi.nlm.nih.gov/pmc/articles/PMC2694864/

Shen, L. (2014*). Culture and stigma: Social exclusion of families of children with cerebral palsy in China.* Retrieved from https://www.researchgate.net/publication/266784978_Culture_and_stigma_Social_exclusion_of_families_of_children_with_cerebral_palsy_in_China

Shields, C. M. (2007). *Can case studies achieve the "gold standard"? Or when methodology meets politics.* Paper presented at the Annual Meeting of the American Educational Research Association, Chicago, IL.

Sidebe, M., & Singh, P. K. (2016). *Thailand eliminates mother-to-child transmission of HIV and syphilis.* Retrieved from http://www.searo.who.int/about/administration_structure/cds/piis0140673616307875.pdf?ua=1

Simon, M. A., Chen, R., Chang, E., & Dong, X. (2014). The association between filial piety and suicidal ideation: Findings from a community-dwelling Chinese aging population. *The Journals of Gerontology: Series A, 69*(Suppl. 2), 90–97. doi:10.1093/gerona/glu142 PMID:25378454

Singh, S. K., Yap, K.-H., Reidpath, D. D., & Allotey, P. (2017, August). Binge drinking and associated risk behaviours among youth in three ethnic groups in Malaysia. *Paper presented at 31st annual conference of the European Health Psychology Society*, Padua, Italy, August 29th-September 2.

Sin, S. (2010). Considerations of quality in phenomenographic research. *International Journal of Qualitative Methods, 9*(4), 305–319. doi:10.1177/160940691000900401

Sman, C. (2017, April 16). SPWCA seeks greater awareness on CP. *Borneo Post Online.* Retrieved from http://www.theborneopost.com/2017/04/16/scpwa-seeks-greater-awareness-on-cp/

Solis, C. M., Meyers, J., & Varjas, K. M. (2004). A qualitative case study of the process and impact of filial therapy with an African American parent. *International Journal of Play Therapy, 13*(2), 99–118. doi:10.1037/h0088892

Sorensen, M. (2018). What is Low Self-Esteem? *The Self-Esteem Institute.* Retrieved from http://getesteem.com/about/

Sourander, A. (2002). Refugee Families During Asylum Seeking. *Nordic Journal of Psychiatry, 57*(3), 203–207. doi:10.1080/08039480310001364 PMID:12775295

Sowislo, J. F., & Orth, U. (2013). Does low self-esteem predict depression and anxiety? A meta-analysis of longitudinal studies. *Psychological Bulletin, 139*(1), 213–240. doi:10.1037/a0028931 PMID:22730921

Springer, P. R., Abbott, D. A., & Reisbig, A. M. J. (2009). Therapy with Muslim couples and families: Basic guidelines for effective practice. *The Family Journal: Counseling and Therapy for Couples and Family, 17*(3), 229–235. doi:10.1177/1066480709337798

Steele, C. M. (1997). A thereat in the air: How stereotypes shape intellectual identity and performance. *The American Psychologist*, *52*(6), 513–629. doi:10.1037/0003-066X.52.6.613 PMID:9174398

Steiger, A. E., Allemand, M., Robins, R. W., & Fend, H. A. (2014). Low and decreasing self-esteem during adolescence predict adult depression two decades later. *Journal of Personality and Social Psychology*, *106*(2), 325–338. doi:10.1037/a0035133 PMID:24467425

Stewart, D. (n.d.). *What Precautions Were Taken to Keep the Tomb of Jesus Secure?* Retrieved October 19, 2017, from https://www.blueletterbible.org/faq/don_stewart/don_stewart_247.cfm

Stocker,, M. (1996). *Valuing Emotions*. New York: Cambridge University Press.

Strupp, H. H. (1980). Humanism and psychotherapy: A personal statement of the therapist's essential values. *Psychotherapy*, *17*(4), 396–400. doi:10.1037/h0085938

Stuntzner, S., & Hartley, M. (2014). Disability and the counseling relationship: What counselors need to know. *Ideas and research you can use: VISTAS 2014*. Retrieved from https://www.counseling.org/docs/default-source/vistas/article_09.pdf?sfvrsn=157ccf7c_12

Suara Rakyat Malaysia. (2014). *Malaysia Human Rights Report*. Retrieved from http://www.suaram.net/wordpress/wp-content/uploads/2015/09/HR2014-lowres.pdf

Suara Rakyat Malaysia. (2015). *Malaysia Human Rights Report*. Retrieved from http://www.suaram.net/wordpress/wp-content/uploads/2017/02/HR2015.pdf

Subramuniyswami, S. (1993). *Dancing with Siva: Hinduism's Contemporary Catechism* (4th ed.). Himalayan Academy.

Sue, D. W., Ivey. A. E., & Pedersen, P. B. (Eds.). (1996). A Theory of Multicultural Counseling and Therapy. Pacific Grove, CA: Brooks/Cole.

Sue, D. W. (2010a). *Microaggressions in everyday life: race gender; and sexual orientation*. Hoboken, NJ: Wiley.

Sue, D. W., & Sue, D. (1977). Barriers to effective cross-cultural counseling. *Journal of Counseling Psychology*, *24*(5), 420–429. doi:10.1037/0022-0167.24.5.420

Sue, D. W., & Sue, D. (2013). *Counseling the culturally diverse: Theory and practice* (6th ed.). New York, NY: John Wiley.

Sue, D. W., & Sue, D. S. (2008). *Counseling the Culturally Diverse: Theory and Practice* (5th ed.). John Wiley & Sons.

Sue, D., Arredondo, P., & McDavis, R. (1992). Multicultural counseling competencies and standards: A call to the profession. *Journal of Multicultural Counseling and Development*, *20*(2), 64–88. doi:10.1002/j.2161-1912.1992.tb00563.x

Sue, S. (1998). In search of cultural competence in psychotherapy and counseling. *The American Psychologist*, *53*(4), 440–118. doi:10.1037/0003-066X.53.4.440 PMID:9572007

Sue, S., & Zane, N. (1987). The role of culture and cultural techniques in psychotherapy: A critique and reformulation. *The American Psychologist*, *42*(1), 35–45. doi:10.1037/0003-066X.42.1.37 PMID:3565913

Sue, S., Zane, N., Nagayama Hall, G. C., & Berger, L. K. (2009). The case for cultural competency in psychotherapeutic interventions. *Annual Review of Psychology*, *60*(1), 525–548. doi:10.1146/annurev.psych.60.110707.163651 PMID:18729724

Sukumaran, T. (2017, May 20). What's causing Malaysia's ethnic Chinese brain drain? *South China Morning Post*. Retrieved from http://www.scmp.com/week-asia/politics/article/2095012/whats-causing-malaysias-ethnic-chinese-brain-drain

Sullivan, G., & Losberg, W. (2003). A study of sampling in research in the field of lesbian and gay studies. In W. Meezan & J. I. Martin (Eds.), *Research methods with gay, lesbian, bisexual, and transgender populations* (pp. 147–162). Binghamton, NY: Harrington Park Press. doi:10.1300/J041v15n01_10

Sumerel,M.B.(1994).Parallelprocessinsupervision.ERICDigest.Retrievedfromhttp://eric.ed.gov/?id=ED372347adresinden elde edildi.

Sundararajan, L. (2015). *Understanding Emotion in Chinese Culture:Thinking Through Psychology*. New York: Springer International Publishing. doi:10.1007/978-3-319-18221-6

Sundararajan, L., Misra, G., & Marsella, A. J. (2013). Indigenous approaches to assessment, diagnosis, and treatment of mental disorders. In F. A. Paniagua & A.-M. Yamada (Eds.), *Handbook of multicultural mental health: Assessment and treatment of diverse populations* (pp. 69–88). London, UK: Elsevier Inc. doi:10.1016/B978-0-12-394420-7.00004-7

Tajfel, H., & Turner, J. C. (1979). An integrative theory of intergroup conflict. In W. G. Austin & S. Worchel (Eds.), *The social psychology of intergroup relations* (pp. 33–47). Monterey: Brooks/Cole.

Tan, J. (2007, October 28). 马来西亚的华人:一个族群,两种观点 [Malaysian Chinese: One Ethnicity, Two Perspectives]. *Sin Chew Jit Poh* [Sin Chew Forum].

Tan, L. E. (2000). Chinese schools in Malaysia: A case of cultural resilience. In Lee. K. H. & Tan. C. B. (Eds.), The Chinese in Malaysia (pp. 228-254).

Tan, C.-B. (2005). Chinese in Malaysia. In M. Ember, C. R. Ember, & I. Skoggard (Eds.), *Encyclopedia of Diasporas: Immigrant and refugee cultures around the world* (pp. 697–706). New York, USA: Springer. doi:10.1007/978-0-387-29904-4_72

Tang, A. (2004). *Understanding the Apostles' Creed.* Retrieved October 19, 2017 from http://www.kairos2.com/Apostles_Creed.pdf

Tang, M. (2002). A comparison of Asian American, Caucasian American and Chinese college students: An initial report. *Journal of Multicultural Counseling and Development*, *30*(2), 124–135. doi:10.1002/j.2161-1912.2002.tb00484.x

Tan, T. J., Ho, W. F., & Tan, J. L. (2005). *The Chinese Malaysian contribution.* Kuala Lumpur: Centre for Malaysian Chinese Studies.

Tappis, H., Biermann, E., Glass, N., Tileva, M., & Doocy, S. (2012). Domestic Violence Among Iraqi Refugees in Syria. *Health Care for Women International*, *33*(3), 285–297. doi:10.1080/07399332.2011.645969 PMID:22325027

Taylor, S. (2017). *Refugee Protection in the Asia Pacific Region*. Retrieved from http://www.refugeelegalaidinformation.org/refugee-protection-asia-pacific-region

The British Psychological Association. (2006). Disciplinary notice: Edward Chan. *The Psychologist*, *19*(10), 619–620.

The Guardian. (2015). *Malaysia Migrant Mass Graves: Police Reveal 139 Sites, Some with Multiple Corpses*. Retrieved from https://www.theguardian.com/world/2015/may/25/malaysia-migrant-mass-graves-police-reveal-139-sites-some-with-multiple-corpses

The Star Online. (2017). *Depression: 40% of Malaysians will suffer from mental health issues in their lifetime.* Retrieved from https://www.thestar.com.my/news /nation /2017/04/02/malaysians-will-suffer-from-mental-health-issues-in-their-lifetime/

The Sun Daily. (2016). *Mental health of Malaysian students worrisome*. Retrieved from http://www.thesundaily.my/news/1967970

Thevadass, L. (2017, May 12). Poor facilities for the disabled. *The Star Online*. Retrieved from https://www.thestar.com.my/metro/community/2017/05/12/poor-facilities-for-the-disabled-study-infrastructure-at-terminals-pose-danger-and-confusion/

Tin, C. S. (2013). *Children with disabilities in Malaysia: Mapping the policies, programmes, interventions and stakeholders*. Family Health Development Division, Ministry of Health Malaysia.

Ting, R. S. K., & Sundararajan, L. (2017). *Culture, Cognition, and Emotion in China's Religious Ethnic Minorities: Voices of Suffering among the Yi*. Palgrave MacMillan Publication.

Ting, S.-K. (2008). *Who am I talking to: The effect of language on bilingual Chinese expression of self-concept and depressive emotion*. Germany: VDM Verlag Dr. Muller.

Ting, S.-K., & Ng, L. O. (2012). Use of Religious Resources in Psychotherapy from a Tradition-Sensitive Approach: Cases from Chinese in Malaysia. *Pastoral Psychology*, *61*(5-6), 941–957. doi:10.1007/s11089-011-0365-4

Tjeltveit, A. C. (1999). *Ethics and values in psychotherapy*. New York: Routledge. doi:10.4324/9780203360453

Todd, P. M., & Gigerenzer, G. (2012). Ecological rationality: Intelligence in the world. OUP USA. doi:10.1093/acprof:oso/9780195315448.001.0001

Trefflich, F., Kalckreuth, S., Mergl, R., & Rummel-Kluge, C. (2015). Psychiatric patients' internet use corresponds to the internet use of the general public. *Psychiatry Research*, *226*(1), 136–141. doi:10.1016/j.psychres.2014.12.037 PMID:25623020

Tribe, R. (2013). Mental Health of Refugees and Asylum Seekers. *Journal of Continuing Professional Development*, *8*, 240–247. doi:10.1192/apt.8.4.240

Trzesniewski, K. H., Donnellan, M. B., Moffitt, T. E., Robins, R. W., Poulton, R., & Caspi, A. (2006). Low self-esteem during adolescence predicts poor health, criminal behavior, and limited economic prospects during adulthood. *Developmental Psychology*, *42*(2), 381–390. doi:10.1037/0012-1649.42.2.381 PMID:16569175

Tuo, L. (2014). 慈悲喜舍的意义与修习方法. Retrieved from http://www.liaotuo.org/fjrw/jsrw/zxjs/66904.html

Turner, J. C. (1985). Social categorization and the self-concept: A cognitive theory of group behaviour. In E. J. Lawler (Ed.), *Advances in group processes*. Greenwich, US: JAI Press.

Turner, J. C., Hogg, M. A., Oakes, P. J., Reicher, S. D., & Wetherell, M. S. (1987). *Rediscovering the social group: A self-categorization theory*. Cambridge, US: Basil Blackwell.

Turner, J. C., Oakes, P. J., Haslam, S. A., & McGarty, C. (1994). Self and collective: Cognition and social context. *Personality and Social Psychology Bulletin*, *20*(5), 454–463. doi:10.1177/0146167294205002

Tyler, T. R., & Blader, S. L. (2000). *Cooperation in groups: Procedural justice, social identity, and behavioral engagement*. New York: Psychology Press.

Ullmann, E., Barthel, A., Tache, S., Bornstein, A., Licino, J., & Bornstein, S. R. (2015). Emotional and Psychological Trauma in Refugees Arriving in Germany in 2015. *Molecular Psychiatry*, *20*(12), 1483–1484. doi:10.1038/mp.2015.164 PMID:26527128

UNHCR. (2017). *Joint statement on the Rohingya refugee crisis.* Retrieved from http://www.unhcr.org/en-my/news/press/2017/10/59e4c17e5/joint-statement-rohingya-refugee-crisis.html

UNICEF. (2012). *Understanding the focus on young people from Key Affected Populations in Concentrated and Low Prevalence HIV Epidemics.* Retrieved from https://www.unicef.org/rosa/20121012_ykap(1).pdf

United Nations High Commissioner for Refugees. (2010). *Convention and Protocol Relating to the Status of Refugees.* Retrieved from: http://www.unhcr.org/en-my/3b66c2aa10

United Nations High Commissioner for Refugees. (2016). *Global Trends Forced Displacement in 2016.* Retrieved from: http://www.unhcr.org/globaltrends2016/

United Nations High Commissioner for Refugees. (2016). *Refugees in Malaysia.* Retrieved from http://www.unhcr.org.my/refugeeMsia.htm

United Nations High Commissioner for Refugees. (2017). *Asia and the Pacific.* Retrieved from http://www.unhcr.org/en-my/asia-and-the-pacific.html

United Nations High Commissioner for Refugees. (2017a). *UNHCR in Malaysia.* Retrieved from: https://www.unhcr.org.my/About_Us-@-UNHCR_in_Malaysia.aspx

United Nations High Commissioner for Refugees. (2017b). *Schools for Refugee Children.* Retrieved from: https://www.unhcr.org.my/Education-@-Schools_For_Refugee_Children.aspx

United Nations High Commissioner for Refugees. (2018a). *UNHCR Population Statistics.* Retrieved from: http://popstats.unhcr.org/en/overview#_ga=2.251604486.1844780328.1522565339-7275457.1483770482

United Nations High Commissioner for Refugees. (2018b). *Figures at a Glance in Malaysia.* Retrieved from: http://www.unhcr.org/en-my/figures-at-a-glance-in-malaysia.html

United Nations Volunteers. (2015). *State of the World's Volunteerism Report 2015.* Retrieved from https://www.unv.org/sites/default/files/2015%20State%20of%20the%20World%27s%20Volunteerism%20Report%20-%20Transforming%20Governance.pdf

University of Florida, Multicultural & Diversity Affairs. (2017). *LGBTQ Terms and Definitions.* Retrieved from https://lgbtq.multicultural.ufl.edu/programs/speakersbureau/lgbtq-terms-definitions/

Urdang, E. (2010). Awareness of Self: A Critical Tool. *Social Work Education, 29*(5), 523–538. doi:10.1080/02615470903164950

Velarde, R. (2009). *What Is the Church?* Retrieved May 31, 2018, from https://www.focusonthefamily.com/faith/the-study-of-god/why-study-god/what-is-the-church

Vijayakumar, L. (2016). Suicide Amongst Refugees – A Mockery of Humanity Crisis. *Journal of Crisis Intervention and Suicide Prevention, 37*(1), 1–4. doi:10.1027/0227-5910/a000385 PMID:27033678

Villalbla, J. A. (2009). Addressing Immigrant and Refugee Issues in Multicultural Counselor Education. *Journal of Professional Counseling: Practice, Theory and Research, 37*(1), 1 – 12. Retrieved from http://ezproxy.help.edu.my:2057/eds/pdfviewer/pdfviewer?vid=33&sid=ef7edb83-181d-48df-8108-368ddbf3b20e%40sessionmgr104

Vogel, S. (2016). Working with People who Identify as Asylum Seekers or Refugees. *Gestalt Journal Of Australia & New Zealand, 12*(2), 83-100. Retrieved from http://ezproxy.help.edu.my:2052/eds/pdfviewer/pdfviewer?vid=1&sid=a0d7a383-ea6a-4ec6-bd990ad8ad602574%40sessionmgr4008&hid=4205

Walker, D. F., Worthington, E. L. Jr, Gartner, A. L., Gorsuch, R. L., & Hanshew, E. R. (2011). Religious commitment and expectations about psychotherapy among Christian clients. *Psychology of Religion and Spirituality*, *3*(2), 98–114. doi:10.1037/a0021604

Walpola, P. L., Walpola, D. Y., Walpola, I. C., & Toneatto, T. (2017). Mapping the Mind: A Model Based on Theravada Buddhist Texts and Practices. *Contemporary Buddhism*, *18*(1), 140–164. doi:10.1080/14639947.2017.1307575

Ward, C., & Hewstone, M. (1985). Ethnicity, language and intergroup relations in Malaysia and Singapore: A social psychological analysis. *Journal of Multilingual and Multicultural Development*, *6*(3-4), 271–296. doi:10.1080/01434632.1985.9994207

Ward, C., & Lin, E. (2010). There are homes at the four corners of the seas: acculturation and adaptation of overseas Chinese. In M. H. Bond (Ed.), *The Oxford handbook of Chinese psychology* (pp. 657–677). New York: Oxford University Press. doi:10.1093/oxfordhb/9780199541850.013.0039

Watson, O. M. (1970). *Proxemic behaviour. A Cross cultural study*. The Hague, The Netherlands: Mouton.

Watson, O. M. (1972). *Symbolic and Expressive Uses of Space: An Introduction to Proxemic behaviour*. Addison: Wesley Modular.

Watters, E. (2011). *Crazy Like Us: The Globalization of the American Psyche*. NY: Free Press.

Wessels, W. K. (2014). *The Refugee Experience: Involving Pre-Migration, In Transit, and Post Migration Issues in Social Services*. Retrieved from: http://sophia.stkate.edu/cgi/viewcontent.cgi?article=1411&context=msw_papers

Williams, D. C., & Levitt, H. M. (2007). A qualitative investigation of eminent therapists' values within psychotherapy: Developing integrative principles for moment-to-moment psychotherapy practice. *Journal of Psychotherapy Integration*, *17*(2), 159–184. doi:10.1037/1053-0479.17.2.159

Worden, J. W. (2009). *Grief Counselling and grief therapy: A handbook for mental health practitioners* (4th ed.). New York: Springer Publishing.

World Atlas. (2017). *People of Malaysia*. Retrieved from, http://www.worldatlas.com/articles/ethnic-groups-of-malaysia.html

World Health Organization. (2011). Malaysia. Retrieved from http://www.who.int/mental_health/evidence/atlas/profiles/mys_mh_profile.pdf

Wubbolding, R. E. (1988). *Using reality therapy*. New York: Harper & Row.

Wubbolding, R. E. (2015). The voice of William Glasser: Accessing the continuing evolution of reality therapy. *Journal of Mental Health Counseling*, *37*(3), 189–205. doi:10.17744/mehc.37.3.01

Wubbolding, R. E. (2015b). *Reality therapy training manual. 16th revision*. Cincinnati: Center for Reality Therapy.

Yaacob, S. N., Juhari, R., Talib, M. A., & Uba, I. (2009). Loneliness, stress, self-esteem and depression among Malaysian adolescents. *Jurnal Kemanusiaan*, *7*, 85–95.

Yeh, K. H., Yi, C., Tsao, W., & Wan, P. (2013). Filial piety in contemporary Chinese societies: A comparative study of Taiwan, Hong Kong, and China. *International Sociology*, *28*(3), 277–296. doi:10.1177/0268580913484345

Yohani, S. C. (2008). Creating An Ecology of Hope: Arts-Based Interventions with Refugee Children. *Child & Adolescent Social Work Journal*, *25*(4), 309–323. doi:10.100710560-008-0129-x

Yuen, T. C.-M. (1997). Filial therapy with immigrant Chinese parents in Canada. *Dissertation Abstracts International. A, The Humanities and Social Sciences*. Retrieved from http://search.ebscohost.com/login.aspx?direct=true&db=psyh&AN=1997-95017-304&site=ehost-live

Yusuff, A. S. M., Tang, L., Binns, C. W., & Lee, A. H. (2014). Prevalence and risk factors for postnatal depression in Sabah, Malaysia: A cohort study. *Women and Birth; Journal of the Australian College of Midwives*, *28*(1), 25–29. doi:10.1016/j.wombi.2014.11.002 PMID:25466643

Zgambo, M., Kalembo, F., He, G., & Wang, H. (2012). Depression among Chinese children and adolescents: A review of the literature. *International Journal of Child, Youth, and Family Studies*, *4*(1), 442–457. doi:10.18357/ijcyfs34.1201211543

Zur, O. (2015). Dual relationships, multiple relationships & boundaries in psychotherapy, counseling & mental health. *Zur Institute*. Retrieved from http://www.zurinstitute.com/dualrelationships.html

About the Contributors

Anasuya Jegathevi Jegathesan earned her Doctorate in Counselling from the University of South Australia. She is a Certified Reality Therapist, a Certified Thanatologist and a Licensed Counsellor in Malaysia. A practitioner and counsellor educator, she conducts individual and Group Therapy privately, specializing in Individual therapy, adolescent and grief counselling. Dr. Anasuya has created her own set of therapy tools called Journeys through Life, and has conducted workshops in Malaysia, Canada, the United States and Australia. Her areas of research are on Grief and Multi-cultural counselling. She works closely with developing counselling centers and programs from NGO's.

Siti Salina Abdullah is a senior lecturer and Head of the Programme for Bachelor of Counseling at the School of Social and Economic Development, University Malaysia Terengganu. She is now appointed as an Associate Fellow of Institute of Tropical Biodiversity and Sustainable Development. She is also a registered counselor with Malaysia Board of Counselor and a Panel Counselor for The National Population and Family Development Board or LPPKN. She holds a Doctorate of Counseling from University of South Australia, Master of Counseling, and Bachelor of Education (Guidance and Counseling) from University Putra Malaysia. Her interest is in multicultural and family counseling. She conducted several research grants that covered areas of delinquent teenagers, non-traditional career, poverty and wellbeing in the community. She actively involves in various programs conducted by LPPKN, YDSM, and others.

* * *

Kiirtaara Aravindhan is a Bachelors of Psychology (Hons) graduate from HELP University and a lifetime member of the Psi Chi International Honors Society. During her time in university, she was actively involved in social work and served as a student leader. She has presented in numerous conferences and has been awarded Best Presenter on several occasions. The abstract of her recent research which focuses on self-cognition and defense response is due to be published in the Malaysian Journal of Psychiatry early 2019. Being an avid observer on social issues, she pens her thought in a weekly column. She is a mental health enthusiast and aims to create a positive difference in the mental health industry. She volunteers on a part-time basis at the Malaysian Mental Health Association (MMHA) and is also a volunteer at a mental health platform known as MY Confidential. Her passion lies in breaking stereotypes.

Diana-Lea Baranovich is a full time associate professor at the University of Malaysia in the department of educational psychology and counselling, She also runs a private psychotherapy practice where she specialises in traumatised children, teenagers and families in transition. Diana holds both a Doctorate of Education from California Coast University and a Doctorate of Clinical Psychology from California Southern University.

Carl Vadivella Belle obtained a Bachelor of Arts degree at the Australian National University, Canberra. Between 1976 and 1979 he served in the Australian High Commission, Kuala Lumpur. He has maintained a long-term interest in Malaysian social, political and religious issues, especially Hinduism in Malaysia, and the histories and traditions of Malaysia's Indian community. His doctoral dissertation, Thaipusam in Malaysia: A Hindu Festival Misunderstood?, was accepted by Deakin University in 2004. Dr Belle has acted as principal consultant to several television and radio productions focussing on the festival of Thaipusam as practiced at Batu Caves, Kuala Lumpur. Between 1992 and 2004 he headed the Barossa, Hills and Plains Rural Counselling Service, and also served as State Secretary of the South Australian Association of Rural Counselling Services. He was appointed inaugural Hindu Chaplain at the Flinders University of South Australia in 2004. He has lectured extensively on Malaysian politics and history, and on South Indian Hindu traditions as well as wider religious issues, and has published numerous papers on these topics. His major study, Tragic Orphans: Indians in Malaysia, was published in 2015, and a companion volume, Thaipusam in Malaysia: A Hindu Festival in the Tamil Diaspora, followed in 2017.

Ming Tik Chia is currently pursuing a master degree in counselling and practicing as the intern counselor at a Buddhist temple and also a Christian church. At the temple, he provides individual counselling and play therapy services, while also acting as a trainer / facilitator for children and youth Buddhist camps as well as a trainer for the social workers. He also helps out in mission work. Ming Tik applies Person-centered, Satir Model and Mindfulness-Based Stress Reduction (MBSR) in his counseling sessions.

Anne Chong graduated with a BA in English and a Master in Guidance and counselling. She has been teaching in colleges for almost 20 years as English teacher and a psychology lecturer. Currently, she is teaching in lodge international school as psychology teacher and a school counsellor.

Tin Fung Chong is a second-year Master student in the Clinical Psychology Program who also completed his bachelor's degree in psychology in HELP University. Previously, he worked as a Cognitive Brain Trainer in Your Brain Academy to provide 1-to-1 brain training to children and adults. Tin Fung has a strong interest in Psychology and co-founded MY Psychology with his peers during his undergraduate years.

Pei Lynn Foo is a clinical psychologist in private practice in Penang, Malaysia. She is an active committee member of the Penang Association of Counselling and Psychology since 2012. Prior to full-time private practice, she headed the School of Psychology at DISTED College Penang and was involved in numerous NGOs for children and mental health. She received her Bachelor of Arts in Psychology from the United States and Master of Clinical Psychology from HELP University Malaysia. Her passion lies in serving the child population and contributing to the growth and development of the field of psychology in Malaysia.

Cheng Chue Han is a professional licensed counselor in Malaysia. Han has worked in school, colleges and universities to provide mental health support to the students for the past 8 years. She strongly believes in systemic approach in helping clients thus works closely with educators and parents as well. Han's research interest is in understanding how to help Malaysian parents to practice therapeutic play with their own children. She has witnessed how therapeutic play has helped troubled children to heal and to grow. Play has tremendous magical power to connect the adults and children. All we need to do is to be mindful and paired with some simple play skills in order to reach out to our children. She will be an advocate of PLAY for life!

Chong Shen Hew is a psychology graduate from HELP University, one of the co-founders of MY Psychology, and is currently holding the position of writer/editor in the company.

Ee Mun Hon is a registered counsellor, with a master degree in Counselling, and bachelor degree in psychology from HELP University. Her foray into counselling began as a psychology intern at Universiti Malaya Medical Centre for two years and then two more years an intern counsellor at a number of centers including private universities, government hospital, vocational boarding center, primary schools and refugee center. Ee Mun is currently practicing in a mental health specialist clinic, providing therapy sessions to individual clients. She is certified in Choice Theory and Reality Therapy (CTRT), which she actively uses in her practice.

Mu Yi Hor is a psychology graduate from HELP University who is now working as a talent acquisition specialist. Mu Yi is also one of the co-founders of MY Psychology and specializes in managing the working team.

Sindusha Darshini Kanna Dasan completed her Bachelor's Degree in Psychology at Sunway University obtaining a dual degree from Lancaster and Sunway University. She is currently pursuing her Masters in Counselling at HELP University. She has a few working experiences related to the field of psychology such as being an assistant teacher at Women's Aid Organisation (WAO) dealing with at risk children from broken homes. She was also a protection assistant in United Nations High Commissioner for Refugees (UNHCR) where as part of the process she was required to interview refugee children and families in order to determine if they can be resettled in a third world country. She also acted as a counsellor to refuges who were disabled, ill, misplaced, estranged from family members and other issues. She also volunteered and worked at the Louis Center for Children with Special Needs for a couple of years. Currently she is doing her internship at Malaysian Mental Health Association (MMHA) where she provides counselling to clients from various backgrounds. She is currently in the process of obtaining a certification in Choice Theory and Reality Therapy (CTRT). Sindusha Darshini resides Malaysia, Kuala Lumpur.

Rajvin Kaur Rhandawa was diagnosed with cerebral palsy when she was just one year old. Today, she is a Bachelor of Communications (Hons) majoring in Public Relations graduate, a motivational speaker, a writer and blogger as well as a cerebral palsy survivor. She is also a Good Will Ambassador for My Mobile University. Her future aspiration is to be more mobile and a successful motivational speaker blogger and writer despite her obstacles under the guidance of her beautiful family, true friends and caregiver.

Gianina Kon was born in a small village in Borneo island. She was inspired to be in a helping profession to help people with mental illness. She is humble, self-driven, self-discipline, self-motivated and persistence individual. She is passionate in the LGBTQ+ population and aspired to help them to live a good quality life. She is a writer by day and a reader by night. She has a bachelor degree in Psychology and Business Management. Gia is also a post-graduate Master in Counselling student. She went on to pursue her PsyD in Neuropsychology to understand the human behaviours and its cognitive functioning.

Jeremy Lim is a 2nd year Master's of Clinical Psychology student at HELP University. Jeremy's approach to therapy is person-centered and systemic, believing that the therapeutic relationship should be built on genuineness, positive regard, and empathy. He believes that we are all part of larger and are made up of smaller systems.

Chuah Siew Mooi is a licensed and registered counsellor from Lembaga Kaunselor Malaysia. She is currently working as a counsellor at HELP University, Malaysia. Chuah has completed a Bachelors in Psychology (Hons) and Masters in Counselling from HELP University, Malaysia. A humanitarian at heart, she has volunteered with various non-profit organizations that work with abuse, gender-based violence, and people living with HIV as well as the LGBTQ+ community. Chuah has presented her research findings about reporting behaviours of children-centric NGO workers on child abuse in the International Conference on Behavioural and Social Sciences in Singapore on August 2017. Her areas on interest include child abuse, trauma, and spirituality in mental health.

Chandana Namal Kumara is a counselor registered with Malaysian Board of Counselors (KB05315). He is the counselor at HELP College of Arts and Technology. He also lectures in psychology program affiliated to the Southern New Hampshire University. Before start working as a counselor, Namal had been a Buddhist monk in Sri Lanka for nearly twenty years. Life as a monk for him was a journey full of experiences that included boredom and excitement, joy and disappointment, successes and failures, and, blames and praises. He considers his experience as a monk is the most important ingredient he brings into the therapy room when he works with people from all walks of life. Master's degree in counseling psychology he earned from HELP University gave a brand name for all his life experiences and license to practice within a structured framework.

Alvin Lai Oon Ng is a clinical psychologist by training with a professional doctorate in clinical psychology from Murdoch University, Western Australia. He practiced as a clinical psychologist and a postgraduate trainer in clinical psychology for 11 years at Universiti Kebangsaan Malaysia (National University of Malaysia) before moving on to focus more on teaching and research at Sunway University where he is an Associate Professor. He currently does not provide clinical consultations per se but is still much into the field of clinical psychology through research and his role as the Vice President of the Malaysian Society of Clinical Psychology (MSCP) which he founded in 2010 as the Founding President. He was also a consultant psychologist, appearing weekly on a breakfast radio show to provide discussions on mental health topics and to answer public questions about mental health issues for two years from 2015 to 2017.

Joo Hou Ng is a registered counsellor in Malaysia. In 2013, he received his certification in Choice Theory Reality Therapy by William Glasser International. Over the last decade, he has mentored many Malaysian youths, helping them cope with life challenges. Joo Hou graduated with a Masters in Counselling in HELP University KL (2015), and a MSc. Social & Organisational Psychology in University of Exeter (2017). Currently, he is pursuing a PhD in Social, Environmental and Organisational Psychology, at The University of Exeter. Besides his PhD research, he is actively mentoring youths from Malaysia, China and UK, and also serving in the area of pastoral care in his local church, Belmont Chapel Exeter.

Ann Nunis is a graduate of the Masters in Counseling program at HELP University, Malaysia. She has worked in various local and international organisations with marginalized communities including survivors of gender-based violence, people living with HIV and refugees. Besides providing counseling and mental health services for tertiary students, she continues to be a volunteer and member for humanitarian causes through NGO work. She believes and continually advocates for improved and accessible mental health and protection services for marginalized communities in Malaysia.

Aaron Page currently works as a Researcher at The University of Exeter Business School. Over the last 4 years he has been awarded a Psychology BSc (2016) and a Social & Organisational Psychology MSc (2017), achieving a first-class and distinction, respectively. While completing his studies, Aaron took pride in producing high quality, innovative research across a range of disciplinary fields including Animal Cognition; Social Psychology; Business Analytics; Social Network Analysis; and Organisational Psychology. Over the course of 2018, Aaron has conducted research on the diversity disclosures of companies listed on the London Stock Exchange and, in addition to this, he has investigated the utility of 'mindfulness training' as an intervention to help improve occupational environments. Moving forward, thanks to the support of the Bateman Family Trust PhD studentship award, Aaron will explore the barriers women encounter as they attempt to climb the cooperate ladder and occupy the most senior positions within organisations.

Kamarul Md Shah is a senior lecturer at the School of Social and Economic Development, Universiti Malaysia Terengganu. He graduated with Bachelor of Education (Guidance and Counseling) from University Putra Malaysia, Master of Education (Guidance and Counseling), from University Malaya and Doctor of Philosophy (Guidance and Counseling) from University Kebangsaan Malaysia. He is a registered counselor with Malaysia Board of Counselor and life member of PERKAMA International. He had presented his research findings at several national and international seminars as well as produced articles on multicultural counseling for journal publications.

Rachel Sing-Kiat Ting is currently teaching at Monash University Malaysia—Department of Psychology. She received her Bachelor of Psychology from National Chung Cheng University, and her Master of Clinical Psychology from Wheaton College. Her PhD in clinical psychology comes from an APA accredited institute (Fuller Graduate School of Psychology) and her post-doc training from University of Southern California. Till date, she holds an active California psychologist license. Since graduating in 2006, she has been teaching in various academic settings of Malaysia, China and the States. She is also an active member of Malaysia Society of Clinical Psychology and American Psychological Association. She advocates for the importance of indigenous psychology for Chinese people through her practice and research.

Gary Yap has a strong interest in psychology and graphic design. He finished his Bachelor's degree at HELP University and is currently completing his Masters studies of Clinical Psychology at the National University of Malaysia. During his undergraduate years, he co-founded MY Psychology with his peers. He believes that psychology knowledge should be made available and accessible to the public community.

Index

A

Abandonment 195
Acculturation 24, 26-29, 48, 132, 136
AIDS 93-94, 96-106, 190
algorithm 55, 57
Arjuna 218-219
Assimilation 23-24, 28, 33, 41, 48, 191
asylum seekers 97-99, 107, 129-131, 133, 140
atman 212, 215, 221
Attachment 85, 88, 193, 212, 219, 238-241
audience 50-61, 218

B

Bhagavad Gita 211, 215, 218, 220-221
bite-sized 58
Bonding 29, 84-85, 88, 90

C

Cerebral Palsy (CP) 150
Chinese in Malaysia 23-24, 48, 191
choice theory 64-67, 186, 197
Church 170, 179, 187, 200-206, 257
Clients 1-19, 28, 33, 35-39, 67, 74, 93, 98-105, 107, 113, 119-120, 134-144, 162, 184, 186-187, 201, 206-207, 213, 216, 219, 223-224, 226, 228-231, 235-236, 242, 245, 254-255, 260-262
Cognitive Therapy 198
Community 4, 16, 19, 24-26, 28-29, 31, 34-42, 52, 54-58, 60, 86, 93-103, 105-108, 119, 129, 131-132, 134, 136-139, 141-143, 151-153, 158, 162, 168-172, 178-179, 184, 187, 192, 202, 204-208, 230, 236-237, 246, 256-257
community service 93-94, 96, 103, 106
Compassion 102-103, 105-106, 190, 193-195, 214, 235, 242-244, 246-247
Competence 1-2, 12-13, 17-18, 24, 36, 221

D

Dependent origination 184, 190-191, 235

F

Facebook 52-53, 55-57, 60, 121, 153
Five Precepts 184, 188-189, 237, 247
Four Noble Truths 184, 188, 238, 245, 247

H

Hinduism 168, 171-173, 177, 211-216, 218, 220-221, 251-252
HIV 93-94, 96-108, 124
Homosexuality 113-114, 120, 177, 214

I

Impermanence 187, 190, 193, 196, 235, 242
Indigenous Psychology 39, 48
Insight 51, 113, 120, 184, 190, 194, 196-197, 200-201, 252
internet 16, 32, 50-51, 76, 101, 107

K

Karma 190-191, 193, 196, 211, 213, 215, 217-218, 221, 244-245, 247, 261

L

LGBTQ+ 112, 114, 120-122, 124-125
Lord Krishna 217-219
Loving-kindness 190, 193-195, 235, 242-243, 246-247

M

magazine 53, 58-59, 160
Malaysia 23-33, 35-38, 40-41, 48, 50-54, 57-59, 79, 84-87, 90, 94-97, 100, 107, 112-113, 120-122, 124-125, 129-130, 133-134, 150-158, 160-161, 165, 169, 171-172, 184-187, 191-192, 200-202, 224, 227, 229, 240, 251-252, 254
Malaysian 10, 23-24, 26, 29-32, 34, 36, 38-41, 50, 54, 64-69, 74, 78-79, 84-86, 90, 120, 152-154, 161, 169, 185, 200, 254
Malaysian secondary schools 64-65, 68, 78-79
Meditation 40, 184-189, 191, 193, 196-197, 207, 211, 216, 219, 235, 239-241
Mental Health 7-10, 14, 16-19, 23-25, 27, 31-32, 34-42, 48, 50-55, 57-59, 62, 66, 84, 90, 93, 95-96, 98-99, 101-108, 124, 129-137, 140, 142-143, 158, 161, 184-186, 192, 197-199, 202, 206, 211, 228, 261-262
messenger 53, 56-58, 60, 225
Mindfulness 40, 140, 186, 188-189, 193, 196-198, 219-220, 235-236, 240, 243, 245
Morality 10, 188-189, 198
Multicultural 1, 4, 13, 24, 36-37, 39, 48, 84, 115, 120, 130, 134, 168, 206, 208, 224, 226, 229-230, 235, 248, 252
Multicultural Competency 4, 24, 36, 39, 48, 229-230
multicultural counselling 120, 168
Multiculturalism 13
Multilingual 23-24, 26, 39-40
Muslim clients 223-224, 226, 228-231

N

NGO 24, 98, 106, 108, 152-153
non-Muslim counsellor 224

P

Psychological Challenges 23, 31, 48
Psychology 8, 23-24, 37-41, 48, 50-62, 67, 142, 165, 183, 185-186, 197, 204-206, 208, 211, 213, 218, 231, 238
Psychotherapy 6, 9, 41, 136, 138-139, 183-185, 187, 192, 196-200, 204-208, 218-219, 236

R

reality therapy 64-70, 72-74, 76, 78-79, 184, 186, 197
refugee 97-104, 128-144, 186
Refugees 8, 93, 95-102, 104-105, 108, 128-136, 138-144
Reincarnation 212, 215, 220-221, 245
Religion 2, 16, 18, 40, 112, 114, 120, 124, 129, 132, 134, 143, 170, 172, 176, 191-192, 199-202, 204, 207, 211-213, 225, 227-229, 231, 235-238, 248, 254, 256, 260-262
Resilience 30-31, 48, 180

S

school guidance counsellor 65, 68-70
self-esteem 64-70, 72, 74, 76, 78-79, 124, 131, 205, 242
Shakthi 213-214, 221
social identity approach 64-65, 67-69
social media 24, 52, 55, 57, 60, 62, 121-122, 132, 135, 152
Society 4, 17-18, 29, 40-41, 59, 62, 64, 93-94, 102-103, 108, 112, 120, 124, 151, 154, 158, 160, 165, 168, 171-172, 179-180, 185, 202, 215, 224, 227-230, 247, 252, 254, 261
Southeast Asia 29, 53, 59-60, 62, 93-97, 100, 102, 106-107, 130-131
Spiritual Bypassing 245, 247
Spirituality 16, 39, 84, 185, 228-229, 254, 262
student 6, 64, 66-67, 69-70, 72, 74, 171, 173-175, 177-178, 186, 230

T

terminology 114, 118, 137
therapeutic 1-7, 9-16, 18-19, 36, 39-40, 66-67, 79, 84-86, 90, 128-129, 135-136, 138-139, 141, 143, 158, 164, 183-184, 193, 207, 211, 221, 224, 230-231, 235-236, 238, 248, 259, 261
Therapist 2-9, 11, 13-19, 39, 66-67, 85-86, 88-89, 122, 124, 138, 141, 156, 161, 193-194, 196, 204-206, 208, 213, 216, 219-221, 230, 238, 245, 260-262
therapists 1-3, 5-6, 8, 10, 12-15, 18-19, 33, 37-40, 66-67, 153, 161, 202, 205-207, 228, 230-231, 242, 254-255, 260-261

Therapy 1-2, 7-19, 33, 35, 38-40, 64-70, 72-74, 76, 78-79, 84-90, 100-101, 103-104, 114, 116, 124, 135-142, 152, 156, 161-162, 184-187, 191, 194, 196-198, 202, 208, 211, 219-221, 228-229, 231, 235, 238, 242, 244, 248, 260
Theravada Buddhism 187, 235-236, 239-240, 244-245, 247-248
translators 40, 137-138
Triple Gems 236-237, 247

U

UNHCR 8, 95, 97, 99, 128-130, 133-134, 142
urban refugees 97, 131, 133-134, 136, 141

V

video 32, 53, 58, 60-61, 76-77

Y

YouTube 52, 58, 60, 76-77, 244

www.ingramcontent.com/pod-product-compliance
Lightning Source LLC
LaVergne TN
LVHW060424300926
849162LV00006B/1518
* 9 7 8 1 5 2 2 5 6 0 7 3 9 *